AMERI
MEDI
ASSOCIA

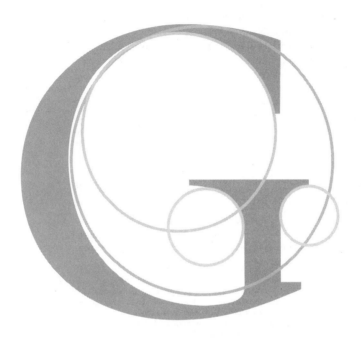

Guide to the Evaluation of
Functional Ability

How to Request, Interpret, and
Apply Functional Capacity Evaluations

Elizabeth Genovese, MD
Jill S. Galper, PT

American Medical Association

Library of Congress Cataloging-in-Publication Data

Guide to the evaluation of functional ability: how to request, interpret, and apply functional capacity evaluations/ [edited] by Elizabeth Genovese and Jill S. Galper.
   p. ; cm.
 Includes bibliographical references and index.
 Summary: "Assists in understanding the components used in functional assessment and their use in postoffer testing, work-injury management, and evaluation of patients with chronic pain"--Provided by publisher.
 ISBN 978-1-60359-001-3
1. Disability evaluation. I. Genovese, Elizabeth. II. Galper, Jill S. III. American Medical Association.
 [DNLM: 1. Disability Evaluation. W 925 G9448 2009]

RC963.4.G815 2009
616.07'5--dc22

                                        2008055513

ISBN 978-1-60359-001-3
BP73:08-P-042:3/09

CONTENTS

CHAPTER

Introduction to Functional Capacity Evaluation   1

Susan Isernhagen, PT

CHAPTER

Approach to Requesting a Functional Evaluation   19

Elizabeth Genovese, MD, MBA, and Susan J. Isernhagen, PT

CHAPTER

General Testing Principles for Functional Capacity Evaluations   41

Susan Isernhagen, PT, and Jill S. Galper, PT, MEd

PREFACE

I SAW MY FIRST functional capacity evaluation (FCE) report in 1987. Because I had already found it difficult to complete physical capacities estimate (PCE) forms with any degree of certainty, and certainly had learned nothing about how to do so during medical school or residency, I was delighted by the prospect of having a tool at my disposal that seemed to provide quantitative information about physical abilities and whether an evaluee was making a "valid" effort. I considered FCEs to be analogous to most other medical tests, ie, I assumed that the information provided was something that could reliably be used as the basis for medical decision making. Although FCEs were not expected to be perfect (no medical tests are perfect), I was under the impression that their contents and the criteria used in interpreting the data they concerned were standardized. Because most of the FCEs I initially reviewed were performed by one of several high-quality providers (including, by 1990, Jill Galper, the coeditor of this book), the information in the reports was relevant to my concerns and generally applicable to my needs.

The FCEs from other providers that I reviewed subsequently were not always as useful. The conclusions about functional ability were often inconsistent with the evaluee's diagnosis or documented objective clinical findings and the criteria incomprehensible, even when raw data were submitted in conjunction with the FCE report. The raw data themselves were impossible to interpret because terminology was not defined and the rationale for classifying a given test as "valid" or "invalid" was unclear. I felt compelled to better understand what I was reading, yet there were no books on the topic and no educational courses for physicians. The solution was to review FCE reports and read all the references cited. Once I had done so, I started reviewing the data from FCE reports and interpreting them myself, only to find that my interpretations were sometimes inconsistent with those of the evaluator. The reason, more often than not, was failure of the evaluator to use his or her clinical judgment when estimating physical capacities and/or do more than "fill in the blanks" when preparing the final report, even when clinical information suggested that this method might lead to an erroneous conclusion. The thought of writing a book to educate others who requested functional testing crossed my mind, but I was too involved in other endeavors.

I subsequently held several consulting positions that required frequent review of FCE reports; this is also something performed by IMX Medical Management Services. The wide variation in the FCEs themselves and in the qualifications (and clinical acumen) of the people who performed them were consistently barriers to their use; one never knew what one was going to get when one ordered an FCE. I was fortunate enough to be able to recruit Jill to work with me; her role included (among other things) performing FCEs, building a network of FCE providers, and reviewing the tests that these providers performed. We lectured on FCEs and continued to bemoan the lack of standardized testing procedures and components and the extent to which many evaluators seemed to have little understanding of what they were doing—their FCEs were formulaic at best. Yet we both thought, correctly or incorrectly, that functional testing, if done appropriately, was a tool that could provide useful information to improve our understanding of a patient's clinical status.

Involvement in the American Medical Association (AMA) *Guides to the Evaluation of Permanent Impairment,* Sixth Edition, reinforced this belief—how does one incorporate functional assessment into an impairment rating if one has no mechanism to use in evaluating it? The FCE could be a potential tool, yet the proliferation of proprietary functional assessment systems and the overall lack of transparency regarding the basis for many of their conclusions made it impossible to endorse FCE as a worthwhile testing procedure in a health care system that was moving further toward evidence-based medicine.

There was still no book available for the use of health care professionals who wanted to gain a deeper understanding of the evidence basis for functional testing or, on a more practical level, help "consumers" understand how best to request, interpret, and apply FCE or functional tests. There were also no detailed guidelines to use in critically evaluating potential FCE providers. I thought that a book was still needed and my subsequent involvement in the *AMA Guides to the Evaluation of Permanent Impairment, Sixth Edition* led the AMA to agree to publish this book and Jill consented to serve as coeditor.

This book is not meant to be an exhaustive technical review of all of the literature germane to functional assessment. It is meant to provide readers from a wide range of professional backgrounds with information that will help them become well-informed consumers of the product. More important, perhaps, is the editors' and chapter-authors' desire for this book to be the first step in advancing an international dialogue—a dialogue about how to improve functional testing to the point where it lives up to its promise as a tool that can provide objective and reliable information about the impact of impairment on function.

E. G.

ABOUT THE EDITORS

Dr. Elizabeth Genovese received her BA magna cum laude, Phi Beta Kappa from Harvard (majoring in Human Behavioral Biology), her MD from the University of Pennsylvania, and her MBA (in Health Care) from the Wharton School. Holding board certifications in Internal Medicine, and Preventative (Occupational) Medicine, she has been Medical Director of two successful multisite occupational medicine clinics prior to (and contemporaneous with) her current position of Medical Director for IMX Medical Management Services. The latter role involves oversight and development of IMX's Independent Medical Examination, file (peer) review, FCE, and occupational medicine consulting programs, although she still performs selected IME and consultative services while maintaining a small private practice focusing primarily on preventive medicine.

Dr. Genovese is Course Director for ACOEM's Musculoskeletal Examination and Treatment course, Co-Director of the ACOEM Clinical Practice Guidelines course, and has lectured for the American College of Occupational and Environmental Medicine (ACOEM), the American Academy of Disability Evaluation Physicians (AADEP), the American Back Society (ABS), the American College of Chiropractic Consultants (ACCC), and various primarily non-medical audiences. She is adjunct professor at the University Of Pennsylvania, School Of Medicine where she lectures on IMEs, Coding, the ACOEM Guidelines, Impairment Ratings, and FCEs for the Occupational Medicine Residency. ACOEM committee memberships include the Coding and Classification Committee (formerly chair), Stay at Work/Return to Work Committee, Evidence-Based Clinical Practice Guideline Committee, and Spine Update Committee. Most recently she has served as lead chair and associate editor for the revision of ACOEM's Chronic Pain Guideline. Other publications include chapters in *Disability Evaluation* (Demeter, ed), *A Physicians' Guide to Return to Work, Guides to the Evaluation of Disease and Injury Causation*, the *ACOEM Clinical Practice Guidelines 2nd edition* (contributing editor), contributing editor for the *AMA Guides to the Evaluation of Permanent Impairment, Sixth Edition* and articles in *Insights* (the ACOEM Guidelines Newsletter), for which she also served as editor.

Jill S. Galper, PT, M.Ed., is a physical therapist and exercise physiologist who has focused her practice on orthopedic and industrial rehabilitation and consultation, which has included performance of work conditioning and functional capacity evaluations, job analyses, ergonomic assessments and work risk assessments. Ms. Galper co-owned and managed a successful physical therapy practice and fitness club for 16 years. She also co-founded a regional physical therapy practice network. She currently is Vice President of Clinical Program Development for IMX Medical Management Services. In addition to the provision of clinical services, Ms. Galper has developed and maintains a national network of qualified FCE providers and provides utilization management services. Ms. Galper received her B.S. in physical therapy from the University of Pittsburgh and her master's degree in exercise physiology from Temple University. She co-authored a chapter in *Fundamentals of Musculoskeletal Assessment Techniques* and a study published in the journal *Work.* She has also lectured nationally about FCEs. Ms. Galper was the American Physical Therapy Association's (APTA) representative for review of the ACOEM Practice Guidelines' second edition and served as a panel member on ACOEM's Occupational Medicine Practice Guidelines Committees for revisions to the Low Back Pain (2007) and Chronic Pain (2008) practice guidelines. Ms. Galper is a member of the APTA and American College of Sports Medicine. She is an associate member of ACOEM and an affiliate member of AADEP. She is a Fellow on the American Board of Disability Analysts. Currently, she is serving as Treasurer of the Pennsylvania Southeast District Physical Therapy Association.

ACKNOWLEDGMENTS

While I first thought of writing this book over ten years ago, I would like to thank the AMA publishing staff for allowing it to become a reality, Jill Galper for her tireless work as coeditor, and my partners, David Dugery and John Sivel, as well as many IMX employees, for supporting my involvement (and that of Jill) in this, and other projects (such as the *AMA Guides Sixth Edition* and ACOEM Clinical Practice Guidelines) that took time away from other endeavors more directly related to the company's immediate activities. I am particularly grateful to all of the chapter authors, whose commitment to improving the design, performance, and application of functional assessment testing is evident not only in the chapters they wrote for this book but in their contribution to the field as a whole. Lastly, I would like to acknowledge my children, Christopher and Jessica Stone—their self-reliance, trustworthiness, and general strength of character have enabled me to engage in a number of professional activities that would have otherwise not been possible.

– EG

This book would not have been written without the effort of many individuals. I am grateful to everyone involved, who either through our professional or personal relationship, helped make this book possible. There are several individuals to whom special mention and thanks are due. I would like to express a huge debt of gratitude to Elizabeth Genovese without whom there would be no book. Her sharp intellect, excellent writing skills, and ability to translate theoretical concepts into practical information are both instructive and amazing. I couldn't have a better mentor. Big thanks to the AMA for agreeing to publish this book. Thanks to all of our contributors, who through this and their other work, continue to provide valuable information to the topic of functional testing. A special thank you to Joan Brown for her many helpful suggestions and contributions after reading text and discussing concepts. Thanks to Sandy Raskin, my wonderful aunt and grammarian, who was always available for consultation. Last but not least, I'd like to acknowledge my colleagues and co-workers at IMX Medical Management Services who have created a wonderful environment in which to work and grow.

– JSG

CONTRIBUTORS

Michael Coupland, CPsych, CRC
AssessAbility, West Palm Beach, FL

Jerry N. Fogel, MS, PT, CHQCM
Imagine Clinical, Coral Springs, FL

Lisa Fore, OTR
PRIDE Research Foundation, Dallas, TX

Douglas P. Gross, PT, PhD
Assistant Professor, Department of Physical Therapy,
University of Alberta, Canada

Mark Hyman, MD, FACP, FAADEP
Associate Clinical Professor of Medicine University
of California, Los Angeles, Los Angeles, California

Ev Innes, PhD, MHPEd, BAppSc(OT),
AccOT, MHFESA
Faculty of Health Sciences, The University of Sydney,
Australia

Susan J. Isernhagen, PT
DSI Work Solutions Inc, Duluth, MN

Janice Keeley, PT
PRIDE Research Foundation, Dallas, TX

Dianna T Kenny, PhD, MA, BA (Hons) Dip Ed
Professor of Psychology, The University of Sydney,
Australia

Phyllis M. King, PhD, OT, FAOTA
Associate Dean, Professor, UWM Center for
Ergonomics, University of Wisconsin-Milwaukee

Cynthia T. Kwasniewski, MS, OTR/L, CHT,
Coordinator, Hand Therapist, MossRehab
Philadelphia, PA

Elaine Labovitz, OTR/L, CHT,
Hand Therapist, MossRehab, Philadelphia, PA

James Lamprakos, DO
VP of Clinical Services, IMX Medical
Management Services, Bala Cynwyd, PA

Tom Mayer, MD
Department of Orthopedics, University of Texas
Southwestern Medical Center at Dallas, Dallas, TX

Margot Miller, PT
VP Provider Solutions, WorkWell, Duluth, MN

Norashikin Mahmud, PhD candidate, BA, MSc
The University of Sydney, Australia

Dale Reese, B.Sc, C.Ped.
PRIDE Research Foundation, Dallas, TX

Michiel Reneman
University Medical Center Groningen, Center for
Rehabilitation, The Netherlands

Eva Schonstein, PhD, MHPEd, AppSc(Phty)
The University of Sydney, Australia

Ryan Shea, MSc.
PRIDE Research Foundation, Dallas, TX

Gwen Simons, PT, JD, OCS, FAAOMPT
Adjunct Professor, University of New England
Physical Therapy Program, Portland, ME
Attorney, Simons & Associates Law, Physical
Therapist, Orthopaedic Physical Therapy Associates,
Scarborough, ME

Bhagwant S. Sindhu, PhD
Assistant Professor, Department of Occupational
Therapy, College of Health Sciences, University of
Wisconsin-Milwaukee, Milwaukee WI

Tim Takken, MD, MSc, PhD
Medical Physiologist, Department of Pediatric
Physical Therapy & Exercise Physiology, Wilhelmina
Children's Hospital, University Medical Center
Utrecht, The Netherlands

Harriët Wittink, PT, MS, PhD
Professor Lifestyle and Health, Faculty of Health
Care, University of Applied Sciences, Utrecht,
The Netherlands

Jasen M. Walker, Ed.D, CRC, CCM
CEC Associates, Valley Forge, PA

Rick Wickstrom, PT, CPE
President, WorkAbility Network, WorkAbility
Wellness Center, West Chester, OH

INTRODUCTION

Physicians and other health care professionals are routinely asked to assess functional ability. One reason may be a desire to prevent injury, as occurs whenever physicians are asked to complete forms or certificates clearing people for participation in work-related or non–work-related activities. The other reason is the determination of disability, ie, the degree to which the functional limitations of people with work-related or non–work-related medical conditions preclude the performance of activities that are needed to meet occupational or non-occupational participatory obligations. While the history, physical examination, and the results of diagnostic testing can generally be used to define the objective manifestations and potential impact of a medical condition on activities of daily living, qualification and quantification of functional limitations are more difficult to obtain.

The relationship between health conditions, disorders, or diseases and disability can be conceptualized by using the World Health Organization's Model of Disablement (Figure 1).

In this model, *activity* is defined as "task execution by the individual" and *activity limitations* as "difficulties the individual may experience carrying out such activities."[1] While patients can be asked to describe the degree to which they are limited by a particular disease or health condition, these perceptions may be inaccurate. And the degree to which health care providers or other interested parties can assess function, especially when it requires the performance of tasks requiring equipment or materials that are not ordinarily used in health-related evaluations, may be limited. Because disability cannot be determined in the absence of knowledge about function, assessment of activity limitations *and* physical capacities can be facilitated by functional capacity evaluations (FCEs) because they help "bridge the gap" between the objective assessment of the physiologic manifestations of disease and disability assessment.

Functional capacity evaluations and other functional test protocols directly measure the ability of persons to perform discreet physical tasks, generally selected to reflect the constructs the evaluator has been asked to assess. An FCE's purported ability to characterize and quantify physical capacities and activity limitations allows identification of the degree to which evaluees are capable of performing

FIGURE 1   ICF Model of Disablement

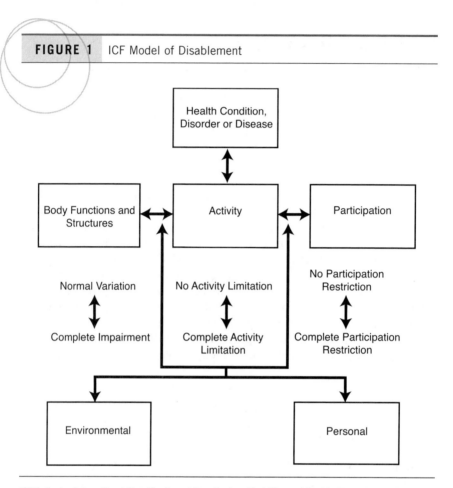

ICF indicates International Classification of Functioning, Disability, and Health. Reproduced with permission from: Rondinelli R, Genovese E, Katz RT, et al, eds. *Guides to the Evaluation of Permanent Impairment*. 6th ed. Chicago, IL: American Medical Association; 2008.

various activities of interest relevant to work capacity (before employees begin a job, during employment, or after injury) and disability evaluations. However, the literature supporting the degree to which the results of functional capacity assessments can be used to predict return to work or the likelihood of injury recurrence is mixed at best.[2-7] This literature also suggests that there is a relationship between improvement in tests of function and psychological measures, which may imply that psychological factors are significant confounders when evaluating function[2,8,9] (see Chapter 18).

On the other hand, it is reasonable to expect there to be some relationship between objectively identified functional abilities and limitations and the ability to perform activities of daily living and work-related tasks. For example, a person identified as incapable of lifting an item weighing 50 lbs during an FCE would not be able to do so at work. And, indeed, functional testing is often useful in situations in which the evaluator wants to assess whether a person who wants to qualify for a particular job can perform physical tasks designed to reflect job demands. Well-designed FCEs are also generally able to identify consistencies and inconsistencies in an evaluee's performance of various tasks, especially in the context of the diagnosis and clinical information obtained from the history, physical examination, and relevant diagnostic testing.

Unfortunately, there has been little content-standardization of various FCE protocols (even when evaluating similar constructs), definitions for some of the terminology used to describe physical abilities, training requirements for evaluators, and criteria to use in classifying an evaluee as failing to exert maximal effort or as inconsistent in his or her performance. This lack of standardization has, in turn, led to wide variation in the degree to which FCEs can reliably and consistently address questions posed by requesting parties, leading many to decide that functional testing is without value. The authors of the chapters in this book, however, many of whom reflect national and international experts in the field of functional assessment, strongly believe that improved standardization of FCE terminology, protocols, and training requirements, concurrent with education regarding the components, applications, interpretation, strengths, and limitations of functional testing, will allow professionals and employers who request and/or apply FCEs to select providers and protocols that will best meet their needs. Furthermore, the editors and chapter authors also believe that providing readers with a comprehensive description of the "science" behind FCEs and how to best apply it toward answering questions regarding evaluee abilities and limitations, coupled with a frank discussion of current test limitations, can allow for the development of an "agenda for the future" to address these limitations.

This book begins with a review of the history and use of functional testing (Chapter 1). Chapters 2 and 3 then help readers understand when different types of functional testing are appropriate; the focus is on fostering development of a systematic, analytic approach to ordering functional testing that will optimize the match between the type of assessment requested and the specific clinical or claims-related issues to be addressed. The next group of chapters (4 through 11) describes the nature, rationale for use, and evidence basis for various functional test components. Chapter 12 focuses specifically on tests used to evaluate upper extremity function, but also describes the upper extremity FCE in general. This discussion of specific "types" of functional assessment continues in Chapters 13 through 15, which discuss their use in postoffer testing, work-injury management, and the evaluation of patients with chronic pain.

By this point, readers should have a thorough understanding of the components used in functional testing and their potential application to generic and specific scenarios. Chapter 16 describes how evaluators should analyze and interpret the information obtained during testing and prepare a report; Chapter 17 discusses the characteristics and qualifications a functional evaluator should possess and identifies considerations when selecting an FCE evaluator. (The appendix provides further help with this process because it describes the components of many currently available FCE systems using information directly provided by their manufacturers.)

The next three chapters (18 through 20) focus on the application of functional test results to specific scenarios. Chapter 18 (Clinician and Insurer Application of Functional Test Results) also briefly reviews some of the literature regarding the application of FCE to return to work and describes how to manage circumstances when the FCE report does not provide adequate guidance. Chapter 19 describes how vocational experts use FCEs, and Chapter 20 discusses legal issues. Chapter 21, which picks up where Chapter 18 left off, summarizes current literature on the scientific status of FCE and is a lead-in to the last chapter, which describes the limitations of FCEs as currently performed and makes recommendations regarding how to best address them, thus providing the agenda for the future.

References

1. Rondinelli R, Genovese E, Katz RT, et al, eds. *Guides to the Evaluation of Permanent Impairment.* 6th ed. Chicago, IL: American Medical Association; 2008:3.
2. Mayer TG, Gatchel RJ, Kishino N, et al. Objective assessment of spine function following industrial injury: a prospective study with comparison group and one-year follow-up. *Spine.* 1985;10:482–493.
3. Takala EP, Viikari-Juntura E. Do functional tests predict low back pain? *Spine.* 2000;25:2126–2132.
4. Gross DP, Battie MC, Cassidy JD. The prognostic value of functional capacity evaluation in patients with chronic low back pain, part 1: timely return to work. *Spine.* 2004;29:914–919.
5. Gross DP, Battie MC. The prognostic value of functional capacity evaluation in patients with chronic low back pain, part 2: sustained recovery. *Spine.* 2004;29:920–924.
6. Gross DP, Battie MC. Functional capacity evaluation performance does not predict sustained return to work in claimants with chronic back pain. *J Occup Rehabil.* 2005;15:285–294.
7. Gross DP, Battie MC. Does functional capacity evaluation predict recovery in workers' compensation claimants with upper extremity disorders? *Occup Environ Med.* 2006;63:404–410.

8. Cutler RB, Fishbain DA, Steele-Rosomoff R, Rosomoff HL. Relationships between functional capacity measures and baseline psychological measures in chronic pain patients. *J Occup Rehabil.* 2003;13:249–258.
9. Geisser ME, Robinson ME, Miller QL, Bade SM. Psychosocial factors and functional capacity evaluation among persons with chronic pain. *J Occup Rehabil.* 2003;13:259–276.

CHAPTER 1

Introduction to Functional Capacity Evaluation

Susan J. Isernhagen, PT

Introduction and Definition

Functional Capacity Evaluation (FCE) is the objective measurement of a person's ability to perform functional work activities. In "ability to work" determinations, functional testing broadens the medical information and provides an objective measure that is useful in determining work placement, accommodation, treatment requirements, case management, or disability eligibility for a worker. It is a foundation for vocational evaluation and employment. The physician or provider may determine diagnosis and medical prognosis, but functional testing is more objective than the current use of estimates, commonly called "restrictions." In an evidence-based medical model, measurements are preferable to estimates. Thus, the objective testing of a worker against work demands (in a reliable and valid manner) provides an evidence base to use in establishing the link between medical diagnosis and gainful employment. When ability to work is limited and disability is questioned, functional and vocational expertise is considered an important component in case determination.

The definition used by Isernhagen[1] in 1988 was the first published definition of FCE that reached a broad audience:

Functional: Meaningful, useful. Functional indicates purposeful activity that is an actual work movement. Functional implies a definable movement with a beginning and an end and a result that can be measured.

Capacity: The maximal ability or capability of a person. Capacity indicates existing abilities for activities that include the maximum function the person is able to perform.

Evaluation: Systematic approach including observation, reasoning, and conclusion. Evaluation is not merely recording test scores but goes further to produce an outcome statement that is explanatory in addition to the objective measurement of the activity.

An FCE is performed on a one-to-one basis for several hours and is an intense physical evaluation of work-related abilities. The purpose is to identify maximum demonstrated capacities and the ability of the evaluee to perform activities for a designated period. The goal of an FCE is to provide information on limitations *and* abilities to help determine the evaluee's safe ability for work.

The FCE is often an integral part of a return-to-work or disability determination process. The FCE provides functional information that complements the medical data applied to return-to-work conclusions and also guides modification of work activities. When used appropriately, it interfaces with information from many professionals on the return-to-work team and, hence, can be an important component of the return-to-work process. The evaluee, who participates in the evaluation process and learns his or her abilities and limitations, is an important member of the team. The FCE has become a basic component of work injury management systems and has been used in the following ways:

- As a stand-alone test to assist in the determination of return-to-work possibilities or to determine whether the absence of abilities to perform the activities involved in gainful employment places the person in a category of disability
- As an entry point to work-related rehabilitation
- As a basis for designing work modifications that allow a person to return to work

A Brief History of Functional Testing

Vocational assessment is routinely used to evaluate the employability of severely injured and physically disabled persons and to ascertain whether training, therapeutic interventions, assistive devices, or accommodations can be developed to promote or support employment. Vocational specialists have developed forms that categorize work activities into a generic list[2] to provide vocational goals. These work-list formats are used in most states in the United States and in many jurisdictions throughout the world. A typical sample of this format is found in Table 1–1.

Occupational therapists and psychologists began using vocationally oriented physical capacity evaluations beginning in 1947. Cranfield[3] and Reuss et al[4] provided various types of assessments of physical capacities, particularly for patients with a combination of physical, psychological, and vocational disability, thus serving to introduce therapists as evaluators of work function.

After World War II, veterans who had suffered injuries returned to the United States and required assistance reintegrating into society and the work world. Rehabilitation and vocational retraining were used intensively for the first time. During the next decades, vocational and functional evaluations broadened to all people with substantive physical limitations interfering with work. In addition to veterans, people with congenital problems or debilitating diseases and people who had traumatic injuries such as amputations or spinal cord injuries were included. Vocational and rehabilitative services were often provided in multidisciplinary rehabilitation centers.

In the mid 1970s, attention turned toward patients in the workers' compensation system with chronic musculoskeletal problems. The cost of having workers

TABLE 1–1 Job Demands

Job Demands	Job Frequencies
Lift	
Carry	
Push	
Grip	Occasionally: 1%–33% of the work day
Fingering [fingers in fine hand-coordination]	
Bend	Frequently: 34%–66% of the work day
Reach	
Squat	Constantly: 67%–100% of the work day
Kneel	
Walk	
Sit	
Stand	
Climb	

unemployed or receiving workers' compensation for long periods was recognized as creating a negative financial effect on industry, state funds, and society. The first Work Capacity Evaluation (WCE) was developed by Leonard Matheson, PhD, at the Work Preparation Center at Rancho Los Amigos Hospital, Downey, CA, in 1975, in response to a change in the workers' compensation law in California. The law required vocational rehabilitation to be provided to a person who could not return to his or her usual and customary job. The determination of whether the person could return to work was based on a structured test battery involving physical and cognitive standardized ability tests. Test results were compared with job analysis data based on the *Handbook for Analyzing Jobs,* which preceded the model later used in the *Revised Dictionary of Occupational Titles.*[2] During the next few years, several rehabilitation facilities in southern California developed similar protocols so that by 1980, WCEs focusing on psychological, functional, and vocational goals were established.[5,6] Matheson's[7-9] early work involved presenting his protocols to occupational therapists, who began to use the psychological-functional-vocational testing in their work.

With the knowledge that work capacities could be measured, state workers' compensation systems in the United States began to provide a form (Table 1–2) to be used by physicians for workers' compensation patients. The form asked physicians to go beyond providing medical information and venture into the realm of return-to-work specifics. The goals of the states' departments of labor and industry were earlier return to work and cost savings for the workers' compensation systems and for the employers that funded the systems. With this new role of determining specific work abilities and limitations, physicians turned to their functional counterparts, physical and occupational therapists, to provide objective information on work function.

TABLE 1–2   Functional Capacity Form

The person will be able to:

Task	Occasionally	Frequently	Constantly
Lift			
Carry			
Push-pull			
Grip			
Fingering [fingers in fine hand-coordination]			
Bend			
Reach			
Squat			
Kneel			
Walk			
Sit			
Stand			
Climb			

MD	Date

Thus, emphasis on vocational evaluation that was initially limited to professionals specializing in vocational rehabilitation or occupational therapy spread to the medical model and resulted in a much broader demand for determining the functional capacity of all workers. The first commercial FCE widely available was the Polinsky Functional Capacity Assessment created for therapists in 1983.[10] Functional capacity testing to reduce lost work time and disability became a viable option as workers' compensation systems focused on trying to use this and similar tests as a tool to control the cost of long-standing injuries. Subsequently, Isernhagen[11] wrote and edited the book, *Work Injury Management and Prevention,* which explored return-to-work issues and specifically addressed FCE development as part of a larger work injury management system.

In the late 1980s FCEs were developed by Glenda Key[12] and Keith Blankenship. Matheson also continued to develop physical capacity evaluations. After 1990, many other commercial FCEs became available. In addition, because FCE providers were usually physical and occupational therapists, many developed their own individualized formats for FCE. Thus, the 1990s saw a proliferation of various types and methods of FCE, which created confusion in the FCE referral base because there was no standard set of criteria to use in determining whether a particular FCE model was suitable to address a particular question or set of questions. The FCE referral base itself continued to grow more diverse, including physicians, vocational counselors, employers, workers' compensation insurers, disability insurers, attorneys, and the patients themselves.

The FCE continues to be used to determine whether evaluees can return to work (and, if so, whether any accommodations or job modifications are required) and to assess whether patients are making progress or need rehabilitative or vocational services.

The nomenclature for FCE is varied. Alternative terms include functional capacity assessment, or FCA; physical capacity evaluation, or PCE; WCE; and functional abilities evaluation, or FAE. In this book, FCE will be used (see Chapter 21 for additional discussion regarding nomenclature).

Use of Functional Capacity Evaluation

When reasonable treatments have been provided and an ill or injured worker is not working, funding via various disability systems can allow persons to sustain themselves even though they are not gainfully employed. These systems include Social Security and private insurance disability for illness and workers' compensation when the disability is attributed to work-related activities.

Disability can also be a result of an auto accident, medical error, or personal injury. In all of these situations, disability determinations are based on the ability (or inability) to work. Knowledge regarding functional capacity is the cornerstone used by the worker, the employer, the insurer (or other relevant party), and the health care professional to establish the degree to which there is a match between the worker and a particular job (or occupation) or the physical abilities required for any form of gainful employment. The FCE, a tool for measuring capability to perform physical work activities, is used to determine the type of work that can be performed and to estimate the time an injured or ill worker can return to or begin work.

When injury or illness has affected a worker or potential worker, there are two issues. The first is that the worker is no longer able to perform his or her original work, causing difficulties for the employer and the worker. The second is that illness and injury are considered medical events, and, thus, medical practitioners become involved in determining when the worker can become productive and return to work. This segue into the medical realm is necessary and important but may result in the transition of "worker" to "patient" when the treatment provided for the medical problem fails to emphasize functional goals, especially return to work.

A medical release is necessary to allow a person to return to work. It is at this juncture that the functional capacity of the worker becomes important. A medical professional must state that the person can return to work without limitations or identify limitations that need to be considered to allow return to work. It is then up to the employer to determine whether the worker can be returned to his or her former job, or any job, with those limitations. For workers whose functional problem is minor or easily accommodated, return to work is relatively quick and uncomplicated. Reinjury does not often occur in these cases because the injury has been resolved and the formerly capable worker has returned to the capable state.

Most FCEs are used when the return to work or placement at work has not been successfully accomplished. In cases in which the diagnosis is complicated or unclear or when the illness or injury interferes with safe work capacity, there often is a delay in productive return to work. The medical provider, the employer, and, more important, the worker can become frustrated at the lack of clarity regarding work ability. It is then that the physician, employer, or case manager refers the worker for an FCE. The test focuses not only on assessing overall work ability and limitation but also on evaluating the worker's effort level and, if needed, job-specific functional capacity. Owing to its roots in work tasks and medical evaluation, the FCE bridges the gap between the medical and employment realms (or, as some have said, between impairment and disability).

Functional Capacity Evaluators

Physical therapists and occupational therapists were the first professionals to work with the initial medical-based FCEs in the late 1980s and early 1990s. Therapists were a logical choice for this role because they have a health care–based education and routinely work closely with physicians to establish ability levels for many types of patients. The transition of therapists into the return-to-work realm fit with the medical-restorative-rehabilitative nature of the health care system. To function in this role, it is necessary for evaluators to understand the primary diagnoses and confounding pathological issues that are often linked to work injury or illness. The educational background that therapists have in neuromusculoskeletal anatomy and pathologies (eg, joint problems, muscle weakness, nerve entrapment, and degenerative conditions) is combined with physiological knowledge of systemic diseases and heart and lung deficiencies. Therapists also have studied movement patterns (kinesiology). This combination of skills allows therapists to interact in return-to-work processes by working with health care professionals and employment case management professionals, including employers.

To maintain quality of FCEs and to create awareness of definition and use, guidelines were developed within the therapy professions performing FCEs. Nevertheless, FCEs are also performed by people who are not therapists and are often unable to provide an equivalent level of clinical assessment. To the extent that performing an FCE and issuing a report require evaluators to analyze test data in the context of his or her clinical impressions, there has been debate regarding the degree to which FCE providers must demonstrate an appropriate base of clinical knowledge to be considered qualified examiners. The guidelines described subsequently assume clinical expertise.

The American Physical Therapy Association developed guidelines[13] for physical therapists who act as evaluators and also defined parameters and uses for referrers and other professionals. Before performing an FCE, evaluators are directed to thoroughly read pertinent medical records, take a history, and perform a physical examination, including musculoskeletal, neurological, and integumentary screening. The FCE itself comprises a comprehensive test related to the *Revised Dictionary of Occupational Titles*[2] and pertinent work definitions. Because it is an evaluation and not just a measurement, the report includes information regarding demonstrated capacities for work-related tasks, answers referral questions, identifies possible activity and task modifications when given job-specific task information, and compares the capacities of the worker and the work demands.

For the American Occupational Therapy Association, practice parameters and definitions have been developed and expressed in guidelines.[14] They apply to occupational therapists who perform FCEs and describe the role of occupational therapy professionals in work evaluation and the use of such evaluations in return to work, job modification, and disability.

Components of FCE Testing

The FCE includes some or all of the following components: patient interview (injury and medical history and current complaints, psychometric questionnaires), musculoskeletal evaluation, movement tests (eg, walking, climbing, and reaching), dynamic material handling tests, static tests, aerobic tests, positional tolerance tests, hand function tests, and job-specific activities. The specific activities included in an FCE for a particular person are determined by consideration of medical safety, the evaluee's diagnoses and functional problems, and the requirement to evaluate the work tasks in a standardized and reproducible manner. The format, Table 1–3, includes reading the medical record for history, taking a personal history from the evaluee, performing a screening physical examination, and proceeding to the formal FCE, which is discussed further in Chapter 4. The models for FCE vary in regard to the specific work task components included in the evaluation process, the specific procedures used to assess activity abilities, and the methods used to score patient participation and performance consistency. This variety necessitates users of and referrers to FCE to consider professional guidelines, intent and method of FCE, accuracy of results, and relationship of the results to real work.

TABLE 1–3 FCE Format

---

1. History and summary of medical records

2. Physical exam and ADL questionnaire

3. Results:

    Level of Effort

    Consistency of Effort

    Physical Demand Level

    Answers to Referral Questions

    Recommendations

TABLE 1–3 FCE Format (continued)

4. FCE grid

Category	Occasionally	Frequently	Constantly
Lift from floor	lbs	lbs	lbs
Lift to shoulder	lbs	lbs	lbs
Lift and carry	lbs	lbs	lbs
Push	lbs	lbs	lbs
Pull	lbs	lbs	lbs
Grip	lbs	lbs	lbs
Pinch	lbs	lbs	lbs
Hand coordination			
Bend			
Reach			
Squat			
Kneel			
Walk			
Sit			
Stand			
Climb			

5. Supporting data

FCE indicates functional capacity evaluation.

Because an FCE acts as a medical evaluation and a vocational assessment tool, and because assessing whether evaluees are truly incapable of performing physical tasks associated with employment (ie, are disabled) may be a consideration, most FCEs have been developed to address multiple factors of work task performance. The following are important in FCE design and are desired by referral sources, case managers, and, in many cases, the evaluees themselves.

    1. *What can a person do safely?* The evaluee has been off work, placed on modified duty, or has a physical problem that has prevented placement

at work. Thus, the question of work ability is paired with the ability to perform work safely. If return to work is a goal, the secondary goal is ability to continue work without reinjury or failure. The evaluator optimally uses physiological measurements, including heart rate and blood pressure, as indicators for continuing or stopping test items. Because there is a medical diagnosis, the evaluator needs to be aware of contraindications to activity aligned with the specific diagnosis. Because evaluees may also have secondary physical issues or diagnoses, the evaluator must note and be aware of other conditions that must be considered in allowing safe performance. Other safety issues in FCE are the level of control of self or objects, balance, coordination, and stability. When maximum effort testing is used on FCE items, the evaluator records a score that indicates the highest level of ability that was demonstrated as safe to perform.

2. *What can the person do repetitiously?* Although information regarding the ability of evaluees to perform high-effort tasks (usually lifting and carrying) is clearly necessary in FCE, the ability to perform repetitious activity is necessary for a full picture of functional capacity in the context of full-time employment. Most FCEs are designed to incorporate repetitions of work tasks, and many also include a "circuit" of repetitious activity so that each task is evaluated more than once. For information on whether the work level can be continued on a day-to-day basis, some FCEs use two- and three-part formats for 2 or more days so that any changes in performance can be noted after the first day of testing. This practice not only solidifies the evaluator's ability to write an FCE work-related report but also allows the evaluee to understand whether day-to-day work can or cannot be accomplished. When work tasks can be repeated on more than 1 day, the evaluee's confidence in the FCE results should increase. This ability of an FCE to evaluate repetitive activity should lead to improved reliability and consistency ratings of the test results.

3. *Did the person give full effort?* Secondary gain is suspected of some persons in the workers' compensation and disability systems. Although this may be true of only a small minority, the possibility that evaluees may intentionally misrepresent their abilities creates the need to verify the level of full effort of most evaluees. Even when measurements or tests are reliable, one can consistently give less than full effort or, conversely, have physical changes when full effort has been exerted. Either of these situations may require the evaluator to adjust the final scores. Thus, the level of effort rating goes beyond consistency. Reliable observational criteria[15-22] have been identified to determine whether an evaluee is at a light-, moderate-, or heavy-effort level.

Referrers and Users of Functional Capacity Evaluations

As noted, work ability information from an FCE is used by a team of stakeholders, including the health care team, vocational or nurse case managers, psychologists, employers, and insurers. Well-designed FCEs are as work-oriented as possible. The FCE report should be written so that all users understand the work ability and limitations of the worker.

The focus of an FCE may differ depending on the referrer and the need for specific questions to be answered. The following are typical referral sources for FCE:

1. A physician or other health care provider: The medical provider is generally responsible for releasing the person back to work. A high-quality FCE provides objective information to assist in decision making regarding the level of work that can be done by the person and also gives some indication of the degree to which work limitations are needed to prevent reinjury (safety). The latter is particularly important given that most medical professionals consider themselves patient advocates and are hesitant to put injured or ill workers back into the workplace who could be reinjured or have their health endangered. They are also concerned about the liability risk of doing so. Thus, the referring medical provider needs to be able to trust that the information in FCEs can be used in return-to-work releases. The functional and medical information combine to allow a release to work or continuance of disability.

2. Case managers: These specialists can be from the vocational or the health care community and can be employed by the insurer or the employer. They prefer FCE language that contains medical information and work task information. The work task information should clearly state the level and specific work tasks that can be performed. Case managers are interested in whether the evaluee can return to the original job and original employer, a new job with the original employer, a new job with a new employer, or to other options, such as self-employment. Clarity in FCEs is extremely important for case managers because they must convey the information to their stakeholders, who then determine whether a return to work in any capacity is warranted. If accommodations cannot be made, case managers can use the information from an FCE to determine the best retraining options. Retraining is often expensive, and FCE information can help determine appropriate use of retraining dollars.

3. Employers: Although employers are interested in returning employees to work as soon and productively as possible to reduce workers' compensation and medical costs and avoid potential disability, they also want the employees to be able to work safely and avoid reinjury. Thus, the standards

are high as employers consider return to work at the highest safe function in the original job, a modification of the original job, or a new job. The FCE information is generic because it comes from a generic list of work activities and, hence, can only give the employer general information on ability levels and possibilities for modification. When the evaluator is provided a detailed objective functional job analysis or description, the FCE information can become more work relevant, with comparison with the job requirements. Employers want return-to-work decisions by medical professionals who will release a person to work at a fair and high level of ability but also limit possibility of the worker being reinjured. This requires confidence in the FCE and the evaluator, in addition to the releasing medical provider.

4. Workplace supervisor: Supervisors' needs are similar to those of case managers or employers, but because they are directly responsible for production and need to deal with the repercussions of reinjuries, they are particularly vested in receiving assurances that workers will come back to work, work their best, work safely, and be productive. The supervisor needs a clearly written FCE report that specifically details the evaluee's ability to perform particular jobs or particular job tasks and identifies potential job modifications that will lead to the highest level of safe productivity. When an FCE is ordered with this application in mind, replacement of the generic FCE with shorter job-specific functional tests that address the employee's original job may be appropriate (Table 1–4). Early return-to-work job-specific testing is a variant of functional testing that is shorter, more logical to the worker, more cost-effective, and better understood as a component of the return-to-work release. Its use, very early in case management, may also contribute to avoiding chronicity, adversarial relations, and lost or restricted time by establishing objective parameters for work release early in a claim.

5. Insurers, including workers' compensation and disability insurer: Both types of insurers are trying to mitigate losses by returning people to work. Their requirement is that an FCE describe the category, level and amount (full- vs part-time) of work, or even specific jobs that can be performed. Because insurers usually want to avoid more lost work or disability, FCE language and information are scrutinized to ascertain if they clearly indicate work abilities and the basis for any identified restrictions, especially if they preclude any form of work. Insurers prefer to know if the worker has worked to his or her full effort level and the anticipated reproducibility of results, although failure to produce full effort does not preclude return to work if the worker has been cleared for some form of full-time employment.

6. Attorneys: Medicolegal issues may arise in complex cases, including workers' compensation, disability, motor vehicle, other personal injury, medical malpractice, divorce, and loss of earning capacity. The capacity

of the person to do activities involved in gainful employment is often of interest because it becomes relevant in many negotiations regarding settlement. In legal hearings, an FCE falls between medical and vocational experts in the following sequence:

- The medical expert discusses pathology and impairment.
- The FCE evaluator discusses physical work ability, functional ability, and limitation related to work or activities of daily living.
- The vocational expert takes the functional work task information and looks for categories of work or specific work that can be found in the geographic area used by that jurisdiction.

Attorneys prefer to use objective evidence as fact to make their case. Because medical opinions of function are subjective, FCEs based on objective testing are used to add to the medical information obtained. Defense attorneys defend the employer and generally order an FCE to show that the person can go back to work, hence minimizing settlement costs for disability. Plaintiff attorneys are interested in maximizing the benefits to plaintiffs who have suffered an illness or injury and prefer to focus on resultant deficiencies in their ability to work. Attorneys who understand the science on which FCE is based and how the choice of components used in an FCE can affect the ultimate determination can analyze these evaluations for potential bias.

William Sommerness, an attorney, has indicated the role of FCEs as being critical in litigation and has used them in his work.[23] He states: "The most important testimony is that from the physical therapist and occupational therapist because they are the ones who have the 'hands on' experience with the client and can do the best job of explaining the client's attitude and performance." The Daubert decision also adds perspective to legal testimony.[24(p.345)] The evaluators and the tests must comply with certain legal conditions. First, the test used must be applicable to the case. Second, it must be backed by scientific rigor of reliability and validity studies. The testifying expert should be an expert in the exact field and the specific use for which testimony is given. This brings FCE to a high level of evidence when test and evaluator credibility are considered, which makes it important for there to be standards regarding their content and interpretation (refer to Chapter 20 for further discussion of the legal implications of FCEs).

In summary, while FCEs should be individualized to meet the needs of the specific referral source, they should be potentially able to fulfill the following requirements:

- Medical basis
- Scientific reliability and validity
- Indications of safety of work performance

- Indications of maximum work performance
- Indications of repetitive work performance
- Clarity of language
- Work task language
- Information that links physical ability with work
- Objective information written in clear and concise terms and based on reliable testing performed by a professional with a background that supports ability to do functional capacity testing

Evidence and Outcomes

Early FCEs were based on the skill of the practitioner, usually therapists, who used their professional background to develop tests within their field of expertise. As physical and occupational therapists traditionally used their skills in pathology, physiology, kinesiology, and anatomy to evaluate function in a wide variety of patients, functional evaluation of work ability was an extension of their work. Given the multiple types of FCEs available, their heterogeneity, and the recent focus on evidence-based medicine, the need for the evidence base of FCEs has grown. King et al[25] rated FCEs in an early article in 1998 on an evidence-based list that has not been updated since its original publication. Many FCEs had no or little evidence base at that time.

Lechner[26] was one of the first to report research on a type of FCE, although the subjects were persons with arthritis, not typical workers' compensation patients for whom FCEs were first developed. Smith[22] reported an early study on the reliability of safe lifting capacities. Isernhagen et al[17] of the United States researched the kinesiophysical Isernhagen Work Systems (IWS) FCE. Reneman[18] and Reneman colleagues[19-21] in the Netherlands have done substantially more work in this method and more thoroughly assessed reliability of several components. Gross and Battie,[16] in Canada, continued work on the moderate to excellent reliability of the IWS system.

Validity studies, in the context of the applicability of the FCE to predict return to work, have demonstrated a weak predictive ability of FCE.[27-29] In these retrospective studies, lifting ability was related to return to work, but weakly. The FCE was considered a stand-alone predictor for these studies, not for its use as part of a return-to-work team assessment as originally intended by most FCE authors. Thus, the primary result of this study may have been to demonstrate that FCE must be used in a larger case management system to have validity. Oesch et al,[30] of Switzerland, evaluated the role of FCE in medical release to work to provide further information on FCE use within a return-to-work system. In this context, the FCE, in conjunction with information from other team members, showed a strong ability to affect and predict return to work. This use of FCE as part of a team approach was the original intended use—FCE was not intended to stand alone but to be used by professionals to facilitate work return and the avoidance of disability. Validity of integrated rather than stand-alone use continues to be evaluated (refer to Chapter 21 for discussion of reliability and validity of FCEs).

Expansion of Functional Evaluation

The FCE will continue to be used in cases in which medical or functional problems are complicated and chronic. Early functional testing has a strong future as employers and medical providers see early return to the original job as a primary goal. Postoffer functional testing offers employer and applicant the opportunity to identify a fit between the work and the worker (refer to Chapter 13 for further discussion). Job-specific functional testing also has applicability in job transfers, after non-illness work absences, and in aging workers (refer to Chapter 14 for further discussion). The inherent differences in comprehensive general FCE tests and shorter job-specific functional tests are found in Table 1–4.

TABLE 1–4   Types of Return-to-Work FCEs

Job-Specific	General FCE
Job-specific	Generic work items (lift)
Short, less expensive	Longer, more expensive
Must be created from job description	Standardized models developed already
Includes unique job tasks (eg, patient transfers or working the molding machine)	Can be used for many jobs
Useful in early and chronic cases	Useful in chronic cases

FCE indicates functional capacity evaluation.

Functional testing should remain objective, a bridge between the health care and the employment communities, and of importance to the patient, the potential worker.

References

1. Isernhagen SJ. Functional capacity evaluation. In: Isernhagen S, ed. *Work Injury Management and Prevention.* Gaithersburg, MD: Aspen Publishers; 1988:Chap 14.
2. US Department of Labor, Employment and Training Administration. *Revised Dictionary of Occupational Titles.* Vol 1 and 2. 4th ed. Washington, DC: US Department of Labor, Employment and Training Administration; 1991.
3. Cranfield HV. Assessment of the working capacity of the physically disabled person. *Am J Occup Ther.* 1997;26:128–131.
4. Reuss EE, Rawe DE, Sundquist AE. Development of a physical capacities evaluation. *Am J Occup Ther.* 1958;12:1–8.
5. Matheson LN. *Work Capacity Evaluation.* Anaheim, CA: California Work Adjustment and Vocational Evaluator Society; 1978.
6. Matheson LN. Evaluation of the work capacity of injured employees' workshop. Presented at the American Occupational Medical Association Annual Scientific Conference; April 1979; Los Angeles, CA.
7. Matheson LN. Work capacity evaluation. Presented at the Occupational Therapy Association of California Annual Conference; October 1981; San Mateo, CA.
8. Matheson LN. Work capacity evaluation. Presented at the Occupational Therapy Association of California Annual Conference; October 1981; San Mateo, CA.
9. Matheson LN. *Work Capacity Evaluation: A Training Manual for Occupational Therapists.* Coto de Caza, CA: Rehabilitation Institute of Southern California; 1982.
10. Polinsky Medical Rehabilitation Center. *Functional Capacity Assessment Manual.* Duluth, MN: Polinsky Medical Rehabilitation Center; 1983.
11. Isernhagen SJ, ed. *Work Injury Management and Prevention.* Gaithersburg, MD: Aspen Publishers; 1983.
12. Work Capacity Analysis. *In: Key G. Physical Therapy.* Philadelphia, PA: JB Lippincott and Co; 1989.
13. American Physical Therapy Association. *Occupational Health Guidelines: Evaluating Functional Capacity.* Alexandria, VA: American Physical Therapy Association; 1999.
14. American Occupational Therapy Association. Functional capacity evaluation. www.aota.org/Practitioners/SISHome/SISs/WPSISS/35117.aspx. Accessed Feb 2, 2008.
15. Brouwer S, Reneman MF, Dijkmstra PU, Groothoff JW, Schnellekens JM. Test-retest reliability of the Isernhagen Work Systems Functional Capacity Evaluation in patients with chronic low back pain. *J Occup Rehabil.* 2003;13:207–218.

16. Gross DP, Battie MC. Reliability of safe maximum lifting determinations of a functional capacity evaluation. *Phys Ther.* 2002;82:364–371.

17. Isernhagen SJ, Hart DL, Matheson LM. Reliability of independent observer judgments of level of lift effort in a kinesiophysical functional capacity evaluation. *Work.* 1999;12:145–150.

18. Reneman MF. *Functional Capacity Evaluation in Patients With Chronic Low Back Pain: Reliability and Validity* [dissertation]. Groningen, the Netherlands: Rijksuniversiteit; 2004.

19. Reneman MF, Brouwer S, Meinema A, Dijkstra PU, Geertzen JH, Groothoff JW. Test-retest reliability of the Isernhagen Work Systems Functional Capacity Evaluation in healthy adults. *J Occup Rehabil.* 2004;14:295–305.

20. Reneman MF, Dijstra PU, Westmaas M, Goeken LN. Test-retest reliability of lifting and carrying in a 2-day functional capacity evaluation. *J Occup Rehabil.* 2002;12:269–275.

21. Reneman MF, Jaegers SM, Westmaas M, Goeken LN. The reliability of determining effort level of lifting and carrying in a functional capacity evaluation. *Work.* 2002;18:23–27.

22. Smith RL. Therapist's ability to identify safe maximum lifting in low back pain patients during functional capacity evaluation. *J Orthop Sports Phys Ther.* 1994;19:277–281.

23. Isernhagen SJ. The attorney's role. In: Isernhagen SJ, ed. *Work Injury Management and Prevention.* Gaithersburg, MD: Aspen Publishers; 1988:chap 24.

24. *Daubert v Merrill Dow Pharmaceuticals, Inc,* 113 S, CT2786, 2795, 125 LE d2d 469 (1993).

25. King PM, Tuckwell N, Barrett TE. A critical review of functional capacity evaluations. *Phys Ther.* 1998;78:852–866.

26. Lechner DE. Reliability and validity of a newly developed test of physical work performance. *J Occup Med.* 1994;38:997–1006.

27. Gross DP, Battie MC. Functional capacity evaluation performance does not predict sustained return to work in claimants with chronic back pain. *J Occup Rehabil.* 2005;15:285–294.

28. Gross DP, Battie MC. Does functional capacity evaluation predict recovery in workers' compensation claimants with upper extremity disorders? *Occup Environ Med.* 2006;63:404–410.

29. Matheson LN, Isernhagen SJ, Hart DL. Relationships among lifting ability, grip force, and return to work. *Phys Ther.* 2002;82:249–256.

30. Oesch P, Devereaux J, Backman S, Kool J. The influence of a functional capacity evaluation on fitness for work certificates in patients with non-specific chronic low back pain. *Work.* 2006;26:3:259–272.

CHAPTER

2

Approach to Requesting a Functional Evaluation

Elizabeth Genovese, MD, MBA, and **Susan J. Isernhagen, PT**

Indiscriminate use of terminology such as "functional capacity evaluation" (FCE) to describe all tests designed to assess function is intrinsically flawed because it creates the impression that there is some standardized "generic" test (or a series of generic tests) applicable to all situations in which there are questions about a person's functional ability. It is therefore unsurprising that many referral sources who have not been educated about the variation in and limitations of FCE individual test components, batteries, and proprietary systems request an FCE without clearly defining, for themselves and whomever they use for this testing, what they are looking for and the context in which the testing is to be applied.

A generic FCE assessing the degree to which a person can perform a wide variety of tasks that are of presumed relevance to a potential work environment is most commonly requested in the context of disability assessment to provide objective information to assist in return-to-work (RTW) issues. It usually consists of lengthy standardized tests of work tasks designed to cover the most common work demands, usually includes some form of "sincerity of effort" testing (see Chapter 11), and is the same for all patients who are tested using a particular FCE model and not job-specific. However, there are alternative patient or job-specific testing options that are applicable to other situations that may be more appropriate to request.

Even when a generic FCE is appropriate, given the wide range of vendor-specific FCE models currently available and the lack of uniformity in their choice of individual test components and the manner in which these components are assimilated in the final report (which is affected by the model and the competence of the evaluator), assumptions regarding the existence of a generic template are totally unfounded. Potential FCE test components are described in the introduction and in Chapters 1 and 3. There is also a description of some of the currently available FCE models in the Appendix; they are clearly quite diverse. There are relatively few published studies supporting the reliability of individual models, but of even greater concern is the tendency of many models to rely on extrapolations of test results to work capacity estimates that have often not been demonstrated in the literature as valid (claims of substantiation by internal, proprietary research may well be correct but are not verifiable). The argument is often made that the lack of evidence supporting the reliability or validity (defined in Chapter 21) of a particular type of FCE is not important given literature supporting the reliability and validity of individual test components. Chapters 5 through 12 will review the available published literature regarding many FCE test components and discuss the degree to which they have been demonstrated to be reliable and/or valid, and Chapter 21 will discuss available evidence about the reliability and validity of FCE as a whole.

Because there is no terminology that has been uniformly accepted for use when referring individuals for functional testing and no standard procedures for assessing physical capacities or restrictions, it is most helpful for people who contemplate ordering a functional assessment to focus on the following:

- Nature of the person on whom the testing is being performed ("who")
- Type of information desired from the testing ("why")
- Context in which the testing is occurring ("where" and "when")

All of these factors will (or at least should) affect the skills assessed, the choice of test components, the length of testing, and the degree to which the evaluator evaluates intratest and intertest consistency of the patient.

Matheson[1] has stated that the reasons for a functional capacity evaluation can be broken into five general categories:

- Functional goal setting: Assess the functional ramifications of an impairment (or impairments) as a prelude to some form of rehabilitation
- Disability rating: Measure loss of ability in key functional areas of work as an estimate of disability
- Job matching: Determine the adequacy of the worker's abilities as they relate to the essential functions of a specific job
- Occupation matching: Determine the adequacy of the worker's abilities as they relate to task demands in a given occupation
- Work capacity evaluation: Evaluate a person's functional capacity in the context of all potential occupations that he or she might hold, which invariably needs to be done in conjunction with a vocational skills and availability assessment

Although this classification system is useful, an alternative is to focus on the medical "reasons" for the evaluations. These can be placed in three overall categories:

- Injury prevention (to avoid or prevent a medical problem)
- Work-related injury or illness management (as an adjunct to treatment of a medical problem)
- Chronic injury or illness evaluation (to assist with the rehabilitation or disposition of persons with chronic medical problems)

The concept of maximal medical improvement (MMI)—the point when "patients are as good as they are going to be from the medical and surgical treatment available to them"[2] or "the date from which further recovery or deterioration is not anticipated, although over time (beyond 12 months) there may be some expected change"[2]—is relevant to the discussion of FCEs as applied to patients in the second and third categories. To elaborate, functional evaluation of people who have not reached MMI is often ordered as part of a treatment plan (including RTW),

CHAPTER 2

whereas the use of FCE is more likely to be "dispositional," ie, aimed at achieving resolution of open claim issues of relevance when performed at or near MMI. The three categories, along with a listing of the different types of testing that fall into each, are listed in Table 2–1. Although there can be some overlap, and some of the testing options fall into more than one category, this structure provides a framework for organizing thoughts regarding who, why, where, and when as a prelude to actually ordering an evaluation.

TABLE 2–1 Medical "Reasons" for Functional Testing

---

1. Injury prevention
   a. Preoffer (physical fitness and agility testing)
   b. Postoffer
   c. Periodic screening
   d. Job transfer
   e. Fitness-for-duty return to work evaluation

2. Work-related injury or illness management (in context of treatment, may or may not be at MMI)
   a. Early return-to-work evaluation
   b. Mini FCE
   c. Return-to-work FCE

3. Chronic injury or illness management (usually at MMI)
   a. Specific job placement–related residual functional abilities assessment
   b. Stand-alone dispositional residual functional abilities assessment
   c. Dispositional FCE as an adjunct to an independent medical evaluation
   d. Special circumstances

FCE indicates functional capacity evaluation; MMI, maximal medical improvement.

Functional Assessment in the Context of Injury Prevention

Functional testing done in the context of injury prevention can occur before a job offer (physical fitness or agility test), after an offer, as a component of periodic screening, in preparation for job transfer, or to assess whether a person with a non–work-related injury or illness can return to some form of work. Even though these evaluations may include tests that screen for specific job skills, the main purpose of requesting them is to minimize the risk that unqualified people will injure themselves or others if hired to work at a level or do tasks for which they are physically unqualified. People who do not have the requisite skills for a job that is not potentially hazardous can simply be eliminated from the position after hire by virtue of not meeting employer expectations. As a consequence, evaluations performed in the context of injury prevention need to include testing and, if cost-effective, clinical assessments that will clearly identify relevant active and, if possible, potential functional deficits, even if occult.

Physical fitness and agility tests and most postoffer functional assessments are usually relatively brief and job-specific. Longer FCEs are often appropriate for people who have been off work, on modified duty, or on disability leave. When performed in the context of evaluating the ability of the worker (with a non–work-related injury or illness) to return to a previously held position, FCEs may be more appropriately classified as a "fitness for duty" FCE (FFD FCE). Return-to-work decisions need clarity and objective information. These tests are lengthy and simulate the physical demands of a specific job. Thus, they are different for each job. Innes and Straker[3,4] were early to describe the differences in job-specific vs generic functional capacity evaluations. Benefits of the generic form of FCE were the ability to perform reliability studies, whereas benefits of the job-specific form of FCE were the ability to define work ability for a particular employer or a particular job or job group. Preoffer and postoffer tests are job-specific.

Preoffer and Postoffer Testing

Preoffer and postoffer testing are used by employers to test applicants against the physical components of the job. They differ in content (postoffer tests are often, but not always, more comprehensive) and, more significantly, in timing and the extent to which medical information can be included as part of the evaluation.

Preoffer functional tests are used to gather nonmedical information specific to a particular skill (as a rule) *before* a job offer is made and are usually used as an adjunct to other preoffer information to offer applicants a job with clearly delineated physical demands. Because these tests are performed at the preoffer stage, no medical information can be obtained or used. They consequently do not include a history or physical examination and can be performed by nonmedical personnel. Preoffer tests can focus on physical fitness or ability, agility, and/or the ability to complete sample job tasks. Title VII of the Civil Rights Act, the Americans with Disabilities Act of 1990 (ADA), and the Age Discrimination Act of 1967 prohibit the use of discriminatory testing, which includes the use of testing that has a "disparate impact on the basis of race, color, religion, sex, or national origin."[5] Employers who use preoffer testing must be certain that the physical requirements of the job and the need for these requirements are clearly described. They should also be prepared to demonstrate that "the selection procedure is job-related and consistent with business necessity,"[5] that there is no "less discriminatory alternative available"[5] (one that could equally predict performance but not disproportionately exclude a protected group), and that the selection procedure is "necessary to the safe and efficient performance of the job."[5]

The term *postoffer* indicates that the employer has made a conditional job offer to a potential employee and the test is being given to determine if the applicant can perform the essential functions of the job. The critical difference between postoffer functional testing and testing done at the preoffer stage is the ability of the employer to include a medical examination as part of postoffer testing. This is because of specification by the ADA that questions about disability cannot be asked and medical examinations cannot be required until after a conditional job offer has been made. The testing must be "job-related and consistent with business necessity"[6] and used as part of the postoffer evaluation of "all individuals entering the same job category."[6]

There is no good reason to obtain a postoffer as opposed to a preoffer evaluation if one is doing so simply to evaluate physical abilities or work-related skills that can be assessed through a nonmedical evaluation. On the other hand, when one needs to assess functional abilities in the context of a prospective employee's physical examination and medical history, a postoffer evaluation is more appropriate. Requirements regarding nondiscrimination and the need to consider the potential worker's request for accommodation, should they occur (the employer does not need to proactively offer accommodation if it is not requested), are virtually identical, regardless of when the evaluation occurred. However, the employer has more information on which to base decisions when data have been obtained postoffer rather than preoffer.

Periodic Screening (Job Transfer) Functional Capacity Evaluations

Although traditionally used as part of the initial hiring process, functional testing similar to that used at the preoffer or postoffer stage can be used to help determine whether a current employee has the skills to move to another job. These *job-transfer evaluations* must be performed for all employees who want to apply for an alternative position. Functional testing that specifically focuses on the ability to perform job-related skills can also be used to periodically screen existing employees to assess whether they continue to meet job requirements. Employers who use this type of testing should have a set list of criteria on which to base the frequency of screening evaluations, generally achieved by requiring that they be performed at regular intervals (hence, the terminology *periodic screening*). To use criteria such as weight gain, age, or other conditions that could be considered as "protected" as the basis for ordering a screening test or evaluation is unwise. There is also little to be gained from arranging these evaluations for workers who are already doing their regular jobs because, regardless of test results, it would be difficult to make the argument that they are not capable of performing essential job functions. However, the evaluations may be of value to use in the assessment of employees such as fire fighters, police officers, and emergency department personnel for whom essential job functions include the sporadic performance of physically taxing activities.

Fitness-for-Duty Functional Capacity Evaluations

On the other hand, if an existing employee has been out of work owing to an illness or injury that is not work-related or the employer suspects that a medical condition may have progressed to the point at which it might interfere with an employee's ability to work safely or pose a hazard to others, an *FFD/return-to-work* medical examination might be warranted. An FFD medical and/or functional evaluation that includes functional testing specific to the position in question is easiest to justify when the employer has already used preoffer screening or postoffer evaluations to initially qualify applicants for the specific position. The ADA, however, states that these evaluations can also be used if the employer has "reasonable belief, based on objective evidence, that the employee will be unable to perform essential job functions or will pose a direct threat because of a medical condition"[5] or received a "request for a reasonable accommodation."[5] Under these circumstances, they can be job-specific or may also be more generic when the potential impact of a new-onset medical condition may preclude an employee from safely or effectively performing activities that ordinarily can be performed by most people. One example would be an employee who has to do somewhat repetitive but not ordinarily arduous work with her right hand but has had breast cancer that required extensive dissection of the lymph nodes in her right arm, resulting in chronic lymphedema. A purely medical evaluation may be all that is required. However, ancillary functional testing may also be useful to demonstrate the development of increased swelling or limb discoloration with the performance of job activities that would preclude doing the job in the way it was done previously. It could also be used to assess whether the essential functions of the job can otherwise be performed with reasonable accommodation or if there are other positions the employee could fill. This situation is one in which judicious proactive use of functional testing will potentially prevent an aggravation of pre-existing disease due to work activities leading to a workers' compensation claim.

Issues Relevant to Selecting, Designing, and Applying Injury Prevention Testing

It is mandatory for an employer to define the essential functions of a job for preoffer or postoffer testing to be performed. An evaluator with clinical experience (such as a physical therapist or occupational therapist) then can, with or without the assistance of other skilled professionals such as ergonomists, perform a job analysis and determine the most appropriate functional tests for the screening or testing process by translating this information to terms that describe the physical activities required. Although there may be typical items such as lifting, pushing, pulling, hand coordination, other portions of the testing are customized to assess the skills or physical capacities required for the specific job for which the applicant is being tested. Therefore, job-specific testing is used in preference to generic testing. As noted earlier, the individual designing the testing regimen must be certain that there is no alternative form of testing that is potentially less discriminatory (particularly relevant when testing women or people with medical conditions that potentially could affect their ability to comprehend testing instructions or other aspects of the testing procedures that do not necessarily translate to ability to perform job requirements). In the case of a qualified applicant with a condition that is covered under the jurisdiction's definition of disability, the evaluator may assist an employer in identifying reasonable accommodations.

When an employer simply wants to assess whether prospective employees have skills that have been clearly delineated as job-related and necessary (see preceding text), preoffer screening tests are often adequate although risk the possibility of missing medical conditions that could affect a person's ability to perform an essential task repetitively, especially when a prospective employee, who is clearly motivated to do his or her best, has a condition that may not become apparent until some time after the task has been performed. (A classic example is a low back problem that may not prohibit performing several 50-lb lifts but would result in severe low back pain, precluding the performance of lifting the next day.) Thus, although these tests can be done by a nonmedical professional, test design should foster identification of occult but relevant medical conditions, which often will mandate that the evaluator be educated about how to discern evidence of fatigue or altered biomechanics that might not be easily discernible.

This issue is potentially less problematic in postoffer functional evaluations because these evaluations are usually performed by professionals such as therapists and often include a history and physical examination performed by the therapist and/or another licensed health care provider such as a physician, physician assistant, or nurse practitioner. The same is the case for FFD/RTW evaluations, which can be more comprehensive (and, thus, provide more information about the patient) than routine postoffer tests when they are evaluating the worker's ability to do a specific job and meet some generic work-related criteria. However, examiner qualifications cannot always compensate for a poorly designed testing regimen and also, obviously, may lead to erroneous conclusions when patients, who clearly want to meet the functional test requirement to be employed, have been less than forthright in providing relevant historical information or describing symptoms that may arise during the course of testing (although, as stated, if the testing is adequate and the evaluator has appropriate clinical training, changes in patient biomechanics or the physical examination may suggest that limitations exist). The evaluator, cognizant of "passing criteria" and the importance of patient safety, must use professional skill in determining how far to proceed with testing and may need to unilaterally stop the testing when clinical evidence suggests that a patient may be at imminent risk of harm if evaluation is continued. The use of tests or combinations of tests to evaluate "consistency of effort" is obviously not required when evaluating people who want to obtain or maintain employment at a particular job because they are motivated to demonstrate ability rather than disability. The employer, on the other hand, is motivated to identify any relevant disability or incapacity that might negatively impact on the employee or others in the workplace.

Outcomes after the use of postoffer testing have been published by Nassau[6] and Gassoway and Flory.[7] The latter study demonstrated significant cost savings and a decrease in injuries and lost time when workers had passed tests for hire. Injuries that occurred in workers who had passed the postoffer or agility tests were less severe or costly compared with injuries that occurred before postoffer test implementation. There also may have been a reduction in turnover. Similar findings were presented by Toeppen-Sprigg and Isernhagen[8] about postoffer testing in a large Goodyear plant in the United States. Decreased injury, decreased cost, decreased lost time, and decreased turnover were measurable after the institution of postoffer testing with savings that were substantiated during a 3-year period.

Functional Assessment as an Adjunct to Work-Related Injury or Illness Management

There is a significant body of literature supporting the benefit of "early RTW" for employees who have sustained on-the-job injuries,[9–13] with employees who have been injured at work most likely to stay at work or have early RTW if they remain in a "worker" rather than a "patient" mode. Liberty Mutual researchers Shaw et al[14] and Pransky et al[15] have documented the benefits of assessing job-relatedness early in a medical case to prevent needless disability. The American College of Occupational and Environmental Medicine has published Stay-at-Work/Return-to-Work guidelines[16] that also discuss the importance of early RTW for the worker and the employer. The general recognition that time away from work can lead to longer, more expensive claims has led occupational medicine–oriented professionals and employers to design proactive programs that allow injured or ill workers to stay at work or RTW early.

The progress of workers receiving rehabilitation toward meeting short- and long-term goals should be routinely assessed by the clinician providing treatment at regular intervals. This assessment should include a clinical evaluation and the use of relevant job-specific functional testing to guide rehabilitation providers and physicians (or other health care providers) in completing employer- and insurer-mandated physical capacity estimates. In situations in which physicians and rehabilitation providers are working closely together and communicate optimally, there is rarely a need for functional assessments other than those that should be routinely included in the therapy re-evaluation. There are, however, situations in which these assessments may not be adequate. The first is when re-evaluations by the rehabilitation provider are not adequately assessing function in the context of job-related tasks (or when an injured employee is not receiving physical or occupational therapy at all) but the employee has injury-related physical limitations that need to be thoroughly assessed and documented to allow health care providers and supervisors to gain an accurate understanding of job-related functional abilities. The second is when the rehabilitation provider (and/or physician) observes a significant discrepancy between objective physical findings (or the nature of the original injury) and self-reported pain, musculoskeletal complaints, or physical limitations but the employee has not been under treatment for a period deemed to be longer than ordinarily required for the initial injury. In the latter situation a *dispositional FCE* (see "Dispositional Functional Capacity Evaluations—Description" and "Dispositional FCEs—Considerations") may be appropriate.

Early Return-to-Work (RTW) Evaluations

Efforts to identify the job tasks that a worker can perform safely and that need to be modified temporarily can be described as *"early RTW evaluations"* because their goal is to optimize the match between current worker abilities and job duties during treatment. Evaluations are brief, job-related, and individualized. They may be repeated often until full duty is reached. Because workers may be in a "healing stage" when testing is performed, therapists must use stopping points for tests that allow opportunities to demonstrate function without having a detrimental effect on healing. When regularly asked to participate in testing focused on objectively delineating their residual functional capacities in the context of the stay-at-work/RTW process, patients are presumably less likely (or able) to use subjective descriptions of their jobs or their own capabilities as grounds for remaining out of work. Thus, as long as they continue to be in the worker mode and believe that the employer desires them to stay or RTW, there is less likelihood of self-limiting performance in early RTW testing. It has been Isernhagen's experience that the majority of workers who have received appropriate medical treatment (stressing the gradual resumption of prior physical activities) perform realistically in the context of early RTW testing.

Mini-Functional Capacity Evaluations

Job-specific physical progress evaluations performed purely to assist in early RTW will not ordinarily include testing protocols that evaluate the level or consistency of effort. However, it has been the experience of Genovese that the initial management of employees who are not meeting expected functional goals or describe symptoms in excess of objective findings is facilitated by the use of brief, focused evaluations that incorporate one or two "sincerity of effort" tests (see Chapter 11). These evaluations can be considered a form of *mini-FCE* because they can alert clinicians to the need to aggressively evaluate patient- and employer-specific factors that may be causing or increasing the risk for "delayed recovery." A list of these factors is given in Table 2–2.[17] Although mini-FCEs are not routinely used as a component of injury management, one can see where the identification and "hard" documentation of submaximal or inconsistent effort can provide an opportunity for physicians (and/or therapists) to frankly discuss results with patients and establish expectations that must be met for treatment to continue.

TABLE 2–2   Risk Factors for Delayed Recovery

Factors
Demographic factor
Age
Historical factors
Previous injuries
Recent prolonged absence from work
Absence from work
Multiple absences from work
Being a victim of past abuse
Social factors
Family history of disability
Change in family role
Family support
Union membership
Personal health
Chemical dependency
Depression
Emotional distress
Employment-related factors
Job satisfaction
Task enjoyment
Adversarial job relationship
Job demands
Alternative work available (absence of modified work)
Perception of work-relatedness
Union agreements
Presence or absence of second injury funds
Injury-related factors
Severity of (self-rated) symptoms and/or health status
Expectations of work capacity
Severity of signs
Delayed presentation
Chronic pain symptoms
Multiple diagnoses
Diagnosis of low back pain or carpal tunnel syndrome
Prior negative treatment experiences
Excessive/inappropriate physical medicine treatment
Economic and legal factors
Income
Education

TABLE 2–2 Risk Factors for Delayed Recovery (continued)

Factors
Compensability
Legal representation
Litigation pending

Reproduced with permission from: Goertz MN. Cornerstones of Disability Prevention and Management. In: Glass LS, ed. *Occupational Medicine Practice Guidelines*. 2nd ed. Elk Grove Village, Ill: American College of Occupational and Environmental Medicine; 2004:75–103.

Return-to-Work Functional Capacity Evaluation

When employees have received treatment for work-related injuries or illness and reach a point where they are failing to make any additional functional progress, an RTW FCE might be warranted. In many situations, patients will be at MMI. In others, they may have just reached the point at which no further benefit can be gained from "conventional" physical therapy and may benefit from referral to a more comprehensive work-conditioning or work-hardening program. The RTW FCE is comprehensive and similar to the FFD FCE previously described. Indeed, the difference between the two may initially be difficult to discern because both are FCEs used to assess whether employees are "fit" for RTW. Nevertheless, it is mandatory that the critical differences between them be understood. Specifically, RTW evaluations that are done after work injuries generally are requested because the employer or insurer is responsible for paying indemnity benefits. They want to help the employee return to work and are motivated to allow him or her to do so even if there are significant physical restrictions and the employee does not want to return to work. Fitness-for-duty evaluations, on the other hand, are performed after non–work-related injuries or illnesses. Employees usually want to return to work but, because the condition was not work-related, the employer has no financial incentive (besides those associated with recruiting and training a new employee) to allow employees who have not fully recovered to return to work if they cannot safely perform the job. In these cases, employers may prefer that the employee not return to work if the job-related activities are deemed to place the employee (or others) at undue risk of injury. Thus, evaluators who perform FFD FCEs are usually testing motivated patients and need to focus test activities on unearthing subtle signs of *disability*, whereas evaluators performing RTW FCEs in the context of workers' compensation injury management may be working with less motivated patients (and motivated employers) and need to carefully evaluate the patient's effort level while focusing on defining his or her *abilities*.

Functional Capacity Evaluations in the Context of Chronic Injury or Disease

People with chronic injuries or disease sent for a functional evaluation often differ markedly from people who are evaluated earlier in the clinical course. In particular, the impact of anatomic and/or physiologic abnormalities on function may have been altered (usually accentuated) by the effect of psychological, social, work-related, and other environmental factors, especially when the disease is accompanied by chronic pain or fatigue. Some people with chronic disease are highly motivated to return to work, have a job (although perhaps not their original job) to return to, and will exert maximal effort during functional testing—the main purpose of this testing is then to develop a reasonably accurate assessment of their physical capacities as a prelude to rehabilitation and/or job placement.

Others may not have a job to return to, may not want to work, or may believe that they are incapable of doing so (see Chapter 15 for a thorough discussion of the relevant issues to be considered and addressed in people with chronic pain). Although this terminology is not ordinarily used, people who request functional testing as part of the management of patients with chronic illness or disease can be thought as doing so to facilitate disposition and the evaluation as a dispositional FCE. In other words, the person sent for the FCE is generally considered to have reached MMI, and the purpose of the FCE is to document residual functional abilities as a prelude to case closure (or claim settlement, or whatever terminology is most appropriate for the situation).

Job Placement–Related Residual Functional Abilities Assessments

Specific *job placement–related residual functional abilities assessments* are useful for motivated people who can no longer perform their former job but want to attempt further rehabilitation or be considered for an alternative position. They are often used in preparation for entrance to a work-conditioning or work-hardening program,[18] and the patient is, consequently, usually *not* at MMI. The FCE gives the rehabilitation team objective information on which to base treatment goals. If the proposed job is available, a comparison can be made between the current functional status and goals that need to be obtained that support RTW. Shorter forms of testing may be repeated during rehabilitation and, unless the patient is fully recovered, followed by a complete FCE at termination of treatment.

Dispositional Functional Capacity Evaluations—Description

As stated previously, the purpose of dispositional FCEs is usually the documentation of residual functional abilities as a prelude to case closure or claim settlement. They can be performed as a *stand-alone* study or as an *adjunct to an independent medical evaluation* (IME). In the latter situation, the FCE may be performed before the IME to provide additional information on which the physician can base his or her opinion. The reverse situation is also encountered, when there is referral for an FCE after an IME is done to confirm, dispute, or more thoroughly describe findings regarding work capacity. Indeed, FCEs are often ordered in conjunction with IMEs for patients with complaints of pain that are disproportionate to objective findings but are not egregiously so to assess residual functional capacities, the level of effort, and the consistency of symptoms, especially in the context of specific physical findings.

A classic illustration of when an FCE would be of value after or in relative temporal relationship to an IME would be when a worker with complaints of back pain (but no objective findings) has been out of work for 5 months owing to a compensable injury needs to be cleared by the physician to return to a job that requires heavy or very heavy lifting. Despite the absence of objective findings, ~~Not true~~ most physicians would be reluctant to return this person to this job without some assurance that the person could perform at the required level. If the FCE cleared the worker for heavy work, the physician would usually agree, whereas if the FCE cleared the worker only for light work, the physician would not release the person to the job but might recommend rehabilitation. However, if the FCE indicated that the person exerted submaximal effort and demonstrated "inconsistencies" in the ability to complete various tasks, the physician might ignore the complaints and return the person to the former position.

An IME and an FCE may describe different capacities for the same person, or the findings might agree. Differences may reflect actual changes in physical abilities in situations when the IME and FCE are temporally separated or reflect inability of the physician to accurately assess physical abilities or the consistency of evaluee reports of incapacitating pain or other symptoms based solely on the history and physical examination. On the other hand, if the individual performing the FCE fails to integrate clinical evaluation of the evaluee into his or her final determinations or the FCE places undue emphasis on symptoms and subjective limitations rather than objective definable limitations (see Chapters 3, 11, 16, and 18), differences between the IME and FCE may also reflect an underestimation of the person's capacity by the FCE. Differences in assessment of work capacities by the physician and therapist can be avoided by integration of information in a combined report, as is done in Switzerland.[19] The physician and FCE evaluator meet to discuss their respective findings and write one report that reflects their mutual opinion. This method has strengthened case management and does not create the need for additional tests to reconcile physician and therapist differences.

The degree to which dispositional FCEs are described as stand-alone studies depends on how one defines them. Most FCEs are ordered to clarify or buttress an IME. Nevertheless, when the results of an FCE are not sent to the IME physician for review, the study can be considered to be independent of the IME. This distinction is important because in the absence of an IME against which to compare FCE results, it is mandatory for the FCE to include a thorough clinical evaluation of the evaluee, which can provide valuable information that can be compared with the medical records and used to interpret FCE test results.

Dispositional FCEs—Considerations

Dispositional FCEs are generally generic rather than job-specific. However, it is still useful for referral sources to be as specific as possible regarding their needs because knowledge of the context in which the examination is being ordered will help the evaluator in the initial choice of test components and in determining how (or whether) evaluee-specific factors should alter testing. It is also recommended that requestors of FCEs determine, if possible, which of the potential FCE components described in the Introduction and in Chapter 1 are relevant to their needs and be certain to specifically ask for their inclusion in any testing that is performed. For example, if the evaluee has a history of chronic pain disproportionate to objective findings, the evaluator should focus on evaluating consistency of effort, sitting, and use of his or her hands (for a possible clearance for sedentary work) and consider use of psychometric questionnaires (see Chapter 15). Alternatively, for an evaluee who claims limitation as a result of hand pain following carpal tunnel surgery, specific tests of hand function (see Chapter 12) should be included in the FCE.

Referral sources who order dispositional FCEs generally want to use the FCE to terminate (or not initiate) benefits or settle a case for as low of a figure as possible by demonstrating that the evaluee is capable of some form of gainful employment. They consequently would like the FCE to demonstrate that the evaluee is capable of at least full-time sedentary work—preferably more. Evaluees, on the other hand, understandably often prefer that FCE results indicate incapacity to return to any form of full-time work (or, at the least, a prior job) to justify continuation (or initiation) of financial benefits or, depending on the circumstances, settlement of the indemnity portion of a case for as high of a figure as possible.

When the dispositional FCE is used as part of the claim settlement process in workers' compensation, long-term disability, Social Security, or other areas in which the extent of a person's residual functional capacities requires clarification, with no need to necessarily demonstrate more than the minimal capacity for full-time work, there is generally no reason to assess highly specific functions or skills relevant to relatively few occupations. The exception is when the FCE is being ordered by a disability carrier at a point in the claim at which a person is entitled to benefits only if he or she cannot meet the physical demands of his or her *own* occupation, in which case it clearly behooves the referral source to make this clear to the evaluator (and include a detailed list of the specific abilities that need to be assessed). Inclusion of tests that evaluate consistency and level of effort, to give guidance on the accuracy of results, is obviously mandatory in dispositional FCEs. Because clinical judgments regarding the consistency of effort are often based not only on raw tests results but also on integrating these results with information obtained from the physical examination and observation of the patient throughout the testing protocol (see Chapters 4–16), the FCE should be performed by an experienced clinician with strong observational skills. Likewise, as noted previously, while all dispositional FCEs should include at least an injury-specific clinical evaluation, this is particularly important for FCEs that are being performed as stand-alone studies.

Regardless of whether a dispositional FCE is ordered as an adjunct to an IME or as a stand-alone study, even under these circumstances there may be situations in which it is optimal for the final results to be interpreted by a physician, skilled therapist, kinesiologist, or ergonomist in the context of information available in the medical record and, at times, surveillance activities. In the latter case, it may be of benefit to arrange for evaluee observation before and after the FCE and to consult with the person who will be reviewing FCE results beforehand. These issues are discussed further in Chapter 18 (Clinician and Insurer Use of FCEs).

Special Circumstances—Functional Capacity Evaluations in the Evaluation of Nonmusculoskeletal Conditions

There are times when the FCE is to be used to evaluate a person claiming incapacity as a result of *fatigue or similar symptoms* that are not easily quantified objectively. The principles described in Chapters 4, 5, 6, 9, 10, 11, 14, 16, and 18 should be reviewed before requesting FCEs for these patients. The FCE should include tests of aerobic capacity—preferably more than one, at different times during the study. The test should also, if possible, be at least 2 days (to assess evaluee status on the day after the study, when many persons state they are extremely debilitated by their disease as a result of the FCE) and make liberal use of activities of daily living and other self-report questionnaires (see Chapter 5).

Summary

Although FCEs share the goal of identifying an evaluee's ability to functionally perform work tasks, there are significant variations among functional evaluations (eg, content, length, "focus," and credentials of evaluator) that must be considered before the test is requested to optimize the test's ability to address the questions of interest. In particular, the degree to which functional evaluations should address specific as opposed to generic job skills and evaluate consistency of effort will depend on the clinical context of the evaluation and evaluee motivation to exert maximal effort, which will be driven in part by the former.

It is therefore mandatory to consider, before requesting a functional evaluation, whether it is being ordered to facilitate injury prevention, for injury or illness management, or for patient "disposition" as part of, or as a preface to, claim resolution (RTW, disability evaluation, or the coordination of legal or insurance benefits; see Chapter 1) and/or requires a focused evaluation of a particular body part (such as the upper extremity; see Chapter 12) or skill set. Failure to appropriately consider the nature of the person on whom the testing is being performed (who), type of information one wants to acquire from the testing (why), and context in which the testing is occurring (where and when) will often lead referral sources to request generic FCEs that may not be equipped to address their specific needs. See Table 2–3 for a summary of FCE purposes and their referral criteria.

TABLE 2–3   Summary of FCE Purposes and Referral Criteria

Purpose of Functional Test	Suggested Name	Usual Source	Length and Components
Injury Prevention			
Assess worker qualifications to perform specific job-related skills before job offer	**Preoffer tests**	Employers	Short and job-specific
Determine if applicant can perform the essential functions of the job after job offer; may include a medical examination	**Postoffer tests**	Employers	Short to moderate length; job-specific
Move employee within the work setting to accomplish a transfer or assess if employee can perform essential functions if the job or worker (eg, aging) has changed	**Periodic screening (job placement) tests**	Employers	Short to moderate length; job-specific
Assess if employee with non–work-related condition (generally with residuals) can return to former job or another available position; may be accompanied by medical evaluation; employee motivated to do well	**Fitness-for-duty FCE**	Employers	Short to moderate; job specificity dependent on context; should include clinical evaluation
Work-related Injury or Illness Management (Early or Noncomplex)			
Job-specific physical progress evaluation performed in the context of ongoing treatment to reduce lost work time or restricted time	**Early return-to-work testing**	Employers, medical providers	Short and job-specific
Physical progress evaluation with addition of tests to assess "sincerity of effort" (usually when patient showing evidence of "delayed recovery")	**Mini FCE**	Medical providers, insurers	Short; might or might not be job-specific; tests for consistency of effort

TABLE 2–3 Summary of FCE Purposes and Referral Criteria (continued)

Purpose of Functional Test	Suggested Name	Usual Source	Length and Components
Assess if employees who continue to be symptomatic (usually at MMI) can return to work at own job or in any capacity, even if there are significant physical restrictions and employee does not want to return; assess consistency (sincerity) of effort	**Return-to-work FCE**	Medical providers, employers, insurers, case managers	Moderate length; generic with or without job-specific components and inclusive of testing to assess sincerity of effort

Chronic Injury or Illness Management

Purpose of Functional Test	Suggested Name	Usual Source	Length and Components
Provide objective information regarding whether employee can return to own job or to alternative position; if not at MMI, may be used in preparation for entrance to a work conditioning or work hardening program (to set treatment goals)	**Residual Functional Abilities Assessment**	Medical providers, insurers, employers, case managers	Moderate length; job- (or work) specific or generic, depending on context; may be repeated
Ordered as a prelude to claim settlement to assess residual functional capacities, the level of effort, and the consistency of symptoms. Results are seen by IME physician and interpreted in the context of the medical record and his or her clinical evaluation	**Dispositional FCE with IME**	Case managers, lawyers, insurers, physicians	Moderate to long; usually generic; includes clinical eval and testing to assess "sincerity of effort"
Also ordered to assess residual functional capacities as a prelude to claim settlement. Results are not interpreted by the IME physician but by other third party (depends on referral source)	**Dispositional FCE–Stand-Alone**	Case managers, lawyers, insurers	As above but long; should include comprehensive clinical evaluation

TABLE 2–3 Summary of FCE Purposes and Referral Criteria (continued)

Purpose of Functional Test	Suggested Name	Usual Source	Length and Components
Assess work capacity in individuals with chronic medical illnesses such as chronic fatigue, multiple sclerosis, etc. Because many of these persons state that they are debilitated by their inability to sustain physical activity, this must be assessed as part of the FCE, preferably by ordering testing over several days	**Special-Purpose FCE**	Insurers, lawyers, medical providers	Long; usually generic (as above) with additional testing for aerobic capacity (endurance) and positional tolerance needed

References

1. Matheson L. The functional capacity evaluation. In: Demeter S, Anderson G, eds. *Disability Evaluation.* 2nd ed. Chicago, IL: Mosby; 2003.
2. Rondinelli R, Genovese E, Katz RT, et al, eds. *Guides to the Evaluation of Permanent Impairment.* 6th ed. Chicago, IL: American Medical Association; 2008:23.
3. Innes E, Straker L. Reliability of work-related assessments. *Work.* 1999;13:107–114.
4. Innes E, Sraker L. Validity of work-related assessments. *Work.* 1999;13:125–136.
5. US Equal Employment Opportunity Commission. Employment Tests and Selection Procedures. www.eeoc.gov/policy/docs/factemployment_procedures.html. Accessed April 20, 2008.
6. Nassau DW. The effects of prework functional screening on lowering an employer's injury rate, medical costs and lost work days. *Spine.* 1999;24(3):269–274.
7. Gassoway J, Flory V. Prework screen: is it helpful in reducing injuries and costs? *Work.* 2000;15:101–108.
8. Toeppen-Sprigg B, Isernhagen S. Fitness for Duty Assessment: Fitness for Duty. Presented at: American Occupational Health Conference; April 29, 1999; New Orleans, LA. Scientific session 115.
9. Labriola M, Lund T, et al. Multilevel analysis of individual and contextual factors as predictors of return to work. *J Occup Environ Med.* 2006;48(11):1181–1188.
10. Atlas SJ, Chang Y, et al. Long-term disability and return to work among patients who have a herniated lumbar disc: the effect of disability compensation. *J Bone Joint Surg Am.* 2000;82(1):4–15.

11. Brooker AS, Cole DC, et al. Modified work: prevalence and characteristics in a sample of workers with soft-tissue injuries. *J Occup Environ Med.* 2001;43(3): 276–284.

12. Bernacki EJ, Guidera JA, et al. A facilitated early return to work program at a large urban medical center. *J Occup Environ Med.* 2000;42(12):1172–1177.

13. Elders LA, van der Beek AJ, et al. Return to work after sickness absence due to back disorders: a systematic review on intervention strategies. *Int Arch Occup Environ Health.* 2000;73(5):339–348.

14. Shaw WW, Pransky G, Patterson W, Winters T. Early disability risk factors for low back pain assessed at outpatient occupational health clinics. *Spine.* 2005;30(5): 572–580.

15. Pransky GS, Verma SK, Okurowski L, Webster BS. Length of disability prognosis in acute occupational low back pain: development and testing of a practical approach. *Spine.* 2006;31(6):690–697.

16. ACOEM Guideline: Preventing needless work disability by helping people stay employed. Elk Grove Village, IL: American College of Occupational and Environmental Medicine; 2006.

17. Goertz MN. Cornerstones of Disability Prevention and Managment. In: Glass LS, ed. *ACOEM Clinical Practice Guidelines.* 2nd ed. Elk Grove Village, IL: American College of Occupational and Environmental Medicine; 2004:84.

18. Darphin L. Work hardening and work conditioning perspectives. In: Isernhagen S, ed. *Comprehensive Guide to Work Injury Management.* Gaithersburg, MD: Aspen Publishers; 1995:450–451.

19. Oliveri M, Hallmark M-L, Hofer H. Rehabilitation of chronic musculoskeletal disorders at the Clinic of Rheumatology, Institute of Physical Therapy, University Hospital Zurich Switzerland. In: Isernhagen S, ed. *Comprehensive Guide to Work Injury Management.* Gaithersburg, MD: Aspen Publishers; 1995:584–595.

CHAPTER

General Testing Principles for Functional Capacity Evaluations

Susan J. Isernhagen, PT, and Jill S. Galper, PT, MEd

A general discussion about functional capacity evaluations (FCEs) is challenging because there is no universally agreed-on standardized protocol used by FCE evaluators to make determinations about an evaluee's work ability. As noted in Chapter 1, the common goal of all FCEs is to provide the FCE requestor with functional information about an evaluee's ability to perform work and functional activities. In the chapters that follow, the various methods used to assess an evaluee's work ability and their respective reliability and validity are discussed in detail. Information about commercially available models is available in the Appendix. Although the specific methods used by an FCE model vary, there are general principles common to all FCEs. These principles include standardization within a specific protocol, evaluee safety, and methods to optimize evaluee cooperation and performance.

Standardization Within a Functional Capacity Evaluation Protocol

Although the methods used to determine an evaluee's physical abilities vary among FCE models, there should be standardized procedures within a specific FCE model regardless of whether the protocol was developed by an individual clinician or is commercially available. Standardization refers to a clearly defined set of procedures for administering and scoring tests.[1] The test procedures should be written in a manual that is easy to use, and each task should be defined and described according to the equipment needed and the procedures to follow.[1] The terminology used in the FCE should be defined in the manual.[1]

The FCE procedure used should be reliable and valid, and the evaluator should be knowledgeable about the research available in support of the FCE method chosen. Chapter 21 reviews the overall scientific status of FCE; the reliability and validity of specific procedures used to assess function are discussed in the relevant chapters of this book.

Evaluee Safety

Primum non nocere, "First, do no harm," applies to FCEs in that all FCE evaluators strive to ensure the safety of evaluees. As used herein, *safety* refers to preventing a new injury or adversely affecting an evaluee's current condition. We do not consider a transient increase in pain symptoms to be unsafe. Safety parameters should be clearly defined in FCE protocols, and evaluators must use sound professional judgment to avoid injury by exceeding an evaluee's musculoskeletal, cardiovascular, or neurologic tolerances.[2] Chapter 21 provides further discussion regarding safety in FCEs.

Medical Contraindications and Precautions

The FCE evaluator should determine that there are no underlying medical conditions that are contraindications or precautions for an evaluee's participation in an FCE.[3,4] Review of the medical record, an evaluee interview, and a clinical examination should identify movements or activities that should be avoided or monitored carefully as indications of when a test should be stopped. Precautions in test procedures should be taken to minimize exacerbation of disease or injury. The FCE evaluator should determine that the evaluee:

- Does not have a diagnosed condition that is in an acute stage or a condition that would worsen by participation in an FCE. With acute conditions, additional injury or exacerbation might occur if healing tissues are stressed too soon in recovery. This includes people who have undergone surgery, sustained a fracture, or experienced a strain or sprain or an inflammation of soft tissue. If referred by a physician, the health status of the evaluee should have been established at the time of the referral.

- Has reached a plateau in medical healing, even if maximum improvement has not been reached. The plateau creates a time in which the person's condition is stationary and work placement can be considered. An FCE is a long and somewhat expensive test, and if the natural history of the condition or further treatment is expected to result in significant improvement in the evaluee's condition that would result in improved function, the FCE outcomes would not be valid beyond a brief period after the FCE. In cases in which the FCE or components of an FCE are used to guide a rehabilitation program or progressive return to work, this would not be a significant concern.

- Has a resting blood pressure or heart rate that allows safe performance of physical test activities. Some evaluators will not proceed with any testing or will limit testing to sedentary activities if the resting blood pressure and/or heart rate equals or exceeds some cutoff criteria. In the American College of Cardiology/American Heart Association Guidelines for Exercise Testing, tachycardia and bradycardia at rest are indicated as relative contraindications for exercise testing, and evaluees with these findings should be monitored carefully.[5] Blood pressure and heart rate are affected by anxiety, stress, caffeine, nicotine, and medication. If an evaluee has an elevation in blood pressure or heart rate, evaluators should help the evaluee relax and try to determine if there was any medication or substance that could account for the increased blood pressure or heart rate. If elevated, these vital signs are usually monitored during the initial stages of the FCE to determine if they decrease enough to allow testing to proceed. If this is not the case, the FCE requestor should be contacted and the test postponed or limited in intensity until blood pressure and heart rate are evaluated and controlled by appropriate medical personnel. The evaluator should be aware of any medication the evaluee is taking that might affect his or her heart rate response to activity (eg, beta-blockers). In these cases, heart rate may not be a good physiologic indicator of effort or physical stress, and this must be taken into account by the evaluator.

- Has a state of endurance that allows evaluation during a multihour (or multiple-day) evaluation.
- Has agreed to participate in the FCE and agrees to cooperate as necessary for accurate evaluation. Evaluees who from the beginning refuse to comply with test instruction are not candidates for FCEs because they are unlikely to fully cooperate with testing, although they could be candidates for testing that would be limited to identifying compliance issues. Chapters 4 and 20 provide information about informed consent.

Body Mechanics During the Functional Capacity Evaluation

The FCE evaluator should assess the evaluee's knowledge of body mechanics during the FCE. Some FCE models promote instruction in optimal body mechanics principles before lifting assessment is done. Other models observe the evaluee and intervene as needed. There is some disagreement about "proper" body mechanics, in part because optimal body mechanics vary depending on the size and/or bulk of the item being handled[6] and are also affected by the evaluee's physical status (eg, limited knee motion). That said, there is wide agreement that horizontal distance (distance from hands to center of feet) should be minimized and trunk rotation (twisting) should be avoided during manual material handling activities (unless specific job simulation conditions apply). Promotion of optimal body mechanics during the FCE should help protect an evaluee who may be performing activities that create stress or discomfort. Evaluators should be knowledgeable in body mechanics and proficient in instruction. Encouraging optimal body mechanics during FCE is considered professionally responsible and diminishes liability.

Test End Points

The FCE protocols should have clearly defined test end points to ensure evaluee safety. The specific parameters may vary depending on the age and medical condition of the evaluee. The evaluator usually calculates the evaluee's maximum allowable heart rate before functional testing is started. The heart rate limit is dependent on the evaluee's medical condition, with values between 70% and 85% of the age-related maximum heart rate. Age-related maximum heart rate (HR_{max}) is often calculated by the formula 220 − age, but Tanaka et al[7] developed a revised formula that may also be used to determine age-related maximum heart rate (HR_{max} = 207 − [0.7 × age]). During activity, an abnormal change in blood pressure or heart rate is an indicator to stop activity, as is the increase in the evaluee's heart rate to a maximal allowable limit. Some evaluators apply the American College of Sports Medicine (ACSM) Guidelines and stop a test activity if the evaluee has a drop in systolic blood pressure of more than 10 mm Hg from baseline blood pressure despite an increase in workload or has a "hypertensive response (systolic blood pressure of > 250 mm Hg and/or a diastolic blood pressure of > 115 mm Hg),"[8(p.106)] which the ACSM Guidelines identify as a relative contraindication to continuing exercise testing. These limits may be reasonable for some patients but unreasonable in the presence of medical conditions in which an excessive rise in blood pressure may place the evaluee at undue risk of an untoward outcome. The blood pressure before the beginning of the evaluation is also of relevance because the relative change in blood pressure often has greater implications with regard to evaluee safety during an FCE than does the baseline level (as acclimatization generally develops). In general, it is best to obtain a complete medical history and monitor all evaluees with elevations in blood pressure above a systolic blood pressure of 180 mm Hg and/or diastolic blood pressure of 115 mm Hg at regular intervals during the evaluation, especially during activities that would be expected to increase blood pressure further. Some evaluators monitor oxygen saturation during testing. The ACSM criteria state that a drop in oxygen saturation of more than 4% is abnormal, but this will depend on the person's baseline (eg, a drop from 98% to 94% may be less significant than a drop from 91% to 87%).[8] Also, the evaluator should terminate testing if there are signs of dizziness, incoordination, or excessive fatigue during a test activity.

Test end points are also related to manifestation of clinical signs or symptoms related to the evaluee's injury or illness. The evaluator should note any effect that an evaluee's condition has on function and determine if an activity exacerbates the evaluee's neuromusculoskeletal problem or illness. This is done by correlating the impact of movement, force, position, and evaluee report on that injury or illness. Activity should be stopped if there is evidence that the evaluee's condition is worsened by that activity. Examples of this are increased numbness in the median nerve distribution or decreased grip strength during tests of hand function in an evaluee with known carpal tunnel syndrome and a test activity that increases lumbar paravertebral muscle spasm in an evaluee with signs and symptoms of a herniated lumbar disk.

Last, test end points may be related to an evaluee's quality of movement and motor control during functional activity. The FCE protocol should have clearly defined operational definitions and standardized procedures about how movement is evaluated and classified, and the FCE evaluator should have good observational skills and a clear understanding of the test protocol's operational definitions and procedures. For example, a lifting test would be stopped when an evaluee demonstrates decreased control of the lumbar spine (eg, loss of stabilization of the lumbar spine and pelvis), because continuing the lifting test would place the spine at risk of injury. These reasons for stopping a test should be clearly documented by the evaluator in the report.

Psychophysical, Physiological, and Kinesiophysical Testing

There are three general approaches in determining the end point of a functional test that are described herein. Many evaluators use a combination of these approaches in performing FCEs.

1. In **psychophysical testing**, the evaluee's opinion determines the test end point. The evaluator asks the evaluee to make a judgment when a certain level of ability or effort is reached. Research studies of workers and/or uninjured subjects use psychophysical criteria to determine an evaluee's perception of his or her ability. This format has been used for lifting and grip and pinch research to obtain normative data. A subject may also be asked to rate "how hard" a test is and the number of repetitions she or he feels capable of performing. Psychophysical testing has significant applicability to identifying ability levels of groups of people categorized by age, sex, or anthropometrics. It has been helpful in static and dynamic research to develop normative data. This approach has less application for evaluees who may not have a clear perception of their own ability, have psychosocial factors (eg, fear-avoidant behavior)

that impact performance, or are suspected of not accurately reporting or demonstrating ability.

2. In **physiologic testing**, indicators of physiologic exertion identify when to stop a test activity. This could include predetermined medical indicators such as blood pressure or heart rate, as discussed. For pace, there may be a metronome or timed rate. The predetermined levels have been set by the protocol and result in test-item termination if reached. Physiologic testing is often integrated with the psychophysical or kinesiophysical approach.

3. In **kinesiophysical testing**, the evaluator uses functional movement criteria to determine the end point of testing. These include safe body mechanics, physiologic end points, and protection of the injured or deficient area from further damage. Observational criteria are used to objectively identify the level of effort: light, moderate, or heavy.[9–15] The evaluee interacts with the evaluator, but it is objective criteria for test performance that are used to determine scores and end points. If an evaluee refuses to perform or to continue and a functional end point has not been reached, this situation will be scored as a self-limited end point, not one determined by the objective criteria. The evaluator uses a combination of the objective criteria, knowledge of safe performance, and precautions related to pathology to determine end points.

Pain vs Function as Evaluation Focus

Before the use of FCEs, many evaluees made their own determination as to how much physical activity they could perform. In patients with low back pain, to determine if a patient's perception of his or her own ability was similar to the capacity tested, Brouwer et al,[16] of the Netherlands, investigated the correlation between FCE outcomes and patient perceptions and found that evaluees significantly underreported their ability levels compared with determinations made using the Isernhagen Work Systems FCE, which relies on objective criteria for test end points.

In many cases, FCE evaluees have reached a chronic stage of recovery. In more acute cases, discomfort and symptoms must be considered because they may indicate that the physical problem could be made worse by activity. Findings from the musculoskeletal-evaluation help identify the signs that should be carefully monitored during testing. However, for an evaluee in the chronic stage, discomfort may be related to numerous problems, including scar tissue, joint degeneration such as arthritis or spurring, or old nerve damage. The history and physical examination almost always reveal that chronic-type pain is present, even before the test starts. It is very helpful to acknowledge and document the evaluee's reports of discomfort. In taking the history, it is often found that physical activity is associated with more discomfort. Statements such as "I hurt more after I do physical activity" are common. These types of symptom reports indicate that although activity can temporarily create more discomfort, this is customary for the evaluee as he or she performs higher levels of activity. The evaluator should determine the evaluee's baseline and usual increase in discomfort with activity. If the evaluee reports more severe discomfort than is typical or reports a different type of discomfort than usual, the evaluator should investigate these complaints further. A person's reaction to pain may affect activity participation in three ways:

1. Pain symptoms are the reason activity is stopped.
2. Pain symptoms are used to gauge the level of activity that can be performed.
3. Function is used as the guide for activity, with little or no attention to pain symptoms.

Because many evaluees with pain symptoms rely on their past reference points for determining "safe" activity limits, there is danger of identifying only subjective beliefs about ability, rather than optimal physical abilities, when professional interactions and criteria are not used during functional testing. The following are examples of what may occur when objective criteria are *not* used as a guide to safe performance:

- An evaluee who uses pain as a guide to stop an activity will perform submaximally because he or she usually quickly stops activity with any discomfort.
- An evaluee who is able to gauge his or her reaction to pain and activity level is usually able to consistently perform activity at a level sustainable for work because the evaluee is able to modify activity levels by using pain as a guide during the course of the day.
- An evaluee who does not use pain as a guide may overexert himself or herself and have consequences such as injury or fatigue. The evaluee often may not be able to reproduce efforts in a multiple-day or multiple-effort FCE or at work. The lack of attention to symptoms may result in harm.

Thus, if pain is used as the test end point, there is limited ability to identify the evaluee's actual maximum safe ability. If the evaluee and evaluator understand that chronic symptoms are part of the condition, optimal functional capability is more accurately determined by objective criteria with the focus on safe performance. The focus away from pain and on productive function may be a new concept for the evaluee and potentially have a positive effect on self-efficacy and self-awareness. With a focus on productive function, the FCE becomes a true functional evaluation and not a pain report.

Evaluator-Evaluee Interactions That Optimize Performance

Interactions between professional evaluators and evaluees are powerful. An example frequently used in educational settings describes the powerful effect of teachers' perceptions and students' performance.[17] When equally matched groups of students were studied and labeled differently, one as "high potential" and the other as "low potential," the outcomes reflected the perception, not the reality. The group for which the teacher had the highest goals (highest potential), scored highest at the end of the study. Conversely the group for which the teacher had lower expectations scored lower despite their equal beginning aptitude. The teaching methods or unintended communication may have resulted in disparate results for the two groups.

For FCE evaluators, the concepts have similar application. If an evaluator begins a test with suspicion or mistrust and is focused on ways to "find the faker," this attitude is communicated to the evaluee. It can create a reactive suspicion of the test process in evaluees, which may result in poor communication, poor compliance, or exaggeration.

Conversely, an evaluee is more likely to cooperate and feel encouraged during the FCE when the evaluator begins each evaluation by communicating a sincere respect for the evaluee, is aware of the evaluee's history, and has an interactive discussion about the test expectations. If the evaluee is a fearful person, the evaluator's professionalism and positive approach can facilitate trust so the evaluee works to her or his best ability. This approach is particularly important when an evaluee has had long-standing and complex physical dysfunction and discomfort, because obtaining useful test results requires the evaluee's cooperation and participation during what can be a physically stressful evaluation. The evaluee's trust in the evaluator will facilitate optimal performance. This trust cannot be mandated; it must be earned. The evaluator has an opportunity to engender this trust at the outset of the FCE by stating her or his professional background, the purpose of the test, the expectation of interaction, and his or her willingness to work with the evaluee during the evaluation process. During the history and physical examination, the evaluee has an opportunity to determine the professional skills of the evaluator and can acquire the respect and trust necessary to go forward with the test.

The FCE evaluator must be aware of his or her personal beliefs and bias and whether they might affect the evaluee's performance. In addition, the evaluator should have good communication and clinical skills. The attributes of FCE evaluators are further discussed in Chapter 17. Aspects of interaction that should also be considered include the following:

■ *Designed instruction set*: Some professionals believe that a structured instruction set creates better test reliability. That belief assumes that the person hearing the instructions does not have her or his attention diverted, does not have a language problem, and can understand language at the speed at which the evaluator speaks. Evaluees who come to an FCE may have one or more of the following: fear, mistrust of the medical or employer community, a long pattern of misunderstanding their own abilities, chronic pain, or intimidation regarding taking a long and difficult test. The ability for an evaluee to concentrate without diversion is not always possible. The evaluator must be able to recognize when there is a need to positively and clearly repeat instructions or use different terminology. Ultimately, the evaluee needs to be fully aware of what is expected and how to correctly execute a task to perform to his or her full ability. One will avoid inconsistencies or poor performance caused by lack of understanding if the evaluator ensures that each item is clearly understood. When language barriers require the presence of an interpreter during the FCE, more attention must be given to ensuring that the evaluee understands the instructions and test purpose. The evaluator also needs to be sensitive to cultural differences that can potentially impact performance or affect how symptoms are communicated.

■ *Interaction about performance*: Some FCE evaluators focus more on "scoring" than "evaluation." In these situations, the evaluator gives instructions and then "scores" the performance with little or no feedback between the evaluee and the evaluator. Other evaluators use interaction between evaluator and evaluee to facilitate full performance and ensure safety. With this type of interaction, an evaluator uses objective scoring criteria but also requires feedback from the evaluee to identify perceptions and symptoms. When the evaluator is open and clear about how the test is progressing, the evaluee is better able to understand his or her abilities and limitations.

■ *Submaximal effort*: Effort levels are part of what the FCE evaluator assesses during the test. If less-than-maximal performance is observed during an FCE, positive confrontation can provide the evaluee with another opportunity to do better. If the purpose of the FCE is to determine full safe functional abilities vs identifying behavioral aberrations, this interactive approach may result in more optimal results. Submaximal effort should also be discussed with the evaluee and the discussion documented, so that the evaluee is not surprised by this determination when it appears in the report. If an evaluee does not put forth full effort in one test, this does not mean that all tests are suspect. For example, the evaluee may be unwilling to put forth full effort during lifting tasks but performs with full effort during walking, hand coordination, or other tasks. The FCE evaluator should document each task and how it was completed and consider the evaluee's overall performance when interpreting test results. This is discussed in more detail in Chapter 16.

- *Exit discussion*: When FCEs are being performed in the context of a treatment program, an exit discussion, in which the evaluator and evaluee discuss the test results, can be helpful to the evaluee. This final discussion assists the evaluee in understanding his or her abilities and cooperation level. It prepares the evaluee for the use of the FCE information by the physician, case manager, employer, and insurer involved in the case. When the FCE is not being performed in the context of ongoing treatment (ie, is a dispositional FCE, discussed in Chapter 2), this discussion might not be appropriate.

CHAPTER 3

Summary

Although FCE models vary in regard to the activities included and the processes by which they are performed and scored, there are basic principles common to all models that are important for consistency within the test process and to ensure patient safety. These common principles were discussed in detail in this chapter and include the need for standardized terminology, operational definitions and instructions, and considerations for patient safety. Considerations for patient safety include ensuring that the evaluee is medically stable and has no absolute contraindications for the FCE. During the FCE, the evaluator should monitor the evaluee's posture, physiologic response, and movement patterns during activity. If the evaluee has preexisting medical problems, more frequent monitoring of vital signs may be appropriate. Each FCE protocol should have clearly defined test end points.

The importance of evaluator-evaluee communication as a means of optimizing the evaluee's performance during an FCE has been discussed. The evaluator should be sensitive to the evaluee's feelings and fears (if present) and attempt to establish an interaction that engenders trust, cooperation, and interactive communication. When an evaluee performs fully within his or her safe physical abilities, meaningful and useful data will be obtained. While the FCE may have value in the absence of full effort, it will not represent more than the evaluee's minimal functional ability.

References

1. King PM, Tuckwell N, Barrett TE. A critical review of functional capacity evaluations. *Phys Ther.* 1998;78:852–866.

2. Lechner DE. The well-designed functional capacity evaluation: application in forensic vocational analysis. *J Forensic Vocational Anal.* 2004;7:83–96.

3. American Physical Therapy Association. *Occupational Health Guidelines: Evaluating Functional Capacity.* Alexandria VA: American Physical Therapy Association; 1999.

4. American Occupational Therapy Association. Functional Capacity Evaluation. American Occupational Therapy Association website. www.org/practitioners/sishome/sisswpsiss/35117aspx. Accessed October 23, 2007.

5. Gibbons RJ, Balady GJ, Bricker JT, et al. ACC/AHA 2002 guideline update for exercise testing: summary article: a report of the American College of Cardiology/American Heart Association Task Force on Practice Guidelines (Committee to Update the 1997 Exercise Testing Guidelines). *Circulation.* 2002;106:1883–1892.

6. Straker LM. A review of research on techniques for lifting low-lying objects, 2: evidence for a correct technique. *Work.* 2003;20:83–96.

7. Tanaka H, Monahan KD, Seals DR. Age-predicted maximal heart rate revisited. *J Am Coll Cardiol.* 2001;37:153–156.

8. American College of Sports Medicine. *ACSM's Guidelines for Exercise Testing and Prescription.* 7th ed. Philadelphia, PA: Lippincott Williams & Wilkins; 2000.

9. Isernhagen SJ. Functional capacity evaluation. In: Isernhagen S, ed. *Work Injury Management and Prevention.* Gaithersburg, MD: Aspen Publishers; 1988:139–163.

10. Isernhagen SJ, Hart D, Matheson LM. Reliability of independent observer judgments of level of lift effort in a kinesiophysical functional capacity evaluation. *Work.* 1999;12:145–150.

11. Gross DP, Battie MC. Reliability of safe maximum lifting determinations of a functional capacity evaluation. *Phys Ther.* 2002;82:364–371.

12. Reneman MF, Brouwer S, Meinema A, Dijkstra PU, Geertzen JH, Groothoff JW. Test-retest reliability of the Isernhagen Work Systems Functional Capacity Evaluation in healthy adults. *J Occup Rehabil.* 2004;14:295–305.

13. Reneman MF, Dijkstra PU, Westmaas M, Goeken LN. Test-retest reliability of lifting and carrying in a 2-day functional capacity evaluation. *J Occup Rehabil.* 2002;12:269–275.

14. Reneman MF, Jaegers SM, Westmaas M, Goeken LN. The reliability of determining effort level of lifting and carrying in a functional capacity evaluation. *Work.* 2002;18:23–27.

15. Smith RL. Therapist's ability to identify safe maximum lifting in low back pain patients during functional capacity evaluation. *J Orthop Sports Phys Ther.* 1994;19:277–281.

16. Brouwer S, Dijkstra PU, Stewart RE, Goeken LNH, Groothoff JW, Geortzen JHB. Comparing self report, clinical examination and functional testing to measure work limitations in chronic low back pain. *Disabil Rehabil.* Sep 2 2005;27(17):999–1005.

17. Lee J, Eccles J, Madon S. Social perception, social stereotypes, and teacher expectations: accuracy and the quest for the powerful self-fulfilling prophecy. *Advances in Experimental Social Psychology.* 1996;29:281–388.

CHAPTER 3

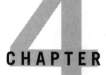

Baseline Functional Capacity Evaluation Components

Jill S. Galper, PT, MEd

The core components of a functional capacity evaluation (FCE) are commonly regarded as positional tolerance assessment, work simulation tasks, and tests to identify material handling, movement, and aerobic ability. Before performing these core tests, the FCE evaluator should review the reason for the FCE referral and any medical records provided, obtain informed consent, interview the evaluee, and perform a musculoskeletal evaluation. In this chapter, these preliminary activities are referred to as baseline FCE components. The use of psychometric tests and questionnaires regarding pain and disability are also considered a baseline component because the evaluee typically completes these questionnaires at the outset of the evaluation, usually before the interview. The use of psychometric testing and similar self-report questionnaires will be discussed further in Chapter 5 and will not be addressed in this chapter. Nearly all FCEs include informed consent and evaluee interview. The inclusion of a musculoskeletal examination in FCEs is more variable. This variability seems dependent on the qualifications of the FCE evaluator and the FCE model used. As will be discussed, the musculoskeletal examination provides valuable information and should be included in all FCEs.

The purposes of informed consent, evaluee interview, and musculoskeletal examination are to:
1. Inform the evaluee about the purpose, procedures, and expectations of the FCE and the associated risks before obtaining his or her decision to consent to or decline participation;
2. Obtain information about the evaluee's current and past symptoms (location, intensity), work and leisure activities, and perceived disability;
3. Identify any potential contraindications or precautions for testing;
4. Determine if the evaluee has medical conditions or takes medication that might impact on performance or response to activity (eg, beta-blockers);
5. Identify what, if any, impairments in strength, motion, and balance, etc, exist and later correlate these findings with functional performance; and
6. Observe the evaluee's sitting tolerance and movements through the completion of these baseline components (although this is not a primary purpose).

This chapter discusses these baseline FCE components, with the exception of the use of pain and psychometric questionnaires, which is discussed in Chapter 5.

Informed Consent

The right of a patient to make an intelligent choice is at the core of informed consent. Delany[1] wrote that there are three broad reasons for obtaining a patient's consent before treatment: (1) The health care practitioner has an ethical duty to respect a patient's autonomy and to act in his or her best interest. (2) The process of providing the patient with information and obtaining consent fosters cooperation and compliance with treatment (or evaluation). (3) There are legal requirements that demand that information be provided so a patient can make an informed decision. The rules for informed consent for physical and occupational therapists are specified in each state's relevant practice act. The use of informed consent in an FCE is recommended by the American Physical Therapy Association (APTA)[2,3] and the American Occupational Therapy Association (AOTA).[4] The APTA *Guide to Professional Conduct*[5] states: "A physical therapist shall respect the patient's/client's right to make decisions regarding the recommended plan of care, including consent, modification, or refusal." Similarly, the AOTA Code of Ethics requires that occupational therapists obtain informed consent before initiating evaluation.[4]

The informed consent should explain what an FCE is, identify the risks associated with the test, and discuss what is expected of the evaluee. The FCE evaluator should respond to any questions the evaluees have and ensure that they understand their right to decline to perform any requested activity, although the evaluator will likely ask the reason for the refusal. Although the consent can be obtained verbally, it is recommended that the consent be written and that evaluees sign and date it. The evaluator should have procedures in place for illiterate and for non–English speaking evaluees. The unwillingness of an evaluee to sign an informed consent is reason to abort further evaluation.

CHAPTER 4

Evaluee Interview

Most FCEs begin with an interview of the evaluee about current symptoms; work and leisure activities; exercise program; medications; treatment performed for the relevant diagnosis and the evaluee's response to it; and medical, surgical, and work history. Some FCE evaluators also inquire about an evaluee's educational history. If the FCE is job-specific, the evaluator should not rely only on the evaluee's description of the job; a detailed job analysis should have been made available to the evaluator before the FCE. Chapter 14 provides further discussion of job-specific testing. The evaluee may also have completed a written medical history and psychometric and pain testing before the interview. Goodman and Snyder[6] wrote: "It is generally agreed that 80 per cent of the information needed to clarify the cause of symptoms is contained within the subjective assessment" and recognized that interviewing is an important clinical skill and evaluation component.

The information obtained from the evaluee interview should include the following:
- The evaluee's physical problem(s)
- Contraindications or precautions for the FCE
- Data to allow the evaluator to compare the evaluee's subjective reports with the following:
  - Results of the psychometric and pain questionnaires
  - The evaluee's behavior, complaints, and performance during testing
  - Observations during distracted activities
- The evaluee's sitting tolerance and use of gestures and movement during conversation

For example, observation of an evaluee with complaints of neck pain and limited motion may demonstrate that the evaluee consistently moves stiffly and guardedly throughout all FCE test components, whereas another evaluee's movement patterns may change during the FCE (less movement during direct examination than during naturalistic observation and activities not directly related to the cervical spine). The evaluator can then use this information in analyzing the evaluee's level of effort and performance consistency during the FCE. Chapter 11 provides further discussion about determining evaluee consistency and level of effort during FCEs.

Musculoskeletal Evaluation

Most FCE protocols include the evaluator's clinical examination of the evaluee. The evaluator should have the appropriate knowledge base, skills, and qualifications to perform the examination. The examination should include baseline measurement of blood pressure, heart rate, height, and weight and should also include a focused clinical examination appropriate to the evaluee's diagnosis and/or area of complaint. A comprehensive discussion regarding musculoskeletal examination is beyond the scope of this chapter, but the examination components may include observation, palpation, girth or volumetric measurement (if appropriate), assessment of range of motion, strength and sensation, and tests specific to the area of involvement (eg, straight leg raise for low back assessment). Some protocols use inclinometers for assessment of spinal range of motion, and some computerized systems determine an impairment rating, based on the rating from the American Medical Association (AMA) *Guides*. Many FCE protocols do not include the AMA impairment rating because this rating, based on active motion, is not regarded as "functional" in terms of the evaluee's ability to perform activities and it is also not consistently used in different editions of the AMA *Guides*. Active motion assessment does not differentiate between evaluees who are unwilling to move (which may be due to a number of factors) and evaluees who are unable to move due to muscle weakness or joint restriction. Passive motion assessment and strength testing of these evaluees should be performed to determine if there are joint restrictions or weakness causing limited movement. Assessment of muscle strength is most often done by manual muscle testing methods, but some evaluators assess muscle strength with a computerized (usually isokinetic) device. These computerized devices permit a number of analyses to be made, including comparison of the involved side with the uninvolved side and computation of agonist/antagonist ratios. Chapter 7 provides discussion about the use of computerized testing for assessment of isolated muscle strength in FCEs.

People with musculoskeletal dysfunction have signs and symptoms specific to that dysfunction. There should be correlation among the findings in medical records (if present), the evaluee's symptoms and signs, the referring physician's diagnosis (if present), and the FCE evaluator's clinical diagnosis. The impairments identified in the clinical examination should correlate with the functional limitations identified during functional testing. For example, a evaluee who had knee surgery may have impairment in knee flexion (decreased motion) and quadriceps weakness that underlies the functional limitations identified for squatting and standing up from lowered positions. In other words, the functional limitations should "make sense" given the examination findings. The FCE evaluator should consider the presence or absence of these correlations when analyzing consistency and level of effort.

If a musculoskeletal examination is not performed as part of an FCE, the evaluator cannot correlate functional performance with an underlying impairment and, instead, can only record the evaluee's performance because there is no clinical context in which to understand it. This is akin to basing a diagnosis on magnetic resonance imaging alone without a clinical examination. Without an examination or other clinical correlation, the FCE evaluator is hard pressed to distinguish between limitations in evaluee performance owing to unwillingness to participate vs limitations due to impairment. The FCE evaluator may not know "why" performance is limited because many factors (eg, fear, pain, and lack of understanding of instructions) affect performance, but functional limitations due to physical impairment can be identified. The correlation between impairment and function is the basis for treatment planning in rehabilitation and is discussed at length in the *Guide to Physical Therapist Practice*.[7]

As noted in Chapter 1, there are a number of commercially available FCE models, as well as FCE protocols developed by individual clinicians. The Appendix provides information about many of the commercially available FCE models in the United States. With two exceptions, all models listed in the Appendix include client history and musculoskeletal evaluation as part of the FCE. The JTech FCE System "strongly encourages" the evaluator to obtain a history and perform an examination. The Medigraph FCE RFC-DOT allows the history to be included in the comment section, but it has no bearing on the outcome of the examination; for musculoskeletal examination, a visual inspection is not required, and movement tests are performed to establish functional ability.

When an evaluee has a constellation of signs and symptoms that do not fit a musculoskeletal dysfunction, other causes (eg, systemic disease and symptom magnification) should be considered by the evaluator. In particular, if the evaluee seems to be in medically stable condition (based on history and clinical information) but appears significantly disabled and pain-focused (based on the results of the interview and pain and disability forms) with objective findings that do not correlate with a neuromusculoskeletal dysfunction, questions have been raised as to whether continuing with the full FCE has value (vs performing a shorter protocol, for example, Functional Assessment Screening Test). This is an area that requires further research. Chapter 15 provides further discussion on the use of FCEs for patients with chronic pain, and Chapter 21 discusses the reliability and validity of FCEs.

Summary

Informed consent, evaluee interview, and performance of a targeted musculo-skeletal examination are components of most FCE models. The information obtained from the FCE has most value when it is analyzed in the context of clinical manifestations and the evaluator's determination of the degree to which the manifestations are consistent with test results. Therefore, the evaluee interview and physical examination are vital testing components.

References

1. Delany C. Informed consent: broadening the focus. *Aust J Physiother.* 2003;49(3):159–161.
2. *Guidelines: Occupational Health Physical Therapy: Evaluating Functional Capacity.* Alexandria, VA: American Physical Therapy Association; 2001; (BOD 03-01-16-54).
3. *Guidelines: Occupational Health Physical Therapy: Legal and Risk Management Issues.* Alexandria, VA: American Physical Therapy Association; 2002; (BOD G02-02-16-21).

4. *Guidelines to the Occupational Therapy Code of Ethics.* Bethesda, MD: American Occupational Therapy Association; 2005.
5. *Guide to Professional Conduct.* Alexandria, VA: American Physical Therapy Association; 2004.
6. Goodman CC, Snyder TEK. *Differential Diagnosis in Physical Therapy.* 2nd ed. Philadelphia, PA: WB Saunders 1995:24.
7. Guide to physical therapist practice. *Phys Therapy Journal.* 2001;18(1).

Activities of Daily Living and Psychometric Questionnaires

Elizabeth Genovese, MD, MBA, and Mark Hyman, MD

All people have a unique response to disease, hence, the term *illness.* Many factors affect a person's performance in a functional capacity evaluation (FCE). Psychological and socioenvironmental factors often have a larger role than physical limitations per se as they can have a significant impact on multiple aspects of the initial illness and the recovery process in injured workers.[1] When synthesizing the final FCE report, the evaluator will accept the evaluee's performance as an accurate representation of ability when acceptable physical effort was obtained. However, when results suggest that the evaluee's limitations were inconsistent or unexplainable by objective physical findings, the examiner is required to interpret the results further.

Definitive assessment of the degree to which psychological, social, and environmental factors have influenced the results of specific FCE components is not possible. Instruments that document self-reported limitations of activities of daily living (ADLs) and instrumental ADLs (IADLs) can be useful tools to apply toward qualifying and quantifying the perceived impact of a given impairment or series of impairments on the ability of the evaluee to perform the tasks required for self-care and the maintenance of customary roles at home and at work.

Psychometrics is the branch of psychology that "deals with the design, administration, and interpretation of quantitative tests for the measurement of psychological variables such as intelligence, aptitude, and personality traits."[2] It has also been applied to the analysis of scored tests used in the measurement of attitudes and beliefs in health-related fields. When used for the latter, the goal of psychometric analysis is to assess to what degree the test is reliable (can be measured consistently) and/or valid (able to accurately measure what it is intended to measure, be sensitive to changes in clinical status, and/or provide meaningful, useful information that can be applied to patient care; Chapter 21 provides further discussion of these terms). A self-report questionnaire is described as being psychometrically validated when formal investigation of that tool demonstrates reliability or validity. These psychometrically validated self-report questionnaires are often referred to as *psychometric questionnaires.* Although some of the psychometric questionnaires used in the context of FCEs concentrate solely on applying a scoring system to listings of self-reported ADLs, many incorporate questions regarding pain, quality of life, and other evaluee characteristics that potentially affect the extent to which a given impairment results in disability.

The ability of a properly constructed tool to provide useful information about psychosocial factors contributing to unemployment depends on the evaluee and the setting in which the tool is used. Although there are many ADL and psychometric questionnaires in the literature, some of which have been regularly used in FCE settings, there have not been any studies of construct validity for their use in FCEs. However, one would expect that tools considered predictive of disability and/or return to work could be reasonably applied in this context.

Although relying heavily on the questionnaires described in this chapter as the sole basis for conclusions reached in the FCE is not recommended, the evaluation of the psychosocial dimension enables the examiner to gain valuable insight into possible reasons why observed limitations may be disproportionate to objective findings.[3]

In addition to alerting the examiner about possible underlying psychological concerns, the use of psychometric and/or ADL questionnaires can assist in the evaluation of discrepancies between expected and submaximal or inconsistent performance during FCEs. This evaluation can be achieved by comparing answers to similar questions on different questionnaires, interpreting answers in the context of the patient's history and demonstrated activity levels, and/or assessing whether observed activities are consistent with described limitations, pain levels, and other relevant factors. Performing analyses such as these is especially important when findings such as fear avoidance behaviors or self-rated perceptions of disability are inconsistent with objective physical examination and test findings. Inconsistencies between performance and psychometric test results should be addressed when interpreting the final FCE results and/or applied as an adjunct to treatment or return-to-work decisions.

There are a host of batteries used to evaluate pain, depression, and job satisfaction. The most useful test batteries would allow identification of significant factors that may be impacting on FCE performance. The presence of one or more factors may prompt additional investigation that could include assessment of the evaluee by a psychologist or psychiatrist. Additional assessment is relevant under these circumstances, given that biopsychosocial models of pain clearly suggest that screening for and addressing psychological factors can influence patient outcomes.[4,5] Regardless, when information other than that purely related to the evaluee's ability to perform various physical tasks will be of little or no relevance (eg, in postoffer FCE testing) or when examiners are comfortable interpreting an FCE based on evaluee performance alone, ancillary use of psychometric questionnaires may not be needed.

The remainder of this chapter reviews practical ADL and psychometric questionnaires that are generally used in many FCE models or can be incorporated into an assessment. Because psychometric questionnaires are being used in the FCE setting for informational purposes only (and not to monitor progress in treatment), only the more relevant literature supporting their use will be cited. Judicious use of these questionnaires by a skilled clinician in the context of functional testing can allow for a more thorough, objectively documented decision process about the impact of self-described deficits in ADLs and psychosocial factors on demonstrated functional abilities. These questionnaires can enhance the FCE evaluator's interpretation of test results and be applied toward treatment considerations, return-to-work prediction,[6] and claim handling. They may also assist with efforts to assess "sincerity of effort" (see Chapter 11). At a minimum, ADL and psychometric questionnaires can be useful as a means of assessing the evaluee's sitting tolerance, which can be evaluated while the questionnaires are being completed.

Activities of Daily Living: Self-reported Questionnaires

The AMA *Guides* is the best known tool for the formal evaluation of impairment and has at its foundation the consideration of ADLs.[7] The common ADLs and IADLs considered are enumerated in the *Guides* and encompass many areas of activity (Table 5–1).

TABLE 5–1 Self-Care
Activities of Daily Living (ADLs)
Bathing, showering
Bowel and bladder management
Dressing
Eating
Feeding
Functional mobility
Personal device care
Personal hygiene and grooming
Sexual activity
Sleep/rest
Toilet hygiene
Instrumental Activities of Daily Living (IADLs)
Care of others (including selecting and supervising caregivers)
Care of pets

CHAPTER 5

TABLE 5–1 Self-Care (continued)

Child rearing
Communication device use
Community mobility
Financial management
Health management and maintenance
Home establishment and maintenance
Meal preparation and cleanup
Safety procedures and emergency responses
Shopping

Source: Youngstrom.[26]

A number of the batteries currently used in ADL evaluation have been designed for application to specific, often geriatric populations[8–13] or for patients with heart disease.[14] Other resources provide guidance and insight into various ADL scales for specific musculoskeletal conditions[15] but do not establish a "gold standard." The *Guides,* Sixth edition, provides a sample ADL questionnaire[7(p483)] that can be adapted for general use and cross-referenced with the results from other questionnaires (Table 5–2).

TABLE 5–2   Activities of Daily Living Questionnaire

Name: _____ Date: _____

Activity	No difficulty	Some difficulty	*Cannot perform*
Self-care, Personal Hygiene Urinating Defecating Brushing teeth Combing hair Bathing Dressing Eating			

TABLE 5–2 Activities of Daily Living Questionnaire (continued)

Activity	No difficulty	Some difficulty	*Cannot* perform
Communication Writing Typing Seeing Hearing Speaking			
Physical Activity Standing Sitting Reclining Walking Climbing stairs			
Sensory Function Hearing Seeing Tactile feeling Tasting Smelling			
Nonspecialized Hand Activities Grasping Lifting Tactile discrimination			
Sexual Function Orgasm			

TABLE 5–2 Activities of Daily Living Questionnaire (continued)

Activity	No difficulty	Some difficulty	*Cannot perform*
Ejaculation Lubrication Erection			
Sleep, Restful Pattern			

Reproduced from: Rondinelli RD, Genovese E, et al. *Guides to the Evaluation of Permanent Impairment.* 6th ed. Chicago, IL: American Medical Association; 2007:p483.

One can also use the questionnaire in Table 5–3 to obtain baseline documentation regarding the degree to which various physical activities lead to improvement or worsening of pain.

The questions about the effects of different positions and activities can help in pain localization and characterization and in determining possible work restrictions. This information can be used to customize the FCE and, later, can be compared with FCE results to assess whether the evaluee's reported limitations were validated. In particular, comparison of the answers between questionnaires and the evaluee's performance can be used to assess whether a musculoskeletal

TABLE 5–3 Alternative ADL Questionnaire

	Effect of Activity or Time of Day		
	Better	**Worse**	**No Effect**
Activity			
Bending			
Squatting			
Crawling			
Climbing			
Crouching			
Kneeling			
Reaching			
Pushing			

TABLE 5–3 Alternative ADL Questionnaire (continued)

	Effect of Activity or Time of Day		
	Better	**Worse**	**No Effect**
Pulling			
Sitting			
Standing			
Rising from sitting			
Rising from lying			
Turning			
Lying on back			
Lying on side			
Lying on stomach			
Having sex			
Sleeping			
Coughing			
Sneezing			
Walking			
Running			
Lifting			
Time of Day			
Morning			
Evening			

injury follows the pattern of normal musculoskeletal experience or if the pain reports are inconsistent with the known pathophysiologic mechanisms of disease. When responses regarding the impact of various activities on pain are inconsistent with normal mechanical musculoskeletal behavior, psychosocial factors may be affecting evaluee performance during the FCE.

Psychometrically Validated Questionnaires

Many questionnaires that ask at least some questions related to pain level, activity level, or specific limitations related to ADLs or IADLs have been psychometrically validated with regard to reliability and/or one or more aspects of validity (especially responsiveness). There are also a number of psychometrically validated questionnaires that specifically screen for psychological problems. These questionnaires may qualify and, perhaps, in some cases, quantify a possible psychological basis for otherwise unexplainable limitations in evaluee function.

No one psychometric questionnaire specific to musculoskeletal dysfunction is consistently used in FCEs. A brief review of this topic can be found in relevant portions of the *Guides*, Sixth Edition.[7(pp482–486)] As stated previously, it is important to recognize that most of these questionnaires were designed to monitor the progress of patients with chronic pain. Although psychometric validation for these tools generally consists of literature supporting their reliability and responsiveness to change in patients' clinical status, it also may include evidence that can assist in differential diagnosis, predicting surgical outcome or return to work, determining disability, and assessing comorbidities (such as anxiety, depression, and other psychological dysfunction). Predictive validity of a given tool thus depends on the outcome being evaluated and the specific tool used. Nevertheless, based, in part, on their use in various FCE models (see Appendix), the following tools are recommended for consideration as potential components in FCEs evaluating musculoskeletal pathology. It is optimal to use the clinical evaluation, in the context of the questions to be addressed by the FCE, to help select a given tool or combination of tools for use. The comments section of Table 5–4 generally includes a Web site where the questionnaire can be obtained at no cost. The Web site www.orthopaedicscore.com is particularly useful because it not only includes a number of questionnaires but also provides scoring information.

CHAPTER 5

TABLE 5–4   Psychometric Questionnaires Used as an Adjunct to Functional Assessment

Focus	Questionnaire	Comments*
General assessment	Pain Numerical Rating Scale[16]	Easy to use; classic form, demonstrated reliability and validity; multiple versions available with little standardization or supportive literature

TABLE 5-4 Psychometric Questionnaires Used as an Adjunct to Functional Assessment (continued)

Focus	Questionnaire	Comments*
General assessment	Pain Drawing[17]	Widely used; may have diagnostic and prognostic value but less useful for psychological screening; online versions available (www1.va.gov/pain_management/docs/paindrawing.pdf and www.spinesource.com/Pain%20Drawing.pdf)
	Visual Analogue Scale[18]	Widely used; many versions
	SF-36[19]	Well-established, psychometrically validated generic health questionnaire; online questions (www.rand.org/health/surveys_tools/mos/mos_core_36item_survey.html) and scoring (www.rand.org/health/surveys_tools/mos/mos_core_36item_scoring.pdf) available
	Pain Disability Questionnaire (PDQ)[20]	Relatively new; used in the *Guides* Sixth edition; online versions available (http://bayareasportstherapy.com/forms/Paindisabilityquestionaire.pdf and http://drbillgallagher.com/Pain_Disability_Questionnaire.pdf)
	Örebro Musculoskeletal Pain Screening Questionnaire[21]	Online questionnaire (www.workcover.vic.gov.au/wps/wcm/resources/file/eb9876059273ff3/Orebro_Musculoskeletal_Pain_Questionnaire.pdf) and scoring (www.workcover.vic.gov.au/wps/wcm/resources/file/eb1a54098670008/Orebro_Scoring_Instructions.pdf) available
	Tampa Scale of Kinesiophobia[22]	Multiple forms available online; original most widely studied (www.worksafe.vic.gov.au/wps/wcm/resources/file/eb5c6742bb4ae48/tampa_scale_kinesiophobia.pdf)
	McGill Pain Questionnaire[23]	Used occasionally; available online (http://hypnosishelpcenter.net/McGillPainQuestionnaire.pdf)

TABLE 5–4 Psychometric Questionnaires Used as an Adjunct to Functional Assessment (continued)

Focus	Questionnaire	Comments*
Back (and neck)	Fear-Avoidance Behavior Questionnaire[24]	Increasingly used to evaluate risk of delayed recovery
	Roland Morris and Modified Roland Morris[25]	Frequently used to track outcomes in studies of interventions for low back pain; available online (www.rmdq.org/)
	Oswestry Disability Index[26]	Most recent version, 2.1a, should be used[27]; available online (www.orthosurg.org.uk/odi/)
	Neck Disability Index[28]	Modification of Oswestry; available online (www.ucclinics.com/Forms/TheNeckPain DisabilityQuestionnaire(BACK).doc and www.chiro.org/forms/NeckDisForm.html)
Upper extremity	DASH and *Quick*DASH[29,30]	Used in the *Guides* Sixth edition; available online (www.dash.iwh.on.ca/)
	UEFI—Upper Extremity Functional Index[31]	Questions similar to DASH; available online (http://apa.advsol.com.au/independent/ documents/outcome_measures/upper extremityfunctionalindex.pdf)
Lower extremity	LEFS—Lower Extremity Functional Scale[32]	Probably best overall scale for lower extremity
	FADI—Foot and Ankle Distress Index[33]	4-point scale for athletes and nonathletes
Psychological	Beck Depression Inventory[34]	Widely used self-report scale used to screen for depression

*The text provides full discussion.

A brief description of each follows.

Pain Numerical Rating Scale and Borg Scale

The Pain Numerical Rating Scale asks evaluees to rate their pain on a numeric scale from 0 (no pain) to 10+ (very, very strong; maximal). This scale is based on a modification of the relative perceived exertion (RPE) scale developed by Borg[35] for the quantitative evaluation of patients with chest pain. His original scale was ordinal, with values from 6 to 20 to describe the chest pain and RPE associated with exercise stress testing. Verbal anchors were used to standardize comparisons between people.[35] As oxygen consumption and heart rate increase linearly with workload, he held that these factors should coincide with ratings of perceived exertion. Thus, ranges from 6 (7 is very, very light) to 20 (19 is very, very hard) were used to denote heart rates ranging from 60 to 200 beats/min, with the scale designed so that the number on the scale multiplied by 10 was the expected heart rate. The RPE scale has been shown to correlate highly with measures such as ventilatory minute volume, carbon dioxide production, and lactate accumulation and has been used as a proxy for stress testing to assess aerobic capacity[36] in healthy people. When used for patients with chronic pain, the RPE seems to be less correlated with physiologic effort,[37] although this lesser correlation seemed to be primarily the case at lower intensity workloads because once the workload was sufficient to induce an aerobic training response, the RPE was an accurate predictor of exercise intensity.[38]

Following development of the RPE scale, Borg developed a "category ratio perceived exertion scale with ratio properties,"[22] the "1 to 10+" pain scale most commonly seen today (referred to as the CR-10). Verbal anchors are again used and evaluees are asked to rate their pain at three distinct times: at the moment of questionnaire completion, at its best during the past 30 days, and at its worst during the past 30 days. The evaluator is to explain in advance that "0" corresponds to "nothing at all," "0.5" to pain that is "very, very weak," "3" to moderate pain at a level that precludes performance of most activities," and "6" or higher ("7" is "very strong") to severe pain that requires a great deal of medication for control. Ratings of "10" (very, very strong) and "10+" (maximal) should be used only to represent pain that is as bad as it could possibly be and would ordinarily require hospitalization. Because all of these ratings were initially linked to the RPE scale (which was, in turn, associated with increases in heart rate), it would seem logical to expect that ratings of 4 or more on the Borg scale should generally be accompanied by some form of objective physical pathology, even if only minimal, whereas pain ratings of 7 to 10+ (indicating very strong to maximal pain, which would presumably preclude showing up for the FCE), would definitely be associated with evidence of pathology consistent with the body part affected.

TABLE 5–5	Borg CR-10 Scale

Rate your <u>major area of pain</u> on the 0–10+ Pain Rating Scale. Write the number of your pain at the <u>present time</u> and your best day and your worst day over the past 30 days. Remember, the numbers refer to your pain, not how strong or weak you feel. For Example: 1 is Very Weak <u>Pain</u> and 7 is Very Strong <u>Pain</u>.

10+	Maximal
10	Very, Very Strong
9	
8	
7	Very Strong
6	
5	Strong
4	Somewhat Strong
3	Moderate
2	Weak
1	Very Weak
0.5	Very, Very Weak
0	Nothing at all

YOUR PAIN RATING

Pain Now _____

Best Day _____ Over the past 30 days

Worst Day _____ Over the past 30 days

Pain at a level of 10 or 10+ would be the worst pain you ever experienced, at a level that would require a visit to the hospital. Pain at a level of 7 would require that you see a doctor. A pain level of 3 or 4 out of 10 would interfere with performing most activities.

Adapted from Borg G. (1998). *Borg's perceived exertion and pain scales.* Stockholm: Human Kinetics.

CHAPTER 5

Although there is literature about the reliability and validity of the classic Borg questionnaire for the evaluation of chest pain, asthma, and muscle fatigue,[39,40] many variations of the original instrument have been developed,[41] with varying degrees of validity. Ratings of perceived exertion have been shown to be influenced by depression and anxiety.[42] Most important, however, is that evaluees to whom the Borg scale is administered are often not fully informed about the meaning of the numbers that represent their pain. Because pain ratings on a 1 to 10 scale are used by many FCE evaluators as one of the psychophysical determinants of whether tasks during an FCE should be terminated (the extent depends on the model), it is highly recommended that evaluees receive verbal instruction regarding the location and significance of the verbal anchors for each level of pain (as described in Table 5–4) before use of the Borg or any numeric scale. It also may be useful to have an evaluee with multiple complaints complete more than one pain rating scale, one per body part affected.

Visual Analogue Scale

The Visual Analogue Pain Rating Scale,[18] generally referred to as the "Visual Analogue Scale" (VAS), is similar to the Borg scale for rating pain because it uses a scale from 0 to 10. However, in this case, the evaluee is usually given a horizontal line on which to indicate the level of pain, with the left side corresponding to no pain and the right side corresponding to "pain as bad as it could be." In the initial version, the line ran vertically rather than horizontally on the page; however, the use of a vertical line vs a horizontal line has not been found to materially affect ratings.[43] The original VAS included no numbers or other marks on the line. See Figure 5–1. Numerous versions of the VAS have appeared in the literature since it was originally developed, varying in length (5–20 cm), the use of demarcations to denote centimeter markings, and the choice of end phrases.[44] Discussion of this topic is beyond the scope of this chapter.

Use of a 10-cm visual analogue scale with an end point of "pain as bad as it could be" is recommended, with scoring achieved by simply placing a ruler along the line and assigning a corresponding number to the area of the line marked. As is the case with the Borg scale, the location and significance of verbal anchors should be clear. The evaluee should be informed that the pain rating of as "bad as it could be" should be used only to characterize pain that is the worst pain imaginable. Again, ratings at this high a level would be expected to require emergency medical care. Some evaluators compare the rating on this scale with ratings on the Borg scale to check for consistency. Blankenship[45] states that the scores on both scales should be within 1 to 1.5 units of each other. This relationship has not been formally studied. A practical limitation of the VAS is that repeated copying of forms often leads to variation in the size of the line and may influence response.

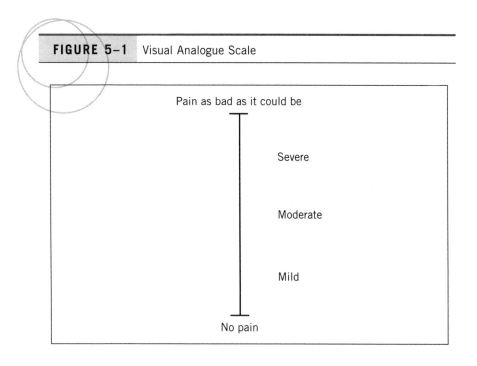

FIGURE 5–1   Visual Analogue Scale

Pain as bad as it could be

Severe

Moderate

Mild

No pain

The Pain Drawing

The Pain Drawing[17] is widely used as part of the evaluation of evaluees with pain and has been demonstrated to have test-retest[46] and interexaminer[47,48] reliability, although evaluators should not have prior knowledge of evaluees that might bias interpretation.[49] The evaluee is asked to localize the pain on a picture of the body, with various symbols used to characterize its quality (aching, burning, stabbing, pins and needless, or numbness). See Figure 5–2. An initial rating scheme used to assign a numeric value to the drawing presumably related to specific psychological disturbances has been questioned.[50–52] Nevertheless, abnormal (nonphysiologic) pain drawings have been shown to be predictive of poor treatment outcome,[53,54] disability,[55,56] and isokinetic functional testing.[57] Use of the pain drawing to document whether pain patterns fit normal anatomic patterns based on the clinical evaluation are useful. The results may also help focus the evaluator on areas that had not been otherwise identified as having potential pathology. Conversely, a diagram characterized by poor anatomic pattern, use of all symbols, pain outside of the diagram, and additional arrows or circles to point out the pain may be indicators of possible psychological disturbance or symptom magnification and would also suggest that the results of functional testing will be pain-limited.

| FIGURE 5–2 | Pain Drawing |

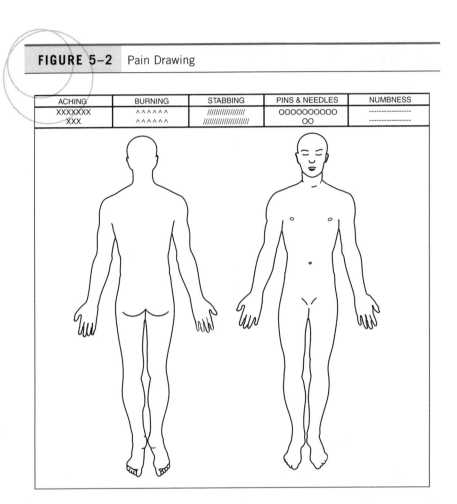

ACHING	BURNING	STABBING	PINS & NEEDLES	NUMBNESS
XXXXXXX	^^^^^^	/////////////////	OOOOOOOOOO	-----------------
XXX	^^^^^^	/////////////////	OO	-----------------

Short Form 36

The Short Form 36 (SF-36), a 36-item questionnaire with multiple subscales, is one of the oldest and most widely used questionnaires in the self-assessment literature and was constructed to survey health status in clinical practice and research, health policy evaluations, and general population surveys. Although later versions of the SF-36 are proprietary, a free version is available on the Rand Web site (see Table 5–4). The SF-36 includes one multi-item scale that assesses eight health concepts: (1) limitations in physical activities because of health problems, (2) limitations in social activities because of physical or emotional problems, (3) limitations in usual role activities because of physical health problems, (4) bodily pain, (5) general mental health (psychological distress and well-being), (6) limitations in usual role activities because of emotional problems, (7) vitality (energy and fatigue), and (8) general health perceptions.

Scoring is somewhat complex (relative to other tools); precoded numeric values are assigned for the answer to each question using a coding key, after which the values for selected questions are averaged to result in the scores for each of the scales. However, scores can be broken into two summary measures representing physical and mental health, with the former often all that is necessary.

The SF-36 is generally preferred to similar generic health care measures such as the SIP (sickness illness profile), NHP (Nottingham Health Profile), and Duke (Duke Health Profile) for measuring general health status.[58] It also (compared with generic measures) has been considered as striking the "best balance between length, reliability, validity, responsiveness, and experience in large populations of patients with back pain," with the "Bodily Pain Scale" often serving as a stand-alone variable providing information (albeit limited) regarding pain intensity and interference with activities.[59]

Pain Disability Questionnaire

While initially used primarily in a rehabilitative setting, the Pain Disability Questionnaire (PDQ)[20] is a relatively new 15-item comprehensive generic evaluation of disability and function. The PDQ is used in the chapters on pain and the spine in the *Guides* Sixth edition. Its psychometrics have been evaluated and have shown strong test-retest reliability, responsiveness, and validity. Answers are provided by putting an "x" on a horizontally oriented, unmarked VAS with cross-hatches corresponding to 0, 2, 4, 6, 8, and 10. Although a version with numbers from 1 to 10 along the horizontal axis is available as well,[60] it is unclear whether this version has been classified as psychometrically equivalent to the original. A "0" connotes the absence of a problem or limitation, and a "10" indicates the opposite. The total possible score is 150, which can be further broken down into functional status (maximum 90 points) and psychosocial status (maximum 60 points) components.

Örebro Musculoskeletal Pain Screening Questionnaire

The Örebro Musculoskeletal Pain Screening Questionnaire[21] was originally developed to assist health care providers in assessing "yellow flags" (psychosocial factors shown to be associated with delayed recovery and/or failure to return to work) as a complement to the standard medical examination for patients with musculoskeletal pain. Although its reliability and validity for predicting absenteeism and functional ability in patients with low back pain was initially described,[61] it has also been shown to predict work disability in patients with a wide range of musculoskeletal pain complaints.[62,63] The instrument has 25 questions; scoring is slightly complex in that there are three ways to score (depending on the question).

Scores range from 0 to more than 202 (scoring for one of the questions is based on the number of painful sites), with low, moderate, and high risk of disability (absence from work) characterized by scores of 105 or less, 105 to 130, and 130 or more, respectively.

Fear-Avoidance Beliefs Questionnaire

The contribution of "fear-avoidance beliefs" to the development of chronic pain states has been increasingly cited in the literature[64–68] and has led to the development of treatment strategies (exercise-based with or without a psychological component) specifically designed to address and ameliorate unrealistic patient concerns about the deleterious effects of physical activity.[69–72] Waddell et al,[73,74] although initially known for writings about the signs[73] and symptoms[74] associated with poor functional outcomes in patients with low back pain, subsequently developed the Fear-Avoidance Beliefs Questionnaire (FABQ) representing a refinement of earlier work.[24] The questionnaire includes 16 questions about the nature and presumed cause of an evaluee's pain and the degree to which the patient believes the pain to preclude physical activity and/or return to work. Scoring is performed by breaking the questions into two sections (scales) and adding the points in each. The final result provides information about "fear-avoidance beliefs about work" (FABQ-W, score range, 0–42) and "fear-avoidance beliefs about physical activity" (FABQ-P, score range, 0–24). An FABQ-P scale score of 29 (using a scoring system that differed slightly from the original) has been shown to be associated with a negative outcome in one group of subjects not receiving workers' compensation and undergoing exercise therapy.[75] Elevations in scores on the FABQ-W scale have been shown to be negatively correlated with return to work in patients with acute low back pain.[67] Although an early study suggested that scores greater than 29 were particularly predictive of poor outcome,[68] a more recent study has indicated that scores as low as 20 are correlated with disability as measured by the Oswestry Disability Index (ODI) at 6 months.[76] Therefore, the information obtained from the FABQ, especially the FABQ-W scale, may be a potentially useful adjunct to FCE. The FABQ was initially developed for use in patients with low back pain, and because weaker associations have been found between fear-avoidance beliefs and disability in patients with cervical pain,[77] its predictive value in evaluees with other musculoskeletal complaints is unclear.

Tampa Scale of Kinesiophobia

The Tampa Scale of Kinesiophobia,[22] available in its original and revised forms, consists of 17 questions scored on a 4-point Likert scale, with higher scores reflecting greater fear of movement, although no specific cutoff points have been described. Because it has been shown to be similar to the FABQ in predicting self-reported disability and poor functional performance[64,78] and to predict future disability and participation compared with other tools,[79,80] it can be considered for use as an alternative or supplement to the FABQ.

McGill Pain Questionnaire

The McGill Pain Questionnaire[23] was designed to provide quantitative measures of clinical pain that could be used in evaluating the impact of treatment and consists of 20 groups of word descriptors. The 20 word groups are further divided into four categories: sensory, affective, evaluative, and miscellaneous. The evaluee is instructed to select up to a maximum of one word per group to describe the subjective pain experience. Because many people may not understand the meanings of some words (eg, lancinating), terms may need to be reviewed with the evaluee. Although the original McGill Pain Questionnaire included an intensity scale and scales evaluating the properties of the pain experience, functional capacity evaluators who use this questionnaire tend to focus only on the number of words chosen (because evaluees are not required to select any words at all) and the total score (obtained by adding the scores from each of the 20 groups, with scoring beginning at 1 and based on the rank of the descriptor in the grouping). A score of more than 30 has been described as indicative of symptom magnification.[45]

Roland Morris Disability Questionnaire

The 24-question Roland Morris Disability Questionnaire (RDQ) is widely used as a tool to monitor functional outcome in studies of interventions for low back pain (as is the ODI). It measures 24 activity limitations, and a positive answer to a question (each question is scored "0" or "1") denotes an adverse effect or problem. The maximum score is 24, and the RDQ is easy to use. In general, a score of 14 or more is described as indicative of a poor outcome.[25] There are 36 available versions of the RDQ. Although some authors have favored its use in specific clinical settings,[81,82] some have suggested that its focus on only a limited range of physical functions does not allow sufficient responsiveness for patients with more severe disability[83] (in other words, it is less responsive on the high end). It has been noted to show only modest correlation with direct measures of physical function.[84]

Oswestry Disability Index

The ODI consists of 10 sections relating to activities of daily living or pain. Each section includes six statements describing increased severity of pain or disability as it pertains to a specific activity, with each section scored from

CHAPTER 5

0 to 5. The scope of questions differs from the scope of questions in the RDQ: in assessing the degree to which pain interferes with physical activities, the tool is more responsive for differentiating between evaluees with greater degrees of disability. The total raw score (a maximum of 50) is added and multiplied by 2 to provide a percentage of disability; adjustments can be made for omitted items. A score of 60% to 80% indicates "bedbound" or "crippled"; scores of 1% to 20%, 20% to 40%, and 40% to 60% represent mild, moderate, and severe disability, respectively.[26] Although the ODI was first developed in 1980, alternative versions, in particular the "revised ODI," have been developed. The latter has been described as leading to "an exaggeration of the treatment effect when compared with other studies," which potentially misleads readers by increasing the proportion of patients meeting criteria based on ODI versions 1.0 and 2.0.[85] Although these issues are of limited relevance in FCE, it would seem best to use the most recent version approved by the authors (v2.1a).[27] As noted, the ODI has a greater range than the RDQ and, hence, may be a better choice for use in populations with higher disability levels, whereas the RDQ is recommended for populations at the "lower end of the disability spectrum."[84]

Neck Disability Index

The Neck Disability Index[28] was modeled after the ODI and is scored and interpreted similarly. Although literature reviewing its psychometric properties is generally favorable,[86-88] it has not been studied as extensively as the ODI.

DASH Outcome Measure

The DASH (Disabilities of the Arm, Shoulder, and Hand) Outcome Measure is a 30-item self-report questionnaire that evaluates physical function and symptoms referable to the upper limbs. The DASH is valid, reliable, and responsive and can be used to study clinical outcomes.[29,30,89,90] A shorter version of the DASH, called the *Quick*DASH[91] and that uses only 11 items to measure physical function and symptoms, is also available. Both versions of the DASH include two optional, four-item modules intended to measure symptoms and function in athletes, performing artists, and other workers whose jobs require a high degree of manual dexterity or upper extremity endurance or strength. Both versions also require evaluees to use a Likert score from 1 to 5 to indicate the presence or absence of pain or ability to perform a given activity; they differ in the number of questions. Scoring instructions are provided with the questionnaire and can be found at www.dash.iwh.on.ca/ and www.orthopaedicscore.com. No scoring interpretation is provided because the primary purpose of the DASH and *Quick*DASH is to monitor progress rather than reach definitive conclusions about the implications of a given score. Nevertheless, the *Quick*DASH was chosen for inclusion in the *Guides*, Sixth Edition; one of the recommendations for use is to compare answers with completed ADL questionnaires. Clearly, the answers from the DASH can also be compared for consistency with demonstrated activities during material handling and other tasks (see Chapter 12 for upper extremity FCE). See Table 5–6.

TABLE 5–6 Comparison Between *Quick*DASH and ADL Questionnaires

Quick DASH question	ADL questionnaire correlate
1. "open a tight or new jar"	Grasping
2. "heavy household chores (eg, wash walls, floors)"	Grasping and lifting
3. "carry a shopping bag or briefcase"	Grasping and lifting
4. "wash your back"	Grasping and bathing
5. "use a knife to cut food"	Grasping and eating (perhaps tactile feeling)
6. "recreational activities"	Grasping, tactile feeling, lifting
7. "social activities"	No correlate; upper limb impairments should not produce social difficulty
8. "work or ADLs"	Writing, typing, tactile feeling, grasping, lifting, and/or tactile discrimination
9. "arm, shoulder, or hand pain"	No direct correlate
10. "tingling"	Tactile feeling and tactile discrimination
11. "sleeping"	Sleep

Note: ADL indicates Activity of Daily Living.
Source: *Quick*DASH questions from Beaton et al, 2005.[7]

Reproduced from: Rondinelli RD, Genovese E, et al. *Guides to the Evaluation of Permanent Impairment.* 6th ed. Chicago, IL: American Medical Association; 2007:p485.

Upper Extremity Function Index

The Upper Extremity Function Index is a 20-item questionnaire about the ability to perform various tasks that emphasize use of the upper extremities. A 0 to 4 Likert scale yields a maximum score of 80. As was the case for the DASH, answers can be compared for consistency with results from material handling tests during the FCE.

CHAPTER 5

Lower Extremity Function Scale

The Lower Extremity Function Scale is also a 20-item questionnaire scored by using a 0 to 4 Likert scale that yields a maximum score of 80. The questions emphasize the ability to use the lower extremities to perform relevant tasks. This scale was validated against the SF-36 and would be the best overall general instrument for lower extremity assessment.

Foot and Ankle Distress Index

The Foot and Ankle Distress Index is a 26-item questionnaire. A 0 to 4 Likert scale yields a maximum score of 104, although the authors recommend reporting the score as a percentage. The much shorter sports version of this instrument has eight items for a total score of 32 points; again, reporting percentages is recommended. These questions ask for responses based on evaluee experiences during the last week rather than the day of evaluation.

Beck Depression Inventory

Although depression frequently accompanies chronic pain and disability, its recognition in an evaluee who is uncomfortable acknowledging depressive symptoms may be challenging. In situations when the evaluator suspects that depression may have a role in clinical manifestations, use of a brief questionnaire such as the Beck Depression Inventory (BDI)[34] may be valuable. There are many versions of the BDI; the most recent is the BDI-II.[92] All are 21-question multiple-choice self-reports, which list an inventory of symptoms consistent with depression. The evaluee is asked to endorse one of four choices for each option (scored 0 to 3), with increased symptoms associated with greater scores. The asymptomatic default position is 0. Greater symptom severity increases from 1 to 3. Healthy people may have symptoms providing a BDI score of 10 or less. Roughly speaking, mild to moderate depression scores are from 11 to 20; severe scores are from 21 to 30; and extreme scores (and exaggerated scores) are more than 30. Older versions of the BDI are widely available; newer versions are proprietary.

Other Tools

There are a number of proprietary questionnaires and tools other than the BDI that may be useful as an adjunct to FCE. Many are sold as part of FCE systems, but some are available separately. The FCE evaluator must assess factors such as the quality and usefulness of the information obtained compared with that obtained by using other methods, convenience of use, applicability to the "usual" evaluee population, usefulness of the information provided to clients, cost, and potential FCE volume before determining whether purchase of any of these tools is appropriate.

Of these tools, the Spinal Function Sort (SFS), which is a variation of the Pictorial and Activity Task Sort[93] and the Hand Function Sort[94] are probably best known. The purpose of the SFS is to quantify the ability to perform work tasks that involve the spine and lower extremities by showing evaluees drawings of specific yet varied tasks and asking them whether they are "able" or "unable" to do them or if they are "restricted" from doing so. The Hand Function Sort works in the same manner but focuses on tasks that require upper extremity use. Each drawing is usually accompanied by a task description.

Use of either tool allows for the reported abilities of evaluees to be compared with their performance during the FCE. There are also validity checks built into the test in which evaluees are asked about their ability to perform tasks that seem different but actually stress identical or similar areas. The computerized version of the SFS allows information to be fed into a program that analyzes 15 physical demand constructs to provide an evaluee's "Whole Body PDC Profile."

The Multidimensional Task Ability Profile (MTAP) was developed as a follow-up to the SFS and Hand Function Sort, drawing elements from both to provide evaluees with a combination of drawings and task descriptions in a self-report format to assess functional capacity. The MTAP was found to be reliable on a test-retest and split-half basis. Comparison of MTAP scores with responses to an established self-report test instrument (the SFS) and performance on a standardized lift capacity test (Epic Lift Capacity) demonstrated good concurrent validity. Citing this, the developer has suggested that after initial calibration with an FCE, the MTAP would be suitable for ongoing monitoring of evaluee progress as a substitute for "more elaborate and expensive performance testing."[95]

There are other, older instruments similar to the SFS, Hand Function Sort, and MTAP available for use in FCEs. The decision about which to use depends on the perceived benefit (vs cost) of each in the context of the evaluator's clinical setting and patient population.

Discussion

This chapter has described some of the options available to assess ADLs and IADLs and obtain evaluee self-reports about general well-being, pain, disability, ability to return to work, and depression. There are a number of other questionnaires from which an FCE evaluator may also choose, some of which may be

CHAPTER 5

superior to those described herein in terms of their ability to predict more narrow outcomes of interest.

The primary purpose of these questionnaires in the contexts of clinical trials and ongoing treatment is generally to allow for quantification of desirable outcomes such as decreased pain or disability, which can then be monitored over time. Their applicability to a "one-time" FCE is predominantly by virtue of their ability to allow the evaluator to qualify, and, to a lesser extent, quantify the degree to which evaluees' self-reported limitations will potentially affect the results of testing. This information can, it turn, be used by the evaluator to customize the FCE through the inclusion of tasks to reflect the abilities and limitations claimed by the evaluee, and also can help the evaluator determine how long to continue the FCE when an evaluee seems to be exerting less than maximal effort. In particular, when evaluees report high levels of pain and disability and initial testing is uniformly self-limited, there is little justification for proceeding with extensive tests of physical strength and ability. Instead, the evaluator should focus on obtaining and documenting information about the consistency of physical complaints, evaluees' ability to tolerate various positions (especially sitting, which can be assessed by providing additional questionnaires to complete), and information relevant to the needs of referral sources that will assist in the constructive application of FCE results. Use of a shorter FCE protocol such as the Functional Assessment Screening Test[96] or short-form FCE[97] could also be considered.

References

1. Gross DP, Battie MC. Factors influencing results of functional capacity evaluations in workers' compensation claimants with low back pain. *Physical Therapy.* 2005;85:315–322.
2. *The American Heritage Medical Dictionary.* Boston, MA: Houghton Mifflin Co; 2007.
3. Lechner DE, Bradbury SF, Bradley LA. Detecting sincerity of effort: a summary of methods and approaches. *Physical Therapy.* 1998;78:867–888.
4. Hays RD, Wells, KB, Sherbourne CD, et al. Functioning and well-being outcomes of patients with depression compared with chronic general medical illnesses. *Archives of General Psychiatry.* 1995;52:11–19.
5. Kroenke K, Spitzer RL, Williams JBW, et al. Anxiety disorders in primary care: prevalence, impairment, comorbidity, and detection. *Annals of Internal Medicine.* 2007;146:317–325.
6. Labriola M, Lund T, Christensen KB, et al. Multilevel analysis of longitudinal and contextual factors as predictors of return to work. *Journal of Occupational Environmental Medicine.* 2006;48:1181–1188.

7. Rondinelli RD, Genovese E, Katz RT, Mayer T, Mueller K, Ranavaya M, eds. *Guides to the Evaluation of Permanent Impairment.* 6th ed. Chicago, IL: American Medical Association; 2007.

8. Bruce B, Fries J. The Stanford health assessment questionnaire (HAQ): a review of its history, issues, progress and documentation. *Journal of Rheumatology.* 2003;30:167–178.

9. Mahoney FI, Barthel D. Functional evaluation: the Barthel index. *Maryland State Medical Journal.* 1965;14:56–61.

10. Katz S, Down TD, Cash HR, et al. Progress in the development of the index of ADL. *Gerontologist.* 1970;10:20–30.

11. Lawton MP, Brody EM. Assessment of older people: self-maintaining and instrumental activities of living. *Gerontologist.* 1969;9:179–186.

12. Linn MW, Linn BS. The rapid disability rating scale-2. *Journal American Geriatric Society.* 1982;30:378–382.

13. Cummings JL, Frank JC, Cherry D, et al. Guidelines for managing Alzheimer's disease, part I: assessment. *American Family Physician.* 2002;65:2263–2272.

14. Rector TS, Cohn JN. Assessment of patient outcome with the Minnesota Living with Heart Failure questionnaire. *Amercian Heart Journal.* 1992;124:1017–1024.

15. Zuckerman J, Park S. Principles of treatment and outcomes assessment. In: Zuckerman JD, Koval KJ. Eds. *Shoulder Fractures: The Practical Guide to Management.* New York, NY: Thieme New York, 2005;1–22.

16. Borg GA. Psychophysical bases of perceived exertion. *Medicine and Science In Sports and Exercise.* 1982;14:377–381.

17. Ransford AO, Cairns D, Mooney V. The pain drawing as an aid to the psychologic evaluation for patients with low back pain. *Spine.* 1976;1:126–134.

18. Huskisson EC, Jones J, Scott PJ. Application of visual-analogue scales to the measurement of functional capacity. *Rheumatology and Rehabilitation.* 1976;15:185–187.

19. Ware JE Jr, Sherbourne CD. The MOS 36-item short-form health survey (SF-36), I: conceptual framework and item selection. *Medical Care.* 1992;30:473–483.

20. Anagnostis C, Gatchel R, Mayer T. The Pain Disability Questionnaire: a new psychometrically sound measure for chronic musculoskeletal disorders. *Spine.* 2004;29:2290–2302.

21. Linton SJ, Hallden K. Can we screen for problematic back pain? a screening questionnaire for predicting outcome in acute and subacute back pain. *Clinical Journal Pain.* 1998;14:209–215.

22. Vlaeyen JW, Kole-Snijders AM, Boeren RG, van Eek H. Fear of movement/ (re)injury in chronic low back pain and its relation to behavioral performance. *Pain.* 1995;3:363–372.

23. Melzack R. The McGill Pain Questionnaire: major properties and scoring methods. *Pain.* 1975;1:277–299.

24. Waddell G, Newton M, et al. A Fear-Avoidance Beliefs Questionnaire (FABQ) and the role of fear-avoidance beliefs in chronic low back pain and disability. *Pain.* 1993;52:157–168.

25. Roland M, Morris R. A study of the natural history of back pain, part I: development of a reliable and sensitive measure of disability in low back pain. *Spine.* 1983;8:141–144.

CHAPTER 5

26. Youngstrom MJ. Occupational therapy practice framework: The evolution of our professional language. *AM J Occup Ther.* 2202;56:609–639.

27. Fairbank JCT, Pynsent PB, Disney S. Owestry Disability Index version 2.1a. Available at: www.orthosurg.org.uk/odi/. Accessed 10/16/08.

28. Vernon H, Mior S. Neck disability index. *Journal of Manipulative and Physiologic Therapeutics.* 1991;14:409–415.

29. Hudak PL, Amadio PC, Bombadier C. Development of an upper extremity outcome measure: the DASH (disabilities of the arm, shoulder, hand). *American Journal Industrial Medicine.* 1996;29:602–608.

30. Jester A, Harth A, Wind G, et al. Disabilities of the arm, shoulder and hand (DASH) questionnaire: determining functional activity profiles in patients with upper extremity disorders. *Journal Hand Surgery.* 2005;30B:23–28.

31. Stratford PW, et al. Development and initial validation of the upper extremity functional index. *Physiotherapy Canada.* 2001;53:259–267.

32. Binkley JM, Stratford PW, Lott SA, et al. The Lower Extremity Functional Scale (LEFS): scale development, measurement properties, and clinical application. *Physical Therapy.* 1999;79:371–383.

33. Hale SA, Hertel J. Reliability and sensitivity of the foot and ankle disability index in subjects with chronic ankle instability. *Journal Athletic Train.* 2005;40:35–40.

34. Beck AT, Guth D, et al. Screening for major depression disorders in medical inpatients with the Beck Depression Inventory for Primary Care. *Behavior Research and Therapy.* 1997;35:785–791.

35. Borg G. Perceived exertion as an indicator of somatic stress. *Scandinavian Journal Rehabilative Medicine.* 1970;2:92–98.

36. Noble BJ. Clinical applications of perceived exertion. *Med Sci Sports Exerc.* 1982;14:406–411.

37. Wallbom AS, Geisser ME, et al. Concordance between rating of perceived exertion and function in persons with chronic, disabling back pain. *Journal Occupational Rehabilitation.* 2002;12:93–98.

38. Barker KL, Dawes H, et al. Perceived and measured levels of exertion of patients with chronic back pain exercising in a hydrotherapy pool. *Archives of Physical Medicine Rehabilitation.* 2003;84:1319–1323.

39. Dedering A, Nemeth G, et al. Correlation between electromyographic spectral changes and subjective assessment of lumbar muscle fatigue in subjects without pain from the lower back. *Clinical Biomechanics (Bristol, Avon).* 1999;14:103–111.

40. Dedering A, Roos af Hjelmsater M, et al. Between-days reliability of subjective and objective assessments of back extensor muscle fatigue in subjects without lower-back pain. *Journal of Electromyography and Kinesiology.* 2000;10:151–158.

41. Mador MJ, Rodis A, Magalang UJ. Reproducibility of Borg scale measurements of dyspnea during exercise in patients with COPD. *Chest.* 1995;107:1590–1597.

42. Knapen J, van de Vliet P, et al. Evaluation of cardio-respiratory fitness and perceived exertion for patients with depressive and anxiety disorders: a study on reliability. *Disability Rehabilitation.* 2003;25:1312–1315.

43. Scott J, Huskisson EC. Vertical or horizontal visual analogue scales [abstract]. *Annals of Rheumatic Disease.* 1979;38:560.

44. Seymour RA, Simpson JM, et al. An evaluation of length and end-phase of visual analogue scales in dental pain. *Pain.* 1985;21:177–185.

CHAPTER 5

45. Blankenship KL. *Industrial Rehabilitation: A Seminar Syllabus.* American Therapeutics, Inc; 1990.
46. Margolis RB, Chibnall JT, et al. Test-retest reliability of the pain drawing instrument. *Pain.* 1988;33:49–51.
47. Bertilson B, Grunnesjo M, et al. Pain drawing in the assessment of neurogenic pain and dysfunction in the neck/shoulder region: inter-examiner reliability and concordance with clinical examination. *Pain Medicine.* 2007;8:134–146.
48. Chan CW, Goldman S, et al. The pain drawing and Waddell's nonorganic physical signs in chronic low-back pain. *Spine.* 1993;18:1717–1722.
49. Reigo T, Tropp H, et al. Pain drawing evaluation: the problem with the clinically biased surgeon; intra- and interobserver agreement in 50 cases related to clinical bias. *Acta Orthopaedics Scandinavia.* 1998;69:408–411.
50. Pande KC, Tripathi S, et al. Limited clinical utility of pain drawing in assessing patients with low back pain. *Journal of Spinal Disorder Technology.* 2005;18:160–162.
51. Pfingsten M, Baller M, et al. Psychometric properties of the pain drawing and the Ransford technique in patients with chronic low back pain [in German] - abstract. *Schmerz.* 2003;17:332–340.
52. Parker H, Wood PL, et al. The use of the pain drawing as a screening measure to predict psychological distress in chronic low back pain. *Spine.* 1995;20:236–243.
53. Takata K, Hirotani H. Pain drawing in the evaluation of low back pain. *International Orthopedics.* 1995;19:361–366.
54. Voorhies RM, Jiang X, et al. Predicting outcome in the surgical treatment of lumbar radiculopathy using the Pain Drawing Score, McGill Short Form Pain Questionnaire, and risk factors including psychosocial issues and axial joint pain. *Spine Journal.* 2007;7:516–524.
55. Toomey TC, Mann JD, et al. Relationship of pain drawing scores to ratings of pain description and function. *Clinical Journal of Pain.* 1991;7:269–274.
56. Ohlund C, Eek C, et al. Quantified pain drawing in subacute low back pain; validation in a nonselected outpatient industrial sample. *Spine.* 1996;21:1021–1031.
57. Ohnmeiss DD, Vanharanta H, et al. The relationship of disability (Oswestry) and pain drawings to functional testing. *European Spine Journal.* 2000;9:208–212.
58. Lurie J. A review of generic health status measures in patients with low back pain. *Spine.* 2000;25:3125–3129.
59. Bombardier C. Outcome assessments in the evaluation of treatment of spinal disorders: summary and general recommendations. *Spine.* 2000;25:3100–3103.
60. Gallagher B. The Pain Disability Questionnaire. Available at: drbillgallagher.com/ Pain_Disability_Questionnaire.pdf. Accessed October 17, 2008.
61. Linton SJ, Boersma K. Early identification of patients at risk of developing a persistent back problem: the predictive validity of the Orebro Musculoskeletal Pain Questionnaire. *Clinical Journal of Pain.* 2003;19:80–86.
62. Dunstan DA, Covic T, et al. Does the Orebro Musculoskeletal Pain Questionnaire predict outcomes following a work-related compensable injury? *International Journal Rehabilitation Research.* 2005;28:369–370.
63. Westman A, Linton SJ, et al. Do psychosocial factors predict disability and health at a 3-year follow-up for patients with non-acute musculoskeletal pain? a validation of the Orebro Musculoskeletal Pain Screening Questionnaire. *European Journal of Pain.* 2008;12:641–649.

CHAPTER 5

64. Crombez G, Vlaeyen JW, et al. Pain-related fear is more disabling than pain itself: evidence on the role of pain-related fear in chronic back pain disability. *Pain.* 1999;80:329–339.

65. Al-Obaidi SM, Nelson RM, et al. The role of anticipation and fear of pain in the persistence of avoidance behavior in patients with chronic low back pain. *Spine.* 2000;25:1126–1131.

66. Buer N, Linton SJ. Fear-avoidance beliefs and catastrophizing: occurrence and risk factor in back pain and ADL in the general population. *Pain.* 2002;99:485–491.

67. Fritz JM, George SZ, et al. The role of fear-avoidance beliefs in acute low back pain: relationships with current and future disability and work status. *Pain.* 2001;94:7–15.

68. Fritz JM, George SZ. Identifying psychosocial variables in patients with acute work-related low back pain: the importance of fear-avoidance beliefs. *Physical Therapy.* 2002;82:973–983.

69. Vlaeyen JW, de Jong J, et al. The treatment of fear of movement/(re)injury in chronic low back pain: further evidence on the effectiveness of exposure in vivo. *Clinical Journal of Pain.* 2002;18:251–261.

70. George SZ, Fritz JM, et al. The effect of a fear-avoidance-based physical therapy intervention for patients with acute low back pain: results of a randomized clinical trial. *Spine.* 2003;28:2551–2560.

71. Klaber Moffett JA, Carr J, et al. High fear-avoiders of physical activity benefit from an exercise program for patients with back pain. *Spine.* 2004;29:1167–1173.

72. Vangronsveld K, Peters M, et al. Applying the fear-avoidance model to the chronic whiplash syndrome. *Pain.* 2007;131:258–261.

73. Waddell G, McCulloch JA, et al. Nonorganic physical signs in low-back pain. *Spine.* 1980;5:117–125.

74. Waddell G, Main CJ, et al. Chronic low-back pain, psychologic distress, and illness behavior. *Spine.* 1984;9:209–213.

75. Al-Obaidi SM, Beattie P, et al. The relationship of anticipated pain and fear avoidance beliefs to outcome in patients with chronic low back pain who are not receiving workers' compensation. *Spine.* 2005;30:1051–1057.

76. George S, Fritz J, et al. Investigation of elevated fear-avoidance beliefs for patients with low back pain: a secondary analysis involving patients enrolled in physical therapy clinical trials. *Journal of Orthopaedic Sports Physical Therapy.* 2008;38:50–58.

77. George SZ, Fritz JM, et al. A comparison of fear-avoidance beliefs in patients with lumbar spine pain and cervical spine pain. *Spine.* 2001;26:2139–2145.

78. Swinkels-Meewisse EJ, Swinkels RA, Verbeek AL, Vlaeyen VA, Oostendorp RA. Psychometric properties of the Tampa Scale for Kinesiophobia and the fear-avoidance beliefs questionnaire in acute low back pain. *Man Ther.* 2003;8:29–36.

79. Swinkels-Meewisse IE, Roelofs J, Verbeek AL, Oostendorp RA, Vlaeyen VA. Fear of movement/(re)injury, disability and participation in acute low back pain. *Pain.* 2003;105:371–379.

80. Swinkels-Meewisse IE, Roelofs J, Shouten EG, Verbeek AL, Vlaeyen VA, Oostendorp RA, et al. Fear of movement/(re)injury predicting chronic disabling low back pain: a prospective inception cohort study. *Spine.* 2006;31:658–664.

81. Ostelo RWJG, de Vet HCW, Knol DL, et al. 24-item Roland Morris disability questionnaire was preferred out of six functional status questionnaires for post-lumbar disc surgery. *Journal of Clinical Epidemiology.* 2004;57:268–276.

CHAPTER 5

82. Patrick DL, Deyo RA, et al. Assessing health-related quality of life in patients with sciatica. *Spine.* 1995;20:1899–1909.

83. Davidson M, Keating JL. A comparison of five low back disability questionnaires: reliability and responsiveness. *Physical Therapy.* 2002;82:8–24.

84. Roland M, Fairbank J. The Roland-Morris disability questionnaire and the Oswestry disability questionnaire. *Spine.* 2000;25:3115–3124.

85. Fairbank JC. Use and abuse of Oswestry Disability Index. *Spine.* 2007;32:2787–2789.

86. McCarthy MJ, Grevitt MP, et al. The reliability of the Vernon and Mior Neck Disability Index, and its validity compared with the Short Form-36 health survey questionnaire. *European Spine Journal.* 2007;16:2111–2117.

87. Cleland JA, Fritz JM, et al. The reliability and construct validity of the Neck Disability Index and patient specific functional scale in patients with cervical radiculopathy. *Spine.* 2006;31:598–602.

88. Cleland JA, Childs JD, et al. Psychometric properties of the Neck Disability Index and Numeric Pain Rating Scale in patients with mechanical neck pain. *Archives of Physical Medicine Rehabilitation.* 2008;89:69–74.

89. Jester A, Harth A, et al. Measuring levels of upper-extremity disability in employed adults using the DASH questionnaire. *Journal of Hand Surgery [Am].* 2005;30:1074 e1–1074 e10.

90. Beaton DE, Katz JN, et al. Measuring the whole or the parts? validity, reliability, and responsiveness of the Disabilities of the Arm, Shoulder and Hand outcome measure in different regions of the upper extremity. *Journal of Hand Therapy.* 2001;14:128–146.

91. Beaton DE, Wright JG, et al. Development of the *Quick*DASH: comparison of three item-reduction approaches. *Journal of Bone and Joint Surgery [Am].* 2005;87:1038–1046.

92. Beck AT, Steer RA, Brown GK. Beck Depression Inventory® II (BDI®-II) Assessment. Oxford, UK: Pearson; 1996. Available at: http://harcourtassessment. com/HAIWEB/Cultures/en-us/Productdetail.htm?Pid=015-8018-370&Mode= summary. Accessed October 17, 2008.

93. Matheson LN. History, design characteristics, and uses of the pictorial activity and task sorts. *Journal of Occupational Rehabilitation.* 2004;14:175–195.

94. Matheson LN, Kaskutas VK, et al. Development and construct validation of the Hand Function Sort. *Journal of Occupational Rehabilitation.* 2001;11:75–86.

95. Mayer J, Mooney V, et al. Reliability and validity of a new computer-administered pictorial activity and task sort. *Journal of Occupational Rehabilitation.* 2005;15:203–213.

96. Ruan CM, Haig AJ, Geisser ME, Yamakawa K, Buchholz RL. Functional capacity evaluations in persons with spinal disorders: predicting poor outcomes on the Functional Assessment Screening Test (FAST). *Journal of Occupational Rehabilitation.* 2001;11:119–132.

97. Gross DP, Battie MC, et al. Development and validation of a short-form functional capacity evaluation for use in claimants with low back disorders. *Journal of Occupational Rehabilitation.* 2006;16:53–62.

CHAPTER 5

6

Dynamic Material Handling Testing

Ev Innes, PhD, MHPEd BAppSc(OT), AccOT MHFESA

Work-related musculoskeletal disorders account for a high proportion of work-related injuries in developed countries. In Australia, for example, "body-stressing" injuries accounted for more than 40% of compensation and work-related injury and disease cases.[1] Approximately half of these body-stressing injuries were the result of some form of manual handling. These figures are similar in other industrially developed nations.

For that reason, the assessment of dynamic material handling is a critical component of all functional capacity evaluations (FCEs). Systems to assess lifting and lowering in particular have been developed as stand-alone evaluations (eg, EPIC Lift Capacity [ELC] Test and Progressive Isoinertial Lifting Evaluation [PILE]) or as components within more extensive FCEs (eg, lifting tests in the Ergo-Kit FCE, Ergoscience Physical Work Performance Evaluation, and Isernhagen Work Systems/WorkWell FCE).

This chapter addresses issues of evaluee safety when assessing dynamic material handling, with an emphasis on lifting capacity. It will also discuss the assessment of lifting using various protocols or systems, the application of these protocols, and their limitations. *Lifting* in this chapter includes lifting and lowering a weight through a vertical distance.

Manual Handling Risk Assessment

The dynamic material handling components within all FCEs are "single manual handling tasks" (ie, lifting, lowering, carrying, pushing, or pulling). They are not "combination manual handling tasks" that require a sequence of single tasks (eg, pulling a box to the edge of a shelf, lifting the box, carrying it to a new shelf, lowering it, and pushing it into place),[2] as would occur commonly in many workplaces.

Given that dynamic material handling is assessed to determine a person's capacity to perform these tasks, usually in a work context, having an understanding of how manual handling tasks are assessed is beneficial when considering how best to assess a person's capacity to perform them. An extensive and thorough review of the literature on manual handling risk assessment was conducted by Straker,[2] in which he examined the various approaches to single and combination manual handling tasks. With regard to single manual handling tasks, the conclusion reached was the following:

...there are a number of approaches and methods available to assess the risk in single manual handling tasks. Although there is often consistency between approaches and methods, there are important differences. It, therefore, appears likely that a range of approaches and methods are needed to adequately capture the risk in any single task manual handling situation.[2(p82)]

The approaches used to assess the risks of manual handling tasks include psychophysical (eg, maximum acceptable weight [MAW]), physiological (eg, heart rate and energy expenditure/oxygen consumption), biomechanical, and other approaches that include psychological methods (eg, discomfort and exertion).[2] These psychological methods are often included as psychophysical approaches.

For example, for low- to moderate-frequency lifts ($\leq$ 6/min), the psychophysical method of determining MAW set for a 20- to 40-minute period seems to reflect reasonable physiological loads for most manual handling tasks. Higher frequencies, however, result in physiological loads exceeding recommended limits.[2] Physiological methods using heart rate and energy expenditure are only useful, however, for repetitive tasks of moderate to high frequency.[2] Discomfort ratings (eg, visual analogue scale) and exertion (eg, Borg Rate of Perceived Exertion [RPE] scale) are useful measures to evaluate tasks performed for short periods and require no sophisticated equipment.[2] However, these methods are "potentially affected to some extent by wider factors such as motivation and social situation,"[2(p65)] as is MAW.

This range of manual handling risk assessment approaches also reflects the methods used to assess dynamic material handling capacity. Various combinations and emphases of these approaches are used in the range of FCEs and lifting assessments currently available and used in clinical practice.

Safety and Lifting Techniques

CHAPTER 6

Safety is considered the most important attribute of work-related assessments, including FCEs.[3-5] Safety is also reported by clinicians to be essential and is the highest rated of any attribute for work-related assessments.[6]

Studies have examined the safety of various FCEs.[7-9] The studies used similar operational definitions of *safety* (ie, the people evaluated did not report any injuries or file any formal complaints, and any increase in symptoms was temporary and returned to pretesting levels).[8,9] Results indicated that although it was not unusual for people to experience an increase in symptoms following testing, this increase was usually mild to moderate, and discomfort returned to pretesting levels within several days to a week in the majority of cases.

Safety also needs to be considered at both ends of the assessment—prescreening before commencing to ensure it is safe to start the assessment, and clear end points to determine when to cease testing. Gibson and Strong[7] reported support for "the screening procedures ... particularly blood pressure measurement, and for the combined approach to monitoring of the person's performance from biomechanical, physiological and psychophysical perspectives."[(p237)]

Clear definitions of what constitutes a "safe lift" also enhance safety. Research has shown that using an operational definition of a safe lift significantly improved therapists' reliability in distinguishing safe from unsafe lifts.[10] This finding is consistent with those of other studies that have recommended the need for clear guidelines for the criteria used in FCEs to evaluate performance.[7,11–13]

However, what constitutes a safe lift is controversial. Most recommendations on lifting technique advocate the use of squat and semisquat lifting techniques; however, stoop lifting is often the technique of choice for many workers. An extensive literature review of lifting low-lying objects by Straker[14] indicates that different lifting techniques are more or less favored depending on whether psychophysical, physiological, biomechanical, psychological, performance, or clinical variables are considered (Table 6–1). There are also varying levels of evidence to support these criteria.

TABLE 6–1   Summary of Evidence for Squat, Semisquat, and Stoop Lifting Techniques[14(p94)]

Criteria	Squat	Semisquat	Stoop
Psychophysical			
MAW	■	■ ■ ■	■ ■
Physiological			
Oxygen consumption	■	■ ■	■ ■ ■
Heart rate	□	□ □	□ □ □
Ventilation	□	□ □	□ □ □
Relative load	□ □	□ □	□ □
Biomechanical			
Lumbar moment	■ ■	□ □	■ ■
Lumbar compression	□ □	□ □	□ □
Lumbar shear	□ □ □	□ □	□
Lumbar erector spinae	□ □	□ □	□ □
Lumbar passive tissues	□ □ □	□ □	□
Quadriceps	□	□ □	□ □ □
Hamstrings	□ □ □	□ □	□
Other joints	□ □	□ □	□ □

TABLE 6–1 Summary of Evidence for Squat, Semisquat, and Stoop Lifting Techniques[14(p94)] (continued)

Criteria	Squat	Semisquat	Stoop
Fatigue kinematics	■	◩ □	■ ■ ■
Strength capacity	◩ □	◩ □	◩ □
Stature loss	□ □	□ □	□ □
Stability	□	□ □	□ □ □
Relative load	□ □ □	□ □	□
Psychological			
General discomfort/exertion	■	◩ □	■ ■ ■
Lumbar discomfort/exertion	□ □ □	□ □	□
Quadriceps discomfort/exertion	□	□ □	□ □ □
Hamstrings discomfort/exertion	□ □ □	□ □	□
	□	□ □	□ □ □
Performance			
Clinical			
Effect of pain	◩ ◩ ◩	◩ ◩	◩
Usual movement	□	□ □	□ □ □
Type of injury	□ □ □	□ □	□
Problem of change	□	□ □	□ □ □

MAW indicates maximum acceptable weight; 3 symbols, most favored technique; 2 symbols, no preference between techniques; 1 symbol, least favored technique; ■, reasonably good evidence; ◩, some evidence; □, minimal evidence.

Straker[14] concluded that a work design approach should be promoted (ie, eliminating manual handling of low-lying objects wherever possible) owing to no clearly favored technique for lifting low-lying objects. He states that "where this is achieved, and objects to be lifted are between knee and shoulder height, the issue of correct technique is nearly obsolete."[14(p93)]

The issue of whether to instruct people and/or correct their lifting techniques before and during assessment is also a vexing one. There is some disagreement between FCE systems when it comes to this issue. Some approaches recommend that evaluees be permitted to use their usual lifting technique and not be corrected during evaluation because a realistic reflection of how they would lift in unsupervised settings, such as at work, is presented. Others believe that it is necessary to ensure that safe manual handling methods are used by instructing evaluees before testing and providing correction throughout if techniques become unsafe. Still others rate the lifting technique used on a number of factors, such as distance of the load away from the body and stance. If the evaluee's technique deteriorates below a predetermined level during testing (ie, the evaluee

CHAPTER 6

demonstrates unsafe practices), the technique is corrected. The assessment is terminated if these techniques do not improve and continue to be unsafe.

Fortunately, given the conflicting evidence in many areas, there is agreement on some aspects of what can be recommended with regard to correct lifting of low-lying objects. The following aspects have strong support from the literature[14]:

- Keeping the load close
- Using a secure grip and a stable base
- Using a smooth movement or moderate pace

Other recommendations have only low-level support from the literature but may be useful in reducing risk.[14] These are as follows:

- Avoiding end-of-range trunk flexion
- Avoiding combining trunk flexion, lateral flexion, and rotation
- Avoiding lifting after prolonged flexion or vibration
- Maintaining bracing of abdominal and trunk muscles
- Stressing muscle rather than ligament

End-Point Determination

Within an FCE it is "necessary to quantify the injured workers' ability to perform the manual materials handling through identifying that component of the functional tasks that serves as the limiting factor in job performance."[15(p183)] This could be considered as determining the end point of the FCE or subtest within the FCE.

Generally, biomechanical, physiological, and psychophysical end points are considered when conducting FCEs. Some systems prefer one approach over another. For example, Jones and Kumar[15] recommend the assessment of isoinertial strength through psychophysical means to determine the maximum weight a person is willing to handle at a freely chosen speed. They consider that "an isoinertial protocol and psychophysical criterion are most appropriately used in an FCE due to the higher correlation between isoinertial techniques and actual work tasks and the ethical demands necessitating the use of psychophysical 'stopping points.'"[15(pp183–184)]

The Progressive Isoinertial Lifting Evaluation (PILE) includes a "safety" end point that is a predetermined anthropometric "safe limit" of 55% to 60% of body weight."[16(p994)] It would seem, however, that this is not necessarily a generally accepted end point. Rainville et al[17] use a lower safe limit of 45% to 55% of body weight for the PILE.

The US National Institute of Occupational Safety and Health (NIOSH) lifting equation is used to calculate a recommended weight limit for bilateral lifts in occupational settings.[18] A lifting index is calculated to determine the physical strain of a specific lifting task: the higher the lifting index, the greater the risk for low back injury. When compared with the floor-to-waist lifting capacity of subjects with chronic low back pain, the NIOSH recommended weight limit produced substantially lower safe lifting weights than the FCE.[19] These differences can potentially result in confusion when making recommendations for safe lifting limits for a person's return to work after injury.

It is widely recommended, however, that biomechanical, physiological, and psychophysical end points that are clearly defined are included in FCEs, particularly when assessing dynamic material handling.[3,7,11,12,20] Several systems incorporate all three approaches to determine the testing end point in their protocols (eg, ELC Test). By doing this, it allows for triangulation of information from different sources to compare responses and determine the most limiting factor. The limiting factors can then be addressed in intervention strategies.

External End-Point Criteria and "No-Lift" Policies

Apart from biomechanical, physiological, and psychophysical end points, there may also be end points set externally. The most common of these external criteria are the following:

- Lifting restrictions imposed by the evaluee's treating medical practitioner or other health care provider; and/or
- Identified physical work demands (eg, the job requires that loads up to 15 kg are lifted once every 30 minutes from floor to bench height [90 cm]).

When there are clearly identified physical work demands, it is not necessary to assess beyond the job requirements. This assumes of course that the evaluee has a job to return to and that a workplace assessment/job analysis has been conducted to determine this end point.

It is also necessary to consider whether no-lift policies have been introduced to workplaces. Some employers, especially in the health and aged-care sectors, have no-lift policies that prohibit employees from lifting. Instead, other manual handling techniques, including the use of manual handling equipment (eg, hoists, sliding/roller sheets, and transfer belts), are enforced. In these situations and others in which there are unusual or unique manual handling requirements, it will be necessary to simulate the job tasks to determine a person's ability to meet the job demands.

CHAPTER 6

Biomechanical End-Point Determination

Determination of a biomechanical end point is also referred to as the *kinesio-physical approach* in the Isernhagen Work Systems (IWS)/WorkWell FCE.[21,22] Results are based on the clinician's evaluation of the evaluee's movement patterns with regard to safety. This approach is associated with the evaluee's capacity to perform the physical demands of the FCE with regard to his or her biomechanical and sensory-motor systems. The criteria used to determine levels of effort include observation of the following[23]:

- Muscle recruitment
- Base of support
- Posture
- Control and movement patterns

In the ELC Test biomechanical end points include the following[24]:

- Lifting restrictions (external criterion)
- Job performance targets (external criterion)
- Body mechanics that demonstrate overloading
- High-risk work style when lifting with regard to the distance between the load and the body and the stance adopted when lifting/lowering

Physiological End-Point Determination

Determination of a physiological end point is also referred to as a cardiovascular or metabolic approach.[3] It relies on measurements such as heart rate, oxygen consumption, and blood pressure to determine the amount of work being performed.[20] This model relates to the capacity to perform the physical demands with regard to cardiovascular, pulmonary, and metabolic systems.[3]

The consensus for an acceptable physiological end point is a heart rate of between 70% and 85% of predicted age-related maximum heart rate (220 beats per minute − age in years). The level selected is dependent on the overall fitness of the evaluee. It is also important to be aware of whether the evaluee is taking any medications that limit heart rate, which would preclude the use of this method for end-point determination. When examining results, consideration is given to whether there is an appropriate heart rate response to increasing activity levels and the recovery time needed to return to resting levels.

Psychophysical End-Point Determination

Determination of a psychophysical end point relates to the evaluee's capacity to perform the physical demands with regard to "the person's cognitive-perceptual systems such as self-perception, beliefs, and expectations."[3(p4)] It includes consideration of the following:

- Perceptions of exertion, load, etc (eg, RPE)
- Maximum acceptable effort or MAW
- Pain location and intensity
- Pain behaviors
- Fear of pain, movement, and/or reinjury

When using the Borg RPE scale, a score of 12 to 14 is considered moderate activity and 15 is considered an appropriate end point on the 6 to 20 scale. This is the equivalent of 7 on the Category Ratio-10 (CR-10) scale. See Chapter 5.

Assessment of Lifting in Functional Capacity Evaluations

Determination of lifting capacity is incorporated into all currently available comprehensive FCEs and is the focus of some specific lifting assessments. Although many FCEs include similar items (eg, lifting and carrying), they determine these in different ways, and so results cannot be used interchangeably or compared.[25] This is demonstrated by the poor correlations between several FCEs measuring apparently the same physical demands.[26-28] It is, therefore, necessary to consider the protocols used and whether there are calculations used to extrapolate the information gained to other areas (eg, using the results of an occasional lifting test to gauge the results of frequent or constant lifting).

Owing to the proprietary nature of many FCEs, it is difficult to compare and contrast the specific protocols used without purchasing the FCE and completing the training required to administer the system. Although general descriptions of the protocols may be included in publications, the detail used in clinical administration of the tests is not available.

Determination of lifting ability through different ranges is included in all FCEs. There is some variation between systems with regard to the start and end points of each range; however, they generally include the following:

- Floor to knuckle/waist—The knuckle/waist level is approximately desk height (between 72 and 76 cm) depending on the height of the evaluee. The apparent difference in height is based on whether the height of the surface (knuckle) to which the load is lifted or the height of the hands (waist) when holding the object lifted is considered.

- Floor to knuckle/waist lifts place stress on the low back and lower limbs (hips, knees, and ankles) in particular.
- Knuckle/waist to chest/shoulder—As with knuckle/waist levels, chest/shoulder level is the height of the surface (chest) or the height of the hands (shoulder).
  - Knuckle/waist to chest/shoulder lifts place stress on the upper limbs and hands/wrists. If the evaluee has reached his or her upper limb strength limit, then there may be low back stress due to the use of compensatory techniques.
- Other ranges include the following:
  - Overhead lifts—These lifts involve lifting above head height and place stress on the upper limbs (especially shoulders) and neck in particular. When placing the load overhead, the wrists may be placed in awkward positions (eg, extreme ulnar deviation).
  - Horizontal lifts—Horizontal lifts occur at knuckle/waist level and require the movement of a load from one surface to another at the same height. Trunk rotation may occur during these lifts if the evaluee does not use appropriate body mechanics.
  - Floor to chest/shoulder or overhead lifts—After determining an evaluee's ability to lift in the floor to knuckle/waist and knuckle/waist to chest/shoulder or overhead ranges, there may be the inclusion of a lift/lower through the full available range.

Some FCEs have limited, if any, published studies regarding their reliability or validity. Although this does not indicate that these systems are unreliable or invalid, it is difficult to make informed decisions about the most appropriate systems to use for the identified purpose. Systems without published reliability studies (as of September 2008) include the Blankenship FCE and Key Method Functional Capacity Assessment (FCA). There are no validity studies published examining the Key Method FCA (as of September 2008).

For the FCEs that have published studies, some deal with the entire system, and others address specific components or subtests within the overall system. Only the FCE systems with studies relevant to manual handling are discussed herein, which include the following: two specific lifting assessments—ELC Test and PILE—and FCEs that incorporate manual handling components—Ergo-Kit FCE, Ergoscience Physical Work Performance Evaluation (PWPE), IWS/WorkWell FCE, and WorkHab FCE.

EPIC Lift Capacity Test

The ELC Test determines the maximum acceptable weight a person can lift and lower on a safe and dependable basis 8 to 12 times per day. It is designed for use with men and women of working age (18–60 years). Potential evaluees are put through a prescreening to ensure their suitability for evaluation. The ELC Test is not designed for people who are significantly obese. Certification is required to conduct the ELC Test.

The ELC Test's precursor was the Progressive Lifting Capacity II test. The ELC Test is included in the California Functional Capacity Protocol and is used as a stand-alone assessment. The test-retest and interrater reliability for the ELC Test are good to excellent. Test-retest reliability was established on a number of different occasions in a variety of settings with large numbers of subjects, strengthening the findings.[9,29-31]

Interrater reliability of evaluators' abilities to determine participants' overall effort levels was good.[32] Although an evaluator's observation and evaluation of effort should not be the sole indicator, it was found to be the best single indicator of determining sincerity of effort.[32] It was possible to determine a subject's level of effort (sincere/insincere) with an overall accuracy of 87%. The indicators of effort used in the study had high positive (0.94) and negative (0.80) predictive values.[32] Although these findings indicate that the construct validity of differentiating between levels of effort is supported, the authors advised that evaluators should err on the side of caution when identifying a person as giving an insincere effort.[32]

Good construct validity was established for the ELC Test's ability to measure change in lifting ability of younger and middle-aged back-injured subjects following treatment.[33] The ability to predict lifting capacity based on subject age, body weight, height, and resting heart rate also supports construct validity.[30] The ELC Test was unable, however, to determine any difference in lifting capacity based on the use of a lumbar support belt.[34]

A study examining aerobic capacity and back strength using a concurrent validation design found that both of these factors contributed to lifting capacity.[35] The authors concluded that the combined use of fitness and back strength training was supported in rehabilitation programs. They also indicated that although tests of aerobic capacity and back strength may be useful for screening purposes in work in which lifting is an important job demand, it was not possible to substitute the measurement of lifting capacity with the measurement of aerobic capacity or back strength.[35]

The concurrent validity of a computerized pictorial activity and task sort (Multidimensional Task Ability Profile) and the occasional lifts of the ELC Test was examined and found to be good to excellent.[36] The correlation coefficient between the two instruments was higher when only the lifting items of the Multidimensional Task Ability Profile were included, rather than all items. The authors indicated that the use of the pictorial activity/task sort could be used as a substitute for aspects of an FCE, such as lifting capacity.[36] This finding is in contrast, however, with a study that compared the perceived and actual lifting capacity of healthy young men using self-report, the Spinal Function Sort, and ELC Test.[37,38] Only one third of subjects were able to accurately (±5 kg) estimate their actual lifting capacity as measured by the ELC Test, whereas approximately one-third overestimated and one-third underestimated their capacity. This finding indicates that knowledge of lifting capacity is limited, even in an uninjured population. Care, therefore, needs to be taken when interpreting discrepancies between self-reported and observed or assessed lifting capacity.

EPIC Lift Capacity Test: Protocol

The six subtests of the ELC Test cover three lifting ranges and two frequencies. It is not necessary to conduct all subtests; however, the order of the subtests must be maintained.[24] The ELC Test uses weight increments throughout the testing, which are the same for males and females. This is in contrast with the PILE, which uses different increments for males and females.

- Lifting Tests and Sequence

1.	Knuckle – shoulder	1×/cycle	start at 4.52 kg (10 lb)
2.	Floor – knuckle	1×/cycle	start at 4.52 kg (10 lb)
3.	Floor – shoulder	1×/cycle	start at 70% of the lesser of No. 1 or No. 2
4.	Knuckle – shoulder	4×/cycle	start at 40% of No. 1
5.	Floor – knuckle	4×/cycle	start at 40% of No. 2
6.	Floor – shoulder	4×/cycle	start at 40% of No. 3

  - Cycle = minimum of 30 seconds
  - Shelves adjusted to suit evaluee's height for knuckle and shoulder levels
- Weight increments
  - Increase by 4.52 kg (10 lb) for each additional load.
  - It is possible to increase by lesser amounts; however, the results cannot be compared with normative data.
- End-point determination
  - Psychophysical
    - Performance-limiting symptoms—Determine if the evaluee's symptoms are new and/or indicate a pathological response to the task or if they are unacceptable to evaluee.
    - RPE (using 0–10 scale)—A rating of 8 or more indicates that testing is discontinued.
    - Appraisal of lifting limits—The evaluee is asked at the end of every cycle if he or she could lift the weight on a safe and dependable basis. The response to the question is considered with other responses (physiological, RPE, and biomechanical limits) to determine whether the test continues or is terminated.

- Physiological
    - Heart rate is monitored throughout the test. If the heart rate exceeds 85% of the predicted maximum heart rate (220 beats per minute – age in years), the test is terminated.
    - The heart rate must be less than 70% of the predicted maximum heart before the subtest or lifting cycle can commence.
- Biomechanical: The ELC Test uses height and sex to set biomechanical load guidelines.
    - High-risk work style—Consider horizontal displacement and stance.
    - Overload body mechanics
- External end points
    - Lifting restrictions imposed by treating physician or other health care professional
    - Job performance targets
- Constant Work Test—This test can be conducted after the standard test battery. The Constant Work Test is performed for a maximum of 2 hours, and results can be compared with methods-time-measurement (MTM) ratings.

Progressive Isoinertial Lifting Evaluation

The PILE is a lifting evaluation that has a lumbar test (floor-to-waist level) and a cervical test (waist-to-shoulder level).

The PILE's interrater reliability is excellent for lumbar (floor-waist) and cervical (waist-shoulder) lifts.[39] This was also the case for test-retest reliability of the cervical lift.[39] However, the test-retest reliability of the lumbar PILE lift varied from moderate for female nursing aides[39] to excellent in subjects with chronic low back pain.[40] This latter study also reported that there should be a change of at least 6 kg for women and 7 kg for men before a true change can be said to have occurred.[40] Test-retest and interrater reliability were considered clinically acceptable in subjects with back or neck pain.[40]

Testing order (ie, whether the PILE was performed before or after other tests in a multidisciplinary assessment) did not affect performance in healthy subjects or subjects with back pain.[41]

No studies were located that specifically examined the validity of the PILE; however, there were a number of studies that used the PILE as an outcome measure or compared PILE results with other measures. These studies are considered to contribute to various aspects of validity of the PILE.

Comparison of the PILE and IWS FCE lifting tests produced significantly different results.[28,42] The study by Schenk et al[28] found that the weights lifted using the PILE were significantly higher than the IWS FCE. This finding was reversed in the study by Soer et al,[42] in which the IWS FCE produced higher lifting results than the PILE. Given the conflicting results from these studies, all that can be said is that the results of these lifting tests are not interchangeable.

When lifting capacity results were compared with job requirements, the workers who met the physical job demands were found to have significantly lower injury rates than the workers who did not.[43] Strength testing alone, however, had no predictive value for determining the incidence of work injuries. Therefore, the authors concluded that "physical evaluation of potential employees is useful for injury prevention only if it can be related to the physical requirements of the job."[43(p306)]

The PILE results had moderate positive correlations with heart rate and perceived exertion, as expected, but also had significant negative correlations with activity avoidance behaviors (ie, increased activity avoidance associated with decreased weight lifted).[44] This finding indicates the importance of addressing activity avoidance in the assessment of functional capacity in people with chronic pain.

Because functional capacity is influenced by psychosocial and physical factors, it is difficult to determine whether maximal effort is exerted in FCEs. The sensitivity and specificity of a number of tests, including the PILE, were examined for their ability to determine maximal effort.[45] Although the combination of tests had reasonable specificity (84%), the sensitivity (65%) was unacceptable because patients giving maximal effort may be incorrectly labeled as exerting submaximal effort.[45] The authors, therefore, urged caution when labeling the efforts of patients.

The PILE was compared with performance on the Functional Assessment Screening Test (FAST), a low-exertion test battery consisting of five subtests for low back pain,[46] contributing to the concurrent validity of the PILE. (Note: None of the FAST subtests involved lifting.) Subjects unable to complete the five subtests in the FAST had significantly lower PILE results for both lifting ranges (ie, lower percentage of expected weight lifted and lower percentage of maximum heart rate achieved) than subjects who completed the FAST.[46]

Construct validity was addressed in a study that attempted to distinguish between subjects with back or neck pain and healthy subjects by using a test battery that included the PILE.[47] There were significant differences between the pain group and healthy control subjects on the PILE; the sensitivity was relatively high (80%–93%), but specificity was much lower (65%–83%) to distinguish between the groups.[47]

Several studies that have used the PILE as an outcome-measure to determine the effectiveness of various treatment programs for subjects with back pain have contributed to our understanding of the construct-validity of the PILE to determine changes in performance following intervention. Following surgery, the performance of subjects with lumbar disc herniation improved significantly, when compared to control subjects, on a number of measures, including the PILE following intensive exercise program, and to a significant but lesser extent following a home exercise program.[48] In a similar study, however, there were no differences found between groups in lifting capacity.[49] This finding is similar to that in a study comparing the effects of a functional restoration program and active individual therapy in which no difference was found in lifting ability between groups, although lifting capacity improved for all subjects.[50] This may be a reflection of the treatment provided to these groups and other factors, rather than the ability of the PILE to detect change.

Progressive Isoinertial Lifting Evaluation: Protocol

The PILE is a lifting evaluation that has two tests (lumbar and cervical) and uses weight increments that differ for males and females[16]:
- Lifting tests
  - Lumbar test—floor to waist (0–76 cm [30 in])
  - Cervical test—waist to shoulder height (76–137 cm [30–54 in]
  - Tests performed separately
- Lifting sequence
  - Perform four lifting/lowering movements in each 20-second interval (ie, lift, lower, lift, lower).
- Starting weight and increments
  - Women—Start at 3.63 kg (8 lb; weight of box + 2.27 kg [5 lb])
    - Increase by 2.27 kg (5 lb) every 20 seconds
  - Men—Start at 5.90 kg (13 lb; weight of box + 4.52 kg [10 lb])
    - Increase by 4.52 kg (10 lb) every 20 seconds
- End-point determination—Continue testing until one of the following end points is reached, and note which was the limiting factor:
  - Psychophysical: Voluntary test termination by subject owing to complaints of fatigue, excessive discomfort, or inability to complete four lifting movements in a 20-second interval
  - Physiological (aerobic): Achievement of a specific aerobic capacity goal, usually 75% to 85% of age-determined maximum heart rate (unless cardiac precautions are in force or heart rate–limiting medications are being taken)[16,17]
  - Safety: A predetermined anthropometric safe limit
    - There are differing views of this limit—the range is from 45% to 55%[17] to 55% to 60%[16] of body weight.

CHAPTER 6

- Results can be expressed as follows:
  - Maximum weight lifted for each range
  - Endurance time to discontinuation of the test
  - Final and target heart rates
  - Total work (force × distance) for each test
  - Power consumption (total work ÷ time)

Ergo-Kit FCE

The Ergo-Kit FCE is a relatively new system and used predominantly in the Netherlands. Intrarater and interrater (4- and 8-day intervals) reliability for seven subtests (five of which were manual handling tests) ranged from high to low levels of reliability when used with uninjured subjects.[51] The back-torso lift and shoulder lift had high levels of intrarater and 8-day interrater reliability; carrying, lower, and upper lifting strength tests had moderate; and forward and lower manipulation tests had low levels.[51] Interrater (4-day) reliability was high for isometric and dynamic lifting tests. There was good interrater reliability for two isometric and three dynamic lifting subtests when subjects with back injuries were assessed.[52]

There was poor concurrent validity between the Ergo-Kit and the IWS FCE for lifting waist-to-overhead in a group of healthy young adults, and so results of these lifting subtests cannot be used interchangeably.[26] Concurrent validity between the ERGOS work simulator static and dynamic lifting strength (panel 1) and the Ergo-Kit was also poor.[27] The study examined occasional, frequent, and constant lifts for low and high levels. There were significant differences between the ERGOS and the Ergo-Kit for each lift, with moderate correlations. The authors concluded that the concurrent validity was poor, with the Ergo-Kit dynamic lifting capacity results significantly higher than for the ERGOS.[27] It was suggested that the ERGOS may be more appropriate when determining functional lifting capacity, but the Ergo-Kit may be used when evaluating ergonomic adaptations for a person at work.[27]

Aspects of the Ergo-Kit's construct validity were reported in a study that examined the extent that self-reports of lifting capacity could replace performance-based testing (ie, waist-to-shoulder lifts).[53] The authors concluded that "correlation coefficients between self-reports and performance tests were too low to be relevant in a clinical situation,"[53(p84)] and, therefore, self-reports should not replace performance tests of lifting waist to shoulder or overhead.

Ergoscience Physical Work Performance Evaluation (PWPE)

The test-retest reliability of nine tasks in the PWPE was studied, using injured workers as subjects.[54] This study included dynamic strength tasks (lifting floor to waist, bilateral carry, pushing), which all demonstrated substantial test-retest reliability.[54]

Interrater reliability for the dynamic strength tests (floor-to-waist lift, waist-to-eye level lift, bilateral and unilateral carry, pushing and pulling) was found to be substantial when used with an injured population.[13] However, interrater reliability when determining subject participation was much more variable and generally lower, particularly in the dynamic strength and mobility sections.[13] The researchers recommended that the criteria for biomechanical end points should be improved.[13]

Contributing to the validity of the PWPE is a study that found work performance to be significantly associated with the dynamic strength subtests of the PWPE that assessed lifting and carrying.[55]

Isernhagen Work Systems FCE

In the past decade, the IWS FCE has become the most intensively researched FCE available. This is primarily because of the work of Dutch (Reneman, Brouwer, and colleagues)[61] and Canadian researchers (Gross and Battié).[62-64] In 2006, the IWS FCE was renamed the WorkWell FCE, version 2.

Test-retest reliability of the IWS FCE has been extensively investigated with healthy subjects and subjects with back pain. When the entire IWS FCE was examined, good to excellent test-retest reliability was found for the material handling tasks in subjects with low back pain[56] and healthy subjects (with the exception of static pushing).[57] Another study, which examined only lifting subtests, had similar results.[58] The lifting subtests are the most reliable of the various sections of the IWS FCE as demonstrated in a number of studies in injured and healthy populations.

The IWS FCE was originally developed to be conducted over 2 days to verify accuracy of results and evaluate the effect of day 1 testing on a person. The test-retest reliability of low and overhead lifts and short carry over a 2-day FCE

CHAPTER 6

was examined.[59] Results indicated good reliability for these subtests for the 2-day FCE, with mean results higher on the second day. The authors concluded "because of good test-retest reliability, the limited relevance of the increase in performance, and cost-containment, we cannot justify the need for a 2-day protocol in a general sense."[59(p273)]

Interrater reliability of the lifting subtests and determining safe maximum limits has also been examined in several studies using healthy and injured subjects.[10,23,60,61] Most studies found interrater reliability to be good to excellent.[23,60, 61] Gardener and McKenna[10] indicated only moderate reliability; however, this was significantly improved when a clear operational definition of a safe lift was provided. Reneman et al[61] found that ratings of effort were more reliable if a CR-10 scale was used, rather than a 4-point categorical scale.

Several studies examined the predictive validity of the IWS FCE.[62–65] Greater lifting ability was weakly related to greater likelihood of returning to work and speedier return to work.[63–65] The floor-to-waist lift was able to predict return to work information from the entire FCE.[64] Further examination of safe return to work found that the IWS FCE was not able to predict recurrence of back injuries.[62,63] The authors concluded that the predictive validity of the IWS FCE to identify people who can safely return to work was not supported.

A number of studies have been conducted comparing the IWS FCE with a range of measures. The IWS and Ergo-Kit FCEs were compared—waist-to-overhead lifts were found to produce different results for the two systems, and so cannot be used interchangeably.[26] The IWS FCE and PILE lifting protocols were also compared, and results differed significantly[28,42] (see previous discussion of this).

The IWS FCE has also been compared with many other measures, including self-report questionnaires related to lifting capacity and disability.[53,66,67] Correlations between self-report and actual lifting capacity were fair to moderate in healthy subjects and negligible to poor in subjects with chronic lower back pain (LBP),[53,66,67] indicating that while performance-based and self-report instruments may measure the same construct, the correlations were too low to be relevant in clinical situations[53] and could not be used interchangeably.

WorkHab FCE

The WorkHab FCE was developed in the mid-1990s and incorporates the monitoring of heart rate, perceived exertion, and pain when various components are tested. Reliability (test-retest, interrater, and intrarater) has been examined for some components, including material handling tasks.[68] These components were part of a pre-employment functional assessment (PEFA) used to determine whether coal miners met the key physical requirements of proposed positions. Results indicate that overall PEFA scores had good to excellent reliability, whereas material handling tests had moderate to good test-retest reliability and good to excellent interrater and intrarater reliability.[68] It should be noted that the PEFA had clearly identified job-related physical demands based on analyses of the various positions.

Predicting Frequent Lifting From Occasional Lifting

Some FCEs extrapolate the weights that can be handled on a frequent or constant basis from other lifting results. The reason may be to allow the recommendation of lifting limits for frequent or constant material handling or to allow comparison with actual lifting performance during testing. Owing to the proprietary nature of almost all FCEs, it is not possible to compare how these extrapolations are calculated, and there is limited research in this area.

One study examined whether it was possible to accurately predict the weight lifted frequently from other data obtained during the FCE and which equations were best to estimate weights for frequent lifting.[69] The FCE used consisted of a 22-hour evaluation conducted over 6 days and included activities that simulated job-specific requirements. The length of this FCE was far in excess of any current commercial FCE. The results indicated that "the best predictor of weight that can be lifted frequently was the amount of weight that can be lifted occasionally at that position."[69(p1723)] However, for some groups of subjects, the amount lifted was much less than predicted, particularly when lifting overhead. The authors seriously questioned the general use of formulae in FCEs and concluded that "the large amount of error in the estimates, however, makes the use of formulas for predicting the weight that can be lifted frequently in clinical practice questionable."[69(p1728)]

Applications and Limitations of Material Handling Components of FCEs

Assessment of manual handling capacity, especially lifting and lowering, in FCEs provides clinicians with a more realistic way of determining an evaluee's ability when the actual workplace and job tasks are not available. This may be because the evaluee does not have a job or employer to return to following an injury, there is difficulty accessing the workplace, or because it is considered unsafe to assess manual handling capacity within the work environment. When possible, however, assessment of job-specific requirements will enable a more focused evaluation of the evaluee's ability to meet the physical demands of the job.

All FCEs have manual handling protocols that use standardized equipment, such as the size and shape of the object lifted, and predetermined lifting ranges. Often the container used is a crate that may have handles attached. Although it is necessary for equipment to be consistent within the assessment, it may be very different from what the evaluee is required to handle in the workplace. Long, narrow pipes and beams, sacks of flour or cement, bags of groceries, sheets of glass or steel, and large trays of baked products all have different manual handling demands. The ranges through which items are lifted or carried may also be different from the ranges within a standardized FCE. It may be necessary, therefore, to include additional manual handling components within the FCE to simulate specific work demands.

Almost all FCEs incorporate a range of end points, including biomechanical, physiological, and psychophysical. Based on the recommendations from several researchers, it is important to have clearly defined end points to enable consistency between assessors and ensure safety during testing. Clinicians are strongly encouraged to use biomechanical, physiological, and psychophysical methods when determining the end point of the assessment. The triangulation of data from various sources allows for the determination of the most limiting factor in the FCE. This enables clearer recommendations for intervention approaches.

Caution needs to be exercised, however, when interpreting results, especially if there are discrepancies between observed and self-reported lifting capacity. Injured workers are known to underestimate their physical capacity.[70] This underestimation may be influenced by fear of pain or reinjury and various other reasons for self-limiting behavior. Clinicians need to be aware, however, that uninjured subjects have also been shown to underestimate their performance.[11,37,38,71] This underestimation may be an indication that injured and uninjured workers are not aware of their actual abilities with regard to work, and although self-report measures are a useful addition to the information obtained, they cannot be relied on to be accurate. Performance-based assessments are, therefore, important to determine actual abilities.

Numerous studies have shown that the manual handling components of various FCEs are not interchangeable. So, although all FCEs incorporate manual handling components, it is not possible to use the results interchangeably.

Manual handling is assessed by all FCEs and several assessments specifically developed to evaluate lifting. Clinicians are encouraged to be familiar with the research conducted using these instruments and select assessments that meet the needs of their evaluees.

References

1. Macdonald W, Evans O. Research on the prevention of work-related musculoskeletal disorders: stage 1: literature review: Australian Safety & Compensation Council; 2006. Available at: http://www.ascc.gov.au/NR/rdonlyres/D0C2EF6D-C027-4BEF-B9A2 -D4F76F50A05A/0/WorkRelatedMusculoSkeletalDisordersStage1LitReviewNov06 .pdf. Accessed January 14, 2009.
2. Straker L. *A Critical Appraisal of Manual Handling Risk Assessment Literature.* Louisville, KY: International Ergonomic Association Press; 1997.
3. Gibson L, Strong J. A review of functional capacity evaluation practice. *Work.* 1997;9(1):3–11.
4. Hart DL, Isernhagen SJ, Matheson LN. Guidelines for functional capacity evaluation of people with medical conditions. *J Orthop Sports Phys Ther.* 1993;18(6):682–686.
5. Matheson LN. Functional capacity evaluation. In: Demeter SL, Andersson GBJ, Smith GM, eds. *Disability Evaluation.* St Louis, MO: Mosby; 1996:168–188.
6. Innes E, Straker L. Attributes of excellence in work-related assessments. *Work.* 2003;20(1):63–76.
7. Gibson L, Strong J. Safety issues in functional capacity evaluation: findings from a trial of a new approach for evaluating clients with chronic back pain. *J Occup Rehabil.* 2005;15(2):237–251.
8. Reneman MF, Kuijer W, Brouwer S, et al. Symptom increase following a functional capacity evaluation in patients with chronic low back pain: an explorative study of safety. *J Occup Rehabil.* 2006;16(2):192–200.
9. Matheson LN, Danner R, Grant J, Mooney V. Effect of computerised instructions on measurement of lift capacity: safety, reliability, and validity. *J Occup Rehabil.* 1993;3(2):65–81.
10. Gardener L, McKenna K. Reliability of occupational therapists in determining safe, maximal lifting capacity. *Aust Occup Ther J.* 1999;46(3):110–119.
11. Reneman MF, Bults MMWE, Engbers LH, Mulders KKG, Göeken LNH. Measuring maximum holding times and perception of static elevated work and forward bending in health young adults. *J Occup Rehabil.* 2001;11(2):87–97.
12. Reneman MF, Joling CI, Soer EL, Göeken LNH. Functional capacity evaluation: ecological validity of three static endurance tests. *Work.* 2001;16(3):227–234.
13. Durand M, Loisel P, Poitras S, Mercier R, Stock S, Lemaire J. The interrater reliability of a functional capacity evaluation: the Physical Work Performance Evaluation. *J Occup Rehabil.* 2004;14(2):119–129.
14. Straker LM. A review of research on techniques for lifting low-lying objects, 2: evidence for a correct technique. *Work.* 2003;20(2):83–96.

15. Jones T, Kumar S. Functional capacity evaluation of manual materials handlers: a review. *Disabil Rehabil.* 2003;25(4–5):179–191.

16. Mayer TG, Barnes D, Kishino ND, et al. Progressive isoinertial lifting evaluation, I: a standardised protocol and normative database. *Spine.* 1988;13(9):993–997.

17. Rainville J, Sobel J, Hartigan C, Monlux G, Bean J. Decreasing disability in chronic back pain through aggressive spine rehabilitation. *J Rehabil Res Dev.* 1997;34(4):383–393.

18. Waters TR, Putz-Anderson V. Revised NIOSH lifting equation. In: Karwowski W, Marras WS, eds. *The Occupational Ergonomics Handbook.* Boca Raton, FL: CRC Press; 1999:1037–1061.

19. Kuijer W, Dijkstra PU, Brouwer S, Reneman MF, Groothoff JW, Geertzen JHB. Safe lifting in patients with chronic low back pain: comparing FCE lifting task and NIOSH lifting guideline. *J Occup Rehabil.* 2006;16(4):579–589.

20. Innes E, Straker L. A clinician's guide to work-related assessments, 3: administration and interpretation problems. *Work.* 1998;11(2):207–219.

21. Isernhagen SJ. Functional capacity evaluation. In: Isernhagen SJ, ed. *Work Injury: Management and Prevention.* Gaithersburg, MD: Aspen Publishers; 1988:139–180.

22. Isernhagen SJ. Advancements in functional capacity evaluation. In: D'Orazio BP, ed. *Back Pain Rehabilitation.* Boston, MA: Andover Medical; 1993:180–204.

23. Reneman MF, Jaegers SMHJ, Westmaas M, Göeken LNH. The reliability of determining effort level of lifting and carrying in a functional capacity evaluation. *Work.* 2002;18(1):23–27.

24. Matheson LN. *EPIC Lift Capacity Examiner's Manual.* St Charles, MO: Employment Potential Improvement Corporation; 2003.

25. Innes E. Reliability and validity of functional capacity evaluations: an update. *Int J Disabil Manage Res.* 2006;1(1):135–148.

26. Ijmker S, Gerrits EHJ, Reneman MF. Upper lifting performance of healthy young adults in functional capacity evaluations: a comparison of two protocols. *J Occup Rehabil.* 2003;13(4):297–305.

27. Rustenburg G, Kuijer PPFM, Frings-Dresen MHW. The concurrent validity of the ERGOS Work Simulator and the Ergo-Kit with respect to maximum lifting capacity. *J Occup Rehabil.* 2004;14(2):107–118.

28. Schenk P, Klipstein A, Spillmann S, Strøyer J, Laubli T. The role of back muscle endurance, maximum force, balance and trunk rotation control regarding lifting capacity. *Eur J Appl Physiol.* 2006;96(2):146–156.

29. Alpert J, Matheson L, Beam W, Mooney V. The reliability and validity of two new tests of maximum lifting capacity. *J Occup Rehabil.* 1991;1(1):13–29.

30. Matheson LN. Relationships among age, body weight, resting heart rate, and performance in a new test of lift capacity. *J Occup Rehabil.* 1996;6(4):225–237.

31. Matheson LN, Mooney V, Grant JE, et al. A test to measure lift capacity of physically impaired adults, part 1: development and reliability testing. *Spine.* 1995;20(19):2119–2129.

32. Jay MA, Lamb JM, Watson RL, et al. Sensitivity and specificity of the indicators of sincere effort of the EPIC Lift Capacity test on a previously injured population. *Spine.* 2000;25(11):1405–1412.

33. Matheson LN, Mooney V, Holmes D, et al. A test to measure lift capacity of physically impaired adults, part 2: reactivity in a patient sample. *Spine.* 1995;20(19):2130–2134.

34. Reyna JR, Leggett SH, Kenney K, Holmes B, Mooney V. The effect of lumbar belts on isolated lumbar muscle: strength and dynamic capacity. *Spine.* 1995;20(1):68–73.

35. Matheson LN, Leggett S, Mooney V, Schneider K, Mayer J. The contribution of aerobic fitness and back strength to lift capacity. *Spine.* 2002;27(11):1208–1212.

36. Mayer J, Mooney V, Matheson LN, et al. Reliability and validity of a new computer-administered pictorial activity and task sort. *J Occup Rehabil.* 2005;15(2):203–213.

37. Bootes M. *Lifting Capacity: A Comparison of Self-report Measures and Functional Capacity Evaluation in Healthy Young Adult Males* [Honors thesis]. Sydney, Australia: School of Occupation & Leisure Sciences, Faculty of Health Sciences, University of Sydney; 2005.

38. Innes E, Hardwick M. Actual versus perceived physical capacity: implications for disability management and injury prevention. Paper presented at: 3rd International Forum on Disability Management; October 8–11, 2006; Brisbane, Queensland, Australia.

39. Horneij E, Holmström E, Hemborg B, Isberg P, Ekdahl C. Inter-rater reliability and between-days repeatability of eight physical performance tests. *Adv Physiother.* 2002;4(4):146–160.

40. Lygren H, Dragesund T, Joensen J, Ask T, Moe-Nilssen R. Test-retest reliability of the Progressive Isoinertial Lifting Evaluation (PILE). *Spine.* 2005;30(9):1070–1074.

41. Haig AJ, Geisser ME, Nicholson C, et al. The effect of order of testing in functional performance in persons with and without chronic back pain. *J Occup Rehabil.* 2003;13(2):115–123.

42. Soer R, Poels BJJ, Geertzen JHB, Reneman MF. A comparison of two lifting assessment approaches in patients with chronic low back pain. *J Occup Rehabil.* 2006;16(4):639–646.

43. Harbin G, Olson J. Post-offer, pre-placement testing in industry. *Am J Ind Med.* 2005;47:296–307.

44. Geisser ME, Haig AJ, Theisen ME. Activity avoidance and function in persons with chronic back pain. *J Occup Rehabil.* 2000;10(3):215–227.

45. Lemstra M, Olszynski WP, Enright W. The sensitivity and specificity of functional capacity evaluations in determining maximal effort: a randomized trial. *Spine.* 2004;29(9):953–959.

46. Ruan CM, Haig AJ, Geisser ME, Yamakawa K, Buchholz RL. Functional capacity evaluations in persons with spinal disorders: predicting poor outcomes on the Functional Assessment Screening Test (FAST). *J Occup Rehabil.* 2001;11(2):119–132.

47. Ljungquist T, Fransson B, Harms-Ringdahl K, Björnham Å, Nygren Å. A physiotherapy test package for assessing back and neck dysfunction: discriminative ability for patients versus healthy control subjects. *Physiother Res Int.* 1999;4(2):123–140.

48. Yílmaz F, Yílmaz A, Merdol F, Parlar D, Sahin F, Kuran B. Efficacy of dynamic lumbar stabilization exercise in lumbar microdiscectomy. *J Rehabil Med.* 2003;35(4):163–167.

49. Filiz M, Cakmak A, Ozcan E. The effectiveness of exercise programmes after lumbar disc surgery: a randomized controlled study. *Clin Rehabil.* 2005;19(1):4–11.

50. Jousset N, Fanello S, Bontoux L, et al. Effects of functional restoration versus 3 hours per week physical therapy: a randomized controlled study. *Spine.* 2004;29(5):487–494.

CHAPTER 6

51. Gouttebarge V, Wind H, Kuijer PP, Sluiter JK, Frings-Dresen MH. Intra- and interrater reliability of the Ergo-Kit Functional Capacity Evaluation method in adults without musculoskeletal complaints. *Arch Phys Med Rehabil.* 2005;86(12):2354–2360.

52. Gouttebarge V, Wind H, Kuijer PP, Sluiter JK, Frings-Dresen MH. Reliability and agreement of 5 Ergo-Kit Functional Capacity Evaluation lifting tests in subjects with low back pain. *Arch Phys Med Rehabil.* 2006;87(10):1365–1370.

53. Kuijer W, Gerrits EHJ, Reneman MF. Measuring physical performance via self-report in healthy young adults. *J Occup Rehabil.* 2004;14(1):77–87.

54. Tuckwell NL, Straker L, Barrett TE. Test-retest reliability on nine tasks of the Physical Work Performance Evaluation. *Work.* 2002;19(3):243–253.

55. Ratzon NZ, Jarus T, Catz A. The relationship between work function and low back pain history in occupationally active individuals. *Disabil Rehabil.* 2007;29(10): 791–796.

56. Brouwer S, Reneman MF, Dijkstra PU, Groothoff JW, Schellekens JMH, Göeken LNH. Test-retest reliability of the Isernhagen Work Systems Functional Capacity Evaluation in patients with chronic low back pain. *J Occup Rehabil.* 2003;13(4):207–218.

57. Reneman MF, Brouwer S, Meinema A, Dijkstra PU, Geertzen JHB, Groothoff JW. Test-retest reliability of the Isernhagen Work Systems Functional Capacity Evaluation in healthy adults. *J Occup Rehabil.* 2004;14(4):295–305.

58. Isernhagen SJ, Hart DL, Matheson LM. Reliability of independent observer judgements of level of lift effort in a kinesiophysical functional capacity evaluation. *Work.* 1999;12(2):145–150.

59. Reneman MF, Dijkstra PU, Westmaas M, Göeken LNH. Test-retest reliability of lifting and carrying in a 2-day functional capacity evaluation. *J Occup Rehabil.* 2002;12(4):269–275.

60. Gross DP, Battié MC. Reliability of safe maximum lifting determinations of a functional capacity evaluation. *Phys Ther.* 2002;82(4):364–371.

61. Reneman MF, Fokkens AS, Dijkstra PU, Geertzen JHB, Groothoff JW. Testing lifting capacity: validity of determining effort level by means of observation. *Spine.* 2005;30(2):E40-E46.

62. Gross DP, Battié MC. The prognostic value of functional capacity evaluation in patients with chronic low back pain, part 2: sustained recovery. *Spine.* 2004;29(8):920–924.

63. Gross DP, Battié MC. Predictive validity of functional capacity evaluation in workers' compensation claimants with upper extremity disorders [Abstract]. *J Pain.* 2005;6(3 suppl 1):S69.

64. Gross DP, Battié MC, Cassidy JD. The prognostic value of functional capacity evaluation in patients with chronic low back pain, part 1: timely return to work. *Spine.* 2004;29(8):914–919.

65. Matheson LN, Isernhagen SJ, Hart DL. Relationships among lifting ability, grip force, and return to work. *Phys Ther.* 2002;82(3):249–256.

66. Brouwer S, Dijkstra PU, Stewart RE, Göeken LNH, Groothoff JW, Geertzen JHB. Comparing self-report, clinical examination and functional testing in the assessment of work-related limitations in patients with chronic low back pain. *Disabil Rehabil.* 2005;27(17):999–1005.

67. Hart DL, Kirk M, Howar J, Mongeon S. Association between clinician-assessed lifting ability and workplace tolerance and patient self-reported pain and disability following work conditioning. *Work.* 2007;28(2):111–119.

68. Legge J, Burgess-Limerick R. Reliability of the JobFit System pre-employment functional assessment tool. *Work.* 2007;28(4):299–312.

69. Saunders RL, Beissner KL, McManis BG. Estimates of weight that subjects can lift frequently in functional capacity evaluations. *Phys Ther.* 1997;77(12):1717–1728.

70. Gatchel RJ. Psychosocial factors that can influence the self-assessment of function. *J Occup Rehabil.* 2004;14(3):197–206.

71. Abdel-Moty AR, Macguire GH, Kaplan SH, Johnson P. Stated versus observed performance levels in patients with chronic low back pain. *Occup Ther Health Care.* 1996;10(1):3–23.

CHAPTER 6

7

Use of Computerized Extremity and Trunk Tests in Functional Capacity Evaluation

Jill S. Galper, PT, MEd, Dale Reese, BSc, C Ped, Ryan Shea, MSc, and Tom Mayer, MD

Computerized assessment of isolated muscle strength has been used in rehabilitation since the early 1960s. It began with use of isokinetic testing and training of athletes following knee injuries, gaining widespread recognition for the concept of "sports medicine rehabilitation." Computerized assessment allows for the objective and quantitative measurement of strength and lifting parameters and can be used to demonstrate progression of muscle performance during treatment. It is particularly valuable when the clinician's subjective manual muscle testing measurement is not a reliable source of information.[1-5] There are a number of assessment units available. Depending on the specific unit, muscle function can be assessed *isokinetically* (constant joint angular or linear speed against accommodating resistance in a prescribed range of motion), *isometrically* (force generated without motion), and/or *isoinertially* (movement against a fixed resistance). Some units evaluate concentric muscle activity (muscle fiber shortening during motion), whereas other units allow concentric and eccentric (muscle fiber lengthening during motion) analysis. The application of isometric (static) testing in functional capacity evaluations (FCEs) is discussed in Chapter 8. This chapter focuses on the use of computerized isokinetic and isoinertial extremity and trunk assessment in FCEs. The application of these devices for trunk and extremity rehabilitation is beyond the scope of this chapter.

Use of Computerized Assessment in Injury Management

The entry of computerized assessment of muscle function into the occupational health world was somewhat indirect. The relevance of trunk strength testing in low back pain (LBP) and early efforts to measure it were studied in the late 1950s.[6] In the 1970s, industrial engineers performed isometric testing of lifting capacity and equated this to "trunk strength," ultimately attempting to use the information in pre-employment screening.[7] The availability of isokinetic dynamometers to evaluate the extremities was followed by the development of specific back testing devices or attachments from multiple manufacturers, such as Cybex (Cybex Inc, Medway, MA), Lido (Loerdan Biomedical, Inc, West Sacramento, CA), Biodex (Biodex Medical Systems, Inc, Shirley, NY), and KinCom (Chattex Corp, Chattanooga, TN), beginning around 1980.[8] The Cybex Back Testing System is composed of three units to assess trunk flexion-extension (TEF), torso rotation (TR), and lifting (LT for Liftask). Investigations of trunk strength using isoinertial and isometric methods led to development of a commercial three-plane isoinertial system, the Isostation B-200 (Isotechnologies, Inc, Hillsborough, NC) and an isometric device (Medex, Ocala, FL).[9-11]

The use of these computerized devices led to development of normative data by testing healthy subjects with adjustments for age, sex, and body weight and noting large differences in comparison with subjects with LBP.[12–14] Normative data are specific to the device and protocol used. Patient inhibition was noted to be a major factor in low torque output by patients with pain, a pattern that had been identified in sports medicine testing, but not to the degree noted in the population with chronic LBP. Subsequently, trunk strength deficits measured using isokinetic devices were found to be closely associated with muscle atrophy and fatty replacement (particularly in postoperative patients) by using imaging techniques that were new at the time (computed tomography and magnetic resonance imaging).[15,16] In addition, substantial improvement in function was identified through serial testing when patients completed a functional restoration rehabilitation program.[17–19] The development of the quantitative functional evaluation with measurement of mobility and strength of an injured joint or spinal region, accompanied by tests of lifting capacity, paralleled the development of the modern-day FCE.[20–23]

Isokinetic testing (fixed speed, measuring the force output) is commonly performed at two velocities, one slow and one fast. The slow speed is thought to reflect muscle strength, whereas the higher speed reflects endurance and muscle recruitment. Performance at different speeds correlates with the type of muscle fiber and demonstrates muscle recruitment.[24]

Studies have demonstrated a relationship between the performance of the type of muscle fiber within a muscular group and isokinetic testing.[25] Substantial differences have been noted between healthy subjects and patients with pain in the ratio of torque output at one speed compared with another and in the agonist-antagonist ratio at a single speed, which have been verified in multiple studies of the trunk and multiple extremity joints. Speeds commonly used for testing include the following:

- Shoulder: 60°/s and 180°/s
- Knee: 60°/s, 180°/s, and 300°/s
- Trunk: 60°/s and 120°/s

Analysis of muscle function in isokinetic tests generally includes computation of the peak force output, which is usually measured as peak torque, because the measurements are generally angular rather than linear. A ratio of torque and/or work to body weight is commonly used, although the correlation is imperfect, particularly in extremely thin or obese people. The *work* is a measure of force times distance, ie, work performed, which is calculated as the area under the torque curve measuring instantaneous torque outputs throughout the range of motion. Other related measures include power output, time to peak torque, angle of peak torque, and a variety of speed and agonist-antagonist ratios.

CHAPTER 7

Consistency of performance and the effort the evaluee puts forth are addressed as a component of the evaluation, and some practitioners have referred to these units as "lie-detectors." Caution must be used in making such inferences, however, because limitation caused by pain can dramatically affect performance. A number of innovative techniques to assess submaximal or inconsistent effort, including use of reactive eccentric capabilities, have been developed.[26-28]

Testing of the trunk is primarily done in the sagittal plane owing to its importance in work and daily activities. A comprehensive discussion of isokinetic and isoinertial testing is beyond the scope of this chapter. Although isokinetic and isoinertial units continue to be used in clinics and laboratories, the only current manufacturers of isokinetic equipment in the United States are Biodex Medical Systems Inc; Computer Sports Medicine Inc (CSMi), Stoughton, MA; and BTE Technologies, Baltimore, MD. The purported advantages of these computerized testing units are their ability to do the following:

1. Identify muscle function within a defined range of motion with graphs of force output plotted against time or joint angle for the purpose of multiple analyses
2. Assess an evaluee's effort through consistency of curve production and reliability of testing
3. Evaluate specific joint-related peri-articular muscle strength in order to:
   - Assess strength (and provide contralateral comparisons) for a putative "weak link," injured area, or compensable body part
   - Assess agonist-antagonist relationships and ratios; and
   - Assess different aspects of strength (and speed relationships to identify degree of dysfunction)
4. Quantify the change over time (progress) and performance of the isolated and functionally deficient link that is limiting global functional capacity
5. Provide measures of muscle endurance once strength levels have been rehabilitated to near-normal levels

These advantages, as applied to FCE, are discussed subsequently in more detail.

The Use of Computerized Testing to Identify Impairment in Functional Capacity Evaluations

Computerized isokinetic and isoinertial testing has been described as an objective, reliable, and valid method to determine isolated muscle strength. The application of these computerized units in FCEs will be discussed in terms of their safety, reliability, validity, and practicality.

Safety

There is agreement in published reports that dynamic testing on all trunk isokinetic and isoinertial units is safe.[1] One of the purported advantages of isokinetic evaluation and exercise is that the resistance is accommodating and dependent on the force applied by the evaluee or subject.

Reliability

A number of studies have investigated the reliability of isokinetic and isoinertial devices; a full review is beyond the scope of this chapter. Acceptable test-retest, interrater, and intrarater reliability have been demonstrated for computerized isokinetic and isoinertial extremity and trunk testing units, with the exception of range-of-motion assessment on the Isostation B-200.[1-7] The literature review by Newton and Waddell[29] of "iso-testing" followed experimental evaluation of trunk strength using the Cybex Back Testing System (TEF, TR, and Liftask) on subjects and patients with chronic LBP.[30-33] Their review included 108 published articles through March 1992 on isokinetic and isoinertial testing of dynamic trunk strength related to LBP. Their review and experimental results provided evidence of reliability for torque and force measurement for isokinetic and isoinertial TEF up to 120°/s, but not at higher speeds. There was limited and conflicting evidence of reliability of trunk or torso rotation (TR) or lateral flexion at any speed. More recently, Karatas et al[33] reported high intrarater and interrater reliability of reciprocal concentric TEF peak torque values for healthy subjects at 60°/s and 90°/s on the Cybex NORM isokinetic dynamometer. Hupli et al[34] investigated intradevice reliability on two models of isokinetic trunk strength test units (Ariel 5000, Ariel Dynamics, Inc, Trabuco Canyon, CA and Lido Multi-Joint II, Loredan Biomedical, Inc., West Sacramento, CA) and found significant differences for the average peak torques between the two devices and low correlations between the two measurements.[34] Others suggested that the results are device-specific and that results obtained from different devices cannot be compared.[35-37] Reliable measures of torque, position, and velocity were reported on the Biodex System 3 for isokinetic speeds up to 300°/s.[35-37] Reliability of isometric torque and position was demonstrated by Drouin et al.[37]

Validity

Because muscular strength is one of the underlying constructs of physical performance, some clinicians advocate the use of computerized strength testing in an FCE to identify the presence of a strength deficit, which is expected to correlate with decreased physical performance. Isokinetic evaluation has been used in sports medicine for many years to help determine an athlete's readiness to safely return to sports. Isokinetic performance indicators include comparison

CHAPTER 7

of the involved limb with the contralateral side, agonist-antagonist relationships, ability to maintain force at higher speeds, and the effect of performance deficits on neighboring joints and muscles.

There is less evidence to support isotesting on injured workers. As noted by Newton and Waddell[29(p807)]: "there is no direct evidence that any iso-measure provides a valid test of trunk muscle strength or objective physical impairment associated with low back pain. There is some evidence that iso-measures may be affected by psycho-physical and behavioral factors." Thus, one's physical performance on computerized machines is subject to the same psychophysical factors that affect performance of functional tasks during an FCE. Isokinetic evaluation has been used by some evaluators in postoffer evaluations. A job applicant, similar to an athlete seeking a position on a team, is usually motivated to perform well and may have a tendency to underreport symptoms. The application of FCE in prehire physical assessments is discussed in Chapter 13.

Another limitation of isokinetic (not isoinertial) testing is that many units record torque only if the subject is able to move at the preset test velocity.[29] More recent technological improvements have corrected this deficiency in the Biodex unit, which measures all force produced throughout the range of motion whether or not the patient or evaluee moves at the set isokinetic speed. Because a certain amount of muscle activity is required to move the trunk, a zero recording is not reflective of a true absence of muscle activity. When a patient develops no force at the slowest speed in the usual protocol, the examiner can substitute a test at an even slower speed (or perform an isometric test) to identify a threshold for muscle activity. Evaluees with limitations due to pain may require other adjustments of initial preset speeds and/or ranges of motion from customary test protocols for the evaluator to evaluate the degree of inhibition or fear-avoidance creating the pain-limited performance.

A challenge when performing trunk as opposed to extremity evaluation is the absence of a contralateral limb measurement within the same person to provide a "gold standard" for comparison. This absence leaves the somewhat less compelling comparison with a normative database as the standard for assessing strength, and the relationship of normative data to function has not been established. With computerized isokinetic devices that can measure concentric and eccentric forces and record forces even before the subject reaches the preset isokinetic speed, some of the trunk testing limitations imposed by first-generation devices have been removed.

Isokinetic evaluation has been criticized as not being "functional" because movements during work activities and activities of daily living are not isokinetic. In addition, testing isolated joint function fails to account for the relationship of multiple joints during a functional activity. Given these limitations, computerized "isotests" should not be performed in isolation when measuring an evaluee's functional abilities. However, these tests can provide valuable information regarding the weak link in the biomechanical chain. Evaluation of isolated joint function can identify strength and movement capability around individual joints or spinal regions that are relevant to force transmission and, therefore, to almost all activities of daily living that involve the involved body part. Computerized testing, therefore, provides an objective and quantifiable measure underlying joint performance that can aid the evaluator in understanding dynamic performance limitations. Rather than being used in isolation, computerized strength tests should be used only in conjunction with other FCE test components.

Dueker et al[38] investigated the usefulness of isokinetic trunk muscle strength to predict lifting ability. Their subject group included 230 consecutive applicants who had applied for a position involving heavy work (100-lb lifting). Isokinetic TEF were measured on a Lido unit (Loredan Biomedical) and results compared with the results of a repetitive isotonic floor to waist height lift (WEST II protocol). They found no relationship between isokinetic trunk muscle performance and isotonic lifting ability to the 100-lb level. Similarly, Curtis et al[39] investigated the physical performance of patients with LBP following participation in a functional restoration program. Testing included isokinetic lifting on the Cybex lifting device at three speeds and an isoinertial lifting examination (PILE protocol). Although the patients demonstrated improvement in both tests following functional restoration treatment, the PILE test demonstrated more significant gains than the isokinetic lift evaluation. The discrepancy between isokinetic performance and lifting ability is likely due to multiple joint contributions involved in lifting that allows a person to compensate for muscular weakness vs isolated muscle performance during computerized testing. The effect of various "links" on strength testing was recognized by ergonomic engineers more than three decades ago and incorporated in the National Institute for Occupational Safety and Health isometric lifting protocols that recognize test methods and normative data for an arm lift, torso lift (straight knee, flexed at waist), and leg lift (straight torso, flexed at hips and knees). Healthy subjects generally demonstrate near equivalence of the leg and torso lifts. However, injured people show amplified differences in one or the other of these tests depending on whether a lower extremity or trunk injury produces the weak link. This finding suggests that a weak link may exist in patients in whom symptoms develop with task repetition (due to decreased local muscle endurance) or in patients who have difficulty performing or are unable to safely perform a given task (owing to decreased strength or neuromuscular control). If a patient barely demonstrates the ability to perform the required manual handling tasks and the weak link remains unidentified, opportunities to prevent injury following new hire employment or postinjury reemployment may be lost. If the person fails to meet minimal job and task demands, computerized testing is an option to further investigate the cause of the performance deficit. In cases in which an evaluee demonstrates the ability to safely and effectively perform the required functional tasks and the musculoskeletal examination does not identify significant muscular weakness, computerized testing would not be necessary or appropriate.

Practicality

There is a learning effect in iso-testing that seems to be greater in patients compared with healthy subjects. Newton and Waddell[29] found that a single test session can significantly underestimate a patient's trunk strength, and they advocate giving the patient a practice session. Providing a practice session would present a logistical problem for evaluees referred for a 1-day FCE. Although this problem can be partly addressed by providing practice repetitions before testing, further research is required to determine if this practice session is sufficient to negate the learning curve.

The number of manufacturers of isomachines decreased with the decline in popularity of isokinetic testing and rehabilitation in the mid 1990s, with Biodex, CSMi, and BTE Technologies the only current manufacturers of isokinetic testing units in the United States. Owners of isounits from other manufacturers may face challenges obtaining necessary parts and repairs to keep their units functioning properly. The decline in manufacturing of computerized devices parallels the elimination of reimbursement for testing on the devices in the late 1980s. The current market is based much more on testing of high-performance athletes and military recruits, for which expense is not as much of a concern. Similar issues are under consideration in developed and emerging markets, and computerized testing devices are available and manufactured in various other parts of the world (eg, Europe, Israel, and China).

The cost of performing an FCE is a consideration for many users of the evaluation, and the addition of isotesting to an FCE process may result in increased cost. Given the validity concerns of isotesting as it relates to lifting performance, it is not clear to what extent the additional cost of these tests adds value. None of the commercial FCE models (listed in the Appendix) currently use computerized isokinetic or isoinertial extremity or trunk testing as part of the FCE process.

Computerized Testing and Evaluee Performance

Computerized evaluation of extremity and trunk muscle performance has been used to assist in the determination of evaluee effort. Consistency of torque production for several repetitions has been used to determine maximal vs submaximal effort. In their review, Newton and Waddell[29] wrote that there was no evidence that isomachines provided a reliable or valid method of effort assessment, citing studies that showed that subjects could consistently produce isokinetic force submaximally. Hazard et al[28] tested 30 healthy subjects instructed to perform with maximal (100%) effort and submaximal (50%) effort on a Cybex TEF unit and the Cybex Liftask (LT) unit. They found that although intercurve variability on the TEF and LT tests distinguished between maximal and submaximal effort, clinical observation by the evaluator was more accurate. In another study published in 1992, Hazard et al[40] noted that a trained observer was better able to distinguish maximal effort than the most accurate physiologic index assessed in their study (heart rate response, average of the maximum distance between curves, and torque–body weight ratios). In contrast, in their review of chronic pain malingering and disease simulation research, Fishbain et al[41] found that isokinetic evaluation techniques might be a viable method for identification of submaximal and malingered efforts.

Dvir,[42,43] Dvir and Keating,[44,45] Dvir et al,[46,47] and Chaler et al[48] have used isokinetic strength testing of the trunk extensors, shoulder flexors, and grip to differentiate between a person's maximal and submaximal efforts by comparing the ratio of eccentric and concentric forces at two velocities, one slow and one fast. The isokinetic testing was performed on a KinCom 125E+ isokinetic dynamometer (Chattanooga Instruments, Chattanooga, TN). This method of assessment is based on the change of concentric and eccentric force at higher velocities of movement. Concentric force decreases at higher velocities, whereas eccentric force increases or is unchanged with increased velocity. In healthy subjects, eccentric force is greater than concentric force at a given velocity, and the eccentric-concentric ratio will increase with increased test velocity. An index termed the DEC represents the difference between these eccentric-concentric ratios at two velocities and has been described as follows: $DEC = (Ecc/Con)_{high} - (Ecc/Con)_{low}$. The test velocities used for assessment are set at a gradient of 1:4, and one set of three repetitions is performed at each velocity. Subjects who were instructed to feign maximal effort were able to decrease concentric force but were less successful in manipulating eccentric force. Cutoff scores have been determined at the 95% and 99% levels of confidence based on the specific joint and plane of motion evaluated. The DEC correctly identified feigned efforts with shortened range of motion of trunk extension and shoulder flexion.[42,43] Dvir[42] cautions that DEC-based validation of weakness should be used with care. The evaluator should consider all factors that affect performance, such as apprehension, cognitive limitation, pain, and unfamiliarity with eccentric contractions. The use of this method and the 95% cutoff level are reserved for people who are in medically stable condition, are able to understand the test instructions, and do not have pain. Therefore, this technique may have limited application given the high number of people who have persistent pain symptoms. The use of this method requires the evaluator to have a Kin-Com unit, which is another barrier to using this method.

CHAPTER 7

One of the current manufacturers of isokinetic equipment, Biodex, has substantially modified its systems since the development of the testing devices used by Newton and Waddell. These current units include measurements of a coefficient of variation that measures performance variance between trials. Up to the present, however, the use of these devices in the athletic world of highly motivated competitors has not provided an impetus for testing consistency of effort. Further research with injured workers and a disabled population is needed to determine if this method is reliable and valid.

Summary

Computerized trunk and extremity testing can provide detailed information about isolated muscle function, but this type of testing should not be used in isolation when determining an evaluee's functional abilities. Although isomeasurements seem to be reliable, research to date has not demonstrated acceptable correlation of isoperformance with dynamic lifting ability. These tests may be a helpful adjunct in some circumstances, particularly to identify whether there is a weak link that underlies an evaluee's functional difficulties or limitations. Although the information from isotesting can be helpful in identifying areas to target in rehabilitation, application in FCE seems somewhat limited based on current research.

References

1. Wadsworth C, Krishnan R, Sear M, Harrold J, Nielsen D. Intrarater reliability of manual muscle testing and hand-held dynametric muscle testing. *Phys Ther.* 1987;67:1342–1347.
2. Hayes K. Reliability of 3 methods for assessing shoulder strength. *J Shoulder Elbow Surg.* 2002;11:33–39.
3. Cuthbert S, Goodheart G. On the reliability and validity of manual muscle testing: a literature review. *Chiropractic Osteopathy.* 2007;15:4–26.
4. Aagaard P, Simonsen E, Magnusson S, Larsson B. A new concept for isokinetic hamstring: quadriceps muscle strength ratio. *Am J Sports Med.* 1998;26:231–237.
5. Kawashima, T, et al. Optimum velocity in isokinetic muscle strength test in relation to closed chain. *Phys Ther.* 1994;74 (2).
6. Flint M. Effective increasing back and abdominal strength in low back pain. *Res Quart.* 1958;29:160–171.
7. Chaffin D, Herrin G, Keyserling W. Preemployment strength testing. *J Occ Med.* 1978;20:403–408.

8. Davies G, Gould J. Trunk testing using a prototype Cybex II dynamometer stabilization system. *J Orthop Sports Phys Ther.* 1982;3:164–170.

9. Hasue M, Masatoshi F, Kikuchi S. A new method of quantitative measurement of abdominal and back muscle strength. *Spine.* 1980;5:143–148.

10. Langrana N, Lee C, Alexander H, et al. Quantitative assessment of back strength using isokinetic testing. *Spine.* 1984;9:287–290.

11. Marras WS, King AL, Joynt RL. Measurements of loads on the lumbar spine under isometric and isokinetic conditions. *Spine.* 1984;9(2):176–187.

12. Smith S, Mayer T, Gatchel R, Becker T. Quantification of lumbar function, part 1: isometric and multispeed isokinetic trunk strength measures in sagittal and axial planes in normal subjects. *Spine.* 1985;10:757–764.

13. Mayer T, Smith SS, Keeley J, et al. Quantification of lumbar function part 2: sagittal plane strength in low back pain patients. *Spine.* 1985;10:765–772.

14. Mayer T, Smith S, Kondraske G, Gatchel R, Carmichael T, Mooney V. Quantification of lumbar function, part 3: preliminary data on isokinetic torso rotation testing with myoelectric spectral analysis in normal and low back pain subjects. *Spine.* 1985;10:912–920.

15. Mayer T, Vanharanta H, Gatchel R, et al. Comparison of CT scan muscle measurements and isokinetic trunk strength in postoperative patients. *Spine.* 1989;14:427–430.

16. Flicker P, Fleckenstein J, Ferry K, et al. Lumbar muscle usage in chronic low back pain: MRI evaluation. *Spine.* 1993;8:582–586.

17. Kohles S, Barnes D, Gatchel R, Mayer T. Improved physical performance outcomes following functional restoration treatment in patients with chronic low back pain: early versus recent training results. *Spine.* 1990;15:1321–1324.

18. Mayer T, Pope P, Tabor J, et al. Physical progress and residual impairment quantification after functional restoration, part I: lumbar mobility. *Spine.* 1994;18:389–394.

19. Brady S, Mayer T, Gatchel R. Physical progress and residual impairment quantification after functional restoration, part II: isokinetic trunk strength. *Spine.* 1994;18:395–400.

20. Kishino N, Mayer T, Gatchel R, et al. Quantification of lumbar function, part 4: isometric and isokinetic lifting simulation in normal subjects and low back dysfunction patients. *Spine.* 1985;10:921–927.

21. Keeley J, Mayer T, Cox R, et al. Quantification of lumbar function, part 5: reliability of range of motion measures in the sagittal plane and an in vivo torso rotation measurement technique. *Spine.* 1986;11:31–35.

22. Curtis L, Mayer T, Gatchel R. Physical progress and residual impairment after functional restoration, part III: isokinetic and isoinertial lifting capacity. *Spine.* 1994;18:401–405.

23. Sawchuk T, Mayer E. Deconditioning. In: Slipman C, Derby R, Simeone F, Mayer T, eds. *Interventional Spine.* London, England: Elsevier Global Publications; 2007:1213–1221.

24. McArdle W, Katch F, Katch L. Exercise training and adaptation. In: *Essentials of Exercise Physiology,* 3rd ed. Philadelphia, PA: Lippincott Williams & Wilkins; 2005: 500.

25. Suter E, Hezog W, Sokolsky J, Wiley J, Macintosh B. Muscle fiber type distribution as estimated by Cybex testing and by muscle biopsy. *Med Sci Sports Exerc.* 1993;25:363–370.

CHAPTER 7

26. Dvir Z. Clinical application of the DEC variables in assessing maximality of muscular effort: report of 34 patients. *Am J Phys Med Rehabil.* 2002;81:921–928.

27. Kaivanto K, Estlander A, Moneta G, Vanharanta H. Isokinetic performance in low back pain patients: the predictive power of the self-efficacy scale. *J Occup Rehab.* 1995;5.

28. Hazard RG, Reid S, Fenwick J, Reeves V. Isokinetic trunk and lifting strength measurements: variability as an indicator of effort. *Spine.* 1988;13:54–57.

29. Newton M, Waddell G. Trunk strength testing with iso-machines. part 1: review of a decade of scientific evidence. *Spine.* 1993;18:801–811.

30. Gaines JM, Talbot LA. Isokinetic strength testing in research and practice. *Biol Res Nurs.* 1999;1:57–64.

31. Delitto A, Rose SJ, Crandell CE, Strube MJ. Reliability of isokinetic measurements of trunk muscle performance. *Spine.* 1991;16:800–803.

32. Newton M, Thow M, Somerville D, Henderson I, Waddell G. Trunk strength testing with iso-machines, part 2: experimental evaluation of the Cybex II Back Testing System in normal subjects and patients with chronic low back pain. *Spine.*1993;18:812–824.

33. Karatas GK, Gogus F, Meray J. Reliability of isokinetic trunk muscle strength measurement. *Am J Phys Med Rehabil.* 2002;81:79–85.

34. Hupli M, Sainio P, Hurri H, Alaranta H. Comparison of trunk strength measurements between two different isokinetic devices used at clinical settings. *J Spinal Disord.* 1997;10:391–397.

35. Montgomery L, et al. Reliability of an isokinetic test of muscle strength and endurance. *J Orthop Sports PT.* 1989;11:315–322.

36. Walmsley RP, Dias JM. Cybex: intermachine reliability of isokinetic concentric measurements of shoulder internal and external peak torque. *Isokinetics Ex Sci.* 1995(5):75–80.

37. Drouin JM, Valovich-McLeod T, Shultz SJ, Gansneder BM, Perrin DH. Reliability and validity of the Biodex System 3 Pro Isokinetic Dynamometer velocity, torque and position measurements. *Eur J Appl Physiol.* 2004;91:22–29.

38. Dueker JA, Ritchie SM, Knox TJ, Rose SJ. Isokinetic trunk testing and employment. *J Occup Med.* 1994;36:42–48.

39. Curtis L, Mayer TG, Gatchel RJ. Physical progress and residual impairment quantification after functional restoration, part III: isokinetic and isoinertial lifting capacity. *Spine.* 1994;19:401–405.

40. Hazard RG, Reeves V, Fenwick JW. Lifting capacity: indices of subject effort. *Spine.* 1992;17:1065–1070.

41. Fishbain DA, Cutler R, Rosomoff HL, Rosomoff RS. Chronic pain disability exaggeration/malingering and submaximal effort research. *Clin J Pain.* 1999;15:244–274.

42. Dvir Z. Reproducibility of performance and certainty of judgment in maximal vs feigned muscular effort. *Percept Mot Skills.* 1999;88(3 pt 2):1078–1080.

43. Dvir Z. Identification of feigned grip effort using isokinetic dynamometry. *Clin Biomech (Bristol, Avon).* 1999;14:522–527.

44. Dvir Z, Keating J. Identifying feigned isokinetic trunk extension effort in normal subjects: an efficiency study of the DEC. *Spine.* 2001;26:1046–1051.

45. Dvir Z, Keating JL. Trunk extension effort in patients with chronic low back dysfunction. *Spine.* 2003;28:685–692.

46. Dvir Z, Prushansky T, Peretz C. Maximal versus feigned active cervical motion in healthy patients: the coefficient of variation as an indicator for sincerity of effort. *Spine.* 2001;26:1680–1688.
47. Dvir Z, Steinfeld-Cohen Y, Peretz C. Identification of feigned shoulder flexion weakness in normal subjects. *Am J Phys Med Rehabil.* 2002;81:187–193.
48. Chaler J, Dvir Z, Diaz U, et al. Identification of feigned maximal shoulder external rotation effort. *Clin Rehabil.* 2007;21:241–247.

8

Static Testing in Functional Capacity Evaluations

Jill S. Galper, PT, MEd, and James Lamprakos, DO

Static strength has been defined as "the capacity to produce torque or force by a maximal voluntary isometric muscular exertion."[1] During an isometric contraction, the muscle maintains a constant length. Measurement of isometric or static force is done by using a force gauge that measures the force in pounds or kilograms. Static testing has been used in functional capacity evaluations (FCEs) to assess an evaluee's risk for future injury, determine material handling capacity, determine strength deficits between extremities, and assess an evaluee's performance consistency and effort level during testing. These applications of static testing are discussed in this chapter.

As noted in the National Institute for Occupational Safety and Health (NIOSH) *Work Practices Guide for Manual Lifting,*[2] the advantages of static testing include simple technique, minimal risk, and reliable measurement. These advantages make static testing attractive to clinicians. These advantages are discussed in more detail in the following list:

1. Simple technique: Body position is controlled, and force, or the magnitude of exertion, is the only measured parameter. In contrast, in dynamic lifting, acceleration and velocity of various body parts must be monitored through the range of motion.

2. Minimal risk: Evaluees develop force slowly, and the amount of force generated is voluntary. Evaluees are instructed to stop the exertion if any abnormal discomfort is felt. Because evaluees are instructed to perform to their maximum tolerable level, the test should be safe. However, there has been some debate as to the safety of static testing. Hansson et al[3] analyzed the loads on the lumbar spine in four healthy volunteers and calculated high compressive loads on L3 during the squat and torso lifts. These elevated compressive loads caused structural failure of the vertebral endplates, but whether this failure would result in damage to the spine in vivo was not demonstrated. Therefore, FCE evaluators should use caution when performing leg lift and torso lift tests on people with documented disc injuries.

3. Reliable measurement: Chaffin[4] reported test-retest coefficients of variance (CVs) of approximately 14%, and other investigators have also documented acceptable inter- and intratester reliability of static testing.[5]

Static Tests Commonly Used in Functional Capacity Evaluations

When static testing is a component of an FCE, one or more of the following tests are typically included based on the static tests listed in the NIOSH Work Practices Guideline.[2] Static testing is performed by using a static testing platform and force gauge that is part of a commercially available FCE system (eg, ERGOs Work Recovery Europa BV; BTE Technologies, Baltimore, MD; JTech Medical, Salt Lake City, UT) or by using a mobile force gauge that can be attached to a platform or used against a wall or other surface. See Figure 8–1. Table 8–1 lists the static tests as listed in the NIOSH manual and the body areas most stressed by a particular test.

FIGURE 8–1	Force Gauge

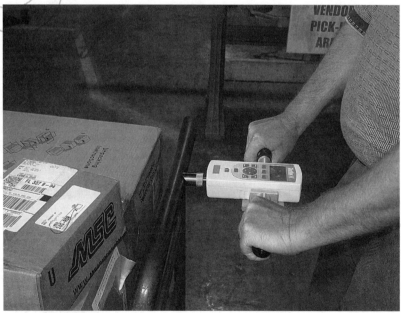

Courtesy of AMTEK

TABLE 8–1 Static Tests for Functional Capacity Evaluation and Their Positions[2]

Lift	Vertical Height, cm	Horizontal Distance, cm	Body Part Most Stressed	Photo
Leg	38	0	Knees, hip, and low back	
Floor	15	25	Knees, hip, and low back	
Torso	38	38	Low back and hips	

TABLE 8–1 Static Tests for Functional Capacity Evaluation and Their
Positions[2] (continued)

Lift	Vertical Height, cm	Horizontal Distance, cm	Body Part Most Stressed	Photo
Arm	90° elbow flexion	Not speci-fied, but photo shows shoulders in neutral	Elbow, wrist, and cervical spine	
High near	152	25	Shoulder girdle, chest wall, and neck	
High far	152	51	Shoulders, elbows, wrist, and neck	

Static testing is frequently used to identify the ability of an evaluee to push and pull. In addition, job-specific tests, in which the position and direction of force are used to simulate a specific job function, can also be performed. The data from these tests are used to assess an evaluee's ability to perform specific job functions or to calculate an evaluee's injury risk (discussed in more detail later in this chapter). Based on the recommendations of Chaffin,[4] the following procedure should be used when performing static testing:

1. The evaluator should review the purpose of the test with the evaluee and provide specific instructions. Chaffin[5] recommends using informed consent, but because static tests are being used as a component of an FCE, the consent should have been obtained before the FCE was initiated (see Chapter 4).

2. Verbal instructions should be objective, meaning that there should not be emotional appeals or encouragement (eg, "Push, push, you can do it") during evaluee performance.

3. Force should be steadily increased to a maximum tolerable level during 1 or 2 seconds (no jerking movements) and held for 3 seconds. The evaluee should understand that there should be no new or increased symptoms during testing but that he or she should work to his or her maximum tolerable level. (Khalil et al[6] coined the term *acceptable maximal effort* to refer to the highest level of force exertion an evaluee can tolerably produce.) Force should be released slowly. The measuring device should be able to record the 3-second average mean, ie, mean force produced over 3 seconds.

4. Each test position should be repeated two to five times, in addition to a practice trial. There should be adequate rest between trials. The rest period between trials varies among protocols but is usually between 30 and 60 seconds.

5. The evaluee's body position should be carefully controlled and monitored throughout the test.

6. Factors that can adversely affect an evaluee's concentration should be minimized (eg, noise and spectators).

Some force gauges can record the peak and average force generated by an evaluee, and this type of gauge is useful when performing FCEs. The *peak force,* which is usually achieved in the first 2 to 3 seconds of a trial, is the maximum force generated. Peak force represents the force required to overcome inertia. For example, when pushing a cart, the peak force represents the force required to put a stationary cart in motion. The average force in a static test trial represents the force the evaluee can sustain and is the measurement usually reported in an FCE. The results of the static tests can be compared with job-specific requirements and with normative data based on sex.[2] Although it had initially been hoped that normative data from static testing could be used to predict evaluee performance, normative data have not predicted or correlated with an evaluee's dynamic lifting ability. For example, if an evaluee's static leg length strength is within the 35th percentile based on sex, the evaluee's ability to lift from floor to waist height is still not known. There are no scientific data that have correlated percentile rankings with an evaluee's ability or disability. The results of static tests still can provide valuable information. The limitations of static testing and the way it can be appropriately used in the FCE setting are discussed in more detail subsequently.

Some commercially available FCE static strength testing systems measure the force generation of each arm when bilateral tests are performed, which permits side-to-side comparison. This comparison identifies whether there is decreased force production on one side during the activity. Comparison can also be made between sides when tests are performed unilaterally. The FCE evaluator should correlate these findings with the results of the previously performed musculoskeletal evaluation to determine if there is consistency in these findings. This consistency is part of the overall assessment of evaluee performance. Chapter 16 provides more information about FCE data analysis.

Static Strength Testing and Postoffer Screening

Historically, static testing was promoted and used by ergonomists as part of a postoffer or preplacement screening evaluation. Chaffin wrote, "From the biomechanical viewpoint, the assessment of static muscular strength of a worker can provide a method of predicting whether the person is capable of performing a physical act in a job without incurring injurious strain."[4(p505)] Chaffin et al[7] found that workers who were not appropriately matched to their job by strength had a higher likelihood and severity of injury. Employee strength rating formulas were developed to quantify a person's risk for back injury (back injury index) or other musculoskeletal injury (musculoskeletal injury index). An evaluee's job-specific static strength was compared with the job strength requirement to determine whether the evaluee was at risk for injury. As discussed by Gallagher et al, the ability of static strength testing to accurately predict risk of future injury or illness for people with physically stressful jobs "depends on the quality of the job evaluation on which the strength tests are based and the care with which the tests are administered."[8(p19)] However, as noted by Dempsey et al,[9] isometric and isokinetic methods should be replaced by isoinertial-based tests that are more representative of the kinematic and kinetic nature of manual material handling tasks. Chapter 13 provides further discussion of FCE application in postoffer evaluations.

Static Strength Testing and Dynamic Lifting Ability

Static strength testing results have not accurately predicted dynamic lifting capability. Garg et al[10] investigated whether static strength tests could be used to predict dynamic lifting capability using a psychophysical method. The static force generated by healthy male subjects was dependent on the horizontal distance and the direction of the generated force, and, depending on the static test position, dynamic ability was overestimated or underestimated (overestimated when hands were close to the body and underestimated in the other two positions studied).[10] In addition, Garg et al[10] noted that the relationship between static and dynamic strength was not well understood. For example, if a movement was highly dynamic with jerking motions, the static predictions might overestimate ability and underestimate lumbar stress. Garg et al[10] consequently stated that a comprehensive biomechanical analysis of a lift is required to develop appropriate static tests that simulate the dynamic lift. In addition, they recommended validation of the static test procedure on incumbent workers to ensure absence of test bias.

Dempsey et al[9] studied the role of muscular power as it relates to the maximal acceptable weight of a lift. Their conclusion was that lifting requires exertion of forces at varying velocities and that, "while isometric strength is appropriate for the pre-liftoff phase of a lift, it becomes a less appropriate measure of capacity as the velocity of the load begins to increase."[9(p1224)] The results of their study suggested that, "dynamic strength is superior to isometric strength for predicting lifting capacity."[9(p1238)]

Static testing is used by a number of FCE evaluators to assess a person's ability to generate push-pull force. An evaluee's ability to initiate force to overcome inertia (peak force) and to sustain push-pull force (average force) is usually measured. The position of the force gauge and the direction of applied force can simulate specific job demands, and the push-pull force generated during the FCE can be matched to the evaluee's work requirements. Evaluating push-pull force through static rather than dynamic testing is considered reasonable because it can be difficult to accurately simulate a dynamic push-pull activity with a weighted cart. The amount of dynamic force expended depends not only on the weight of the object pushed or pulled, but also on the coefficient of friction of the floor surface, the required force to overcome inertia, and the condition and size of the wheels.[11] Use of a force gauge to measure the force required to move a cart or sled, rather than reporting the actual weight on the sled or cart, is recommended for circumstances when pushing and pulling ability are determined dynamically. An exception to this practice is when a job-specific test is performed in which all relevant factors, including wheel size and floor surface, are replicated. The issue in this job-specific test is whether the evaluee can or cannot perform job tasks. Chapter 14 provides further discussion of job-specific FCEs.

Although static testing can be used to assess the initial force needed to push or pull various objects, a static test does not involve walking, which may prevent the impact of an evaluee's lower extremity impairment from becoming apparent. The evaluee is usually positioned with one leg forward and the other back (staggered stance) during the evaluation of static pushing and pulling. The back leg generates most of the force when pushing, and the forward leg generates more force during pulling. Therefore, depending on the position of the lower extremities during static pushing and pulling, dynamic push-pull force might be overestimated. Another disadvantage of static vs dynamic push-pull testing is the inability to assess the evaluee's aerobic response.

Static Strength Testing and Assessment of Performance Consistency and Effort

Some FCE evaluators use the results of static strength testing as indicators of an evaluee's level of effort and/or consistency of performance. A number of methodologies have been used, including calculating the CV of repetitive trials, measuring changes in heart rate during static effort, comparing static force and dynamic performance of related tasks, and determining changes in horizontal strength with static tests. These uses of static tests are discussed subsequently, although there is debate in the literature as to the validity of these methods. This debate is discussed in more detail in Chapter 11.

Use of the Coefficient of Variation

To assess an evaluee's effort and consistency, some FCE evaluators calculate the CV of three to five repetitive trials of static tests. As noted earlier, the commonly performed static tests include the arm lift, push, pull, leg lift, and high near and high far lifts (as described by NIOSH in the *Work Practices Guide for Manual Lifting*[2]). It is expected that the CV should not exceed a cutoff score, usually between 15% and 18%, although identification of a specific cutoff score has not been definitely determined and remains debated. The basis for use of the CV is that evaluees should be able to consistently produce a tolerable level of force (also termed acceptable maximal effort or force until discomfort) as long as the test does not directly involve the impaired component of the biomechanical system, is controlled by the evaluee, has a low error variance, allows short-term replication, and gives the evaluee minimal visual or proprioceptive feedback about the results of his or her effort.[12] Chapter 11 provides further discussion of the use of CVs in determining evaluee effort.

Heart Rate Response During Static Testing

As an evaluee performs a static test, an increase in heart rate is expected (in the absence of illness or medication that would limit the response in the heart rate). Lack of a response in the heart rate is considered an indicator of submaximal effort. Klimek and Strait[13] suggest that an evaluee's heart rate should increase 20 beats per minute from rest or reach 65% of the age-adjusted target maximum during isometric lifting. Although an increased heart rate in response to physical effort during static testing is logical from a physiologic standpoint, there are no studies that have determined the magnitude of response in the heart rate that constitutes maximal vs submaximal effort. Therefore, applying the response in heart rate to effort analysis during static testing is difficult.

Force Curve Analysis

Analysis of force output curves during static tests has been proposed as a method of identifying submaximal effort, but reports are conflicting as to the effectiveness of this method. Most of the available literature about force output curves relates to grip strength, not static strength tests. In regard to force output curves for grip strength, visual inspection of the force curves has not allowed discrimination between maximal and submaximal efforts. It is not known whether visual inspection of force curve output would allow discrimination between maximal and submaximal effort during static strength testing. Shectman et al[14] examined the validity of the slopes of the force-time curve (during force-generation and force-decay phases) as indicative of sincerity of effort in a group of healthy adults, and their findings suggested that this method might be useful, but further study on subjects with hand injury is needed.

Horizontal Strength Change Testing

Horizontal strength change testing has been proposed as a method of assessing evaluee effort. This test refers to repeating a static test in which the vertical distance remains the same but the horizontal distance changes, usually by 10 in. This method is based on biomechanical principles. As the horizontal distance increases, the evaluee's static strength is expected to decrease, and vice versa. Harber and SooHoo[15] briefly discussed horizontal strength change testing as a potentially useful method, and this method was further investigated by Berryhill et al.[16] They studied horizontal strength changes in injured and uninjured groups by using three vertical heights—6, 15, and 60 in. Horizontal distance was changed 10 in at each vertical height. A cutoff score of 33% increase or decrease in isometric force with a respective 10-in decrease or increase was derived from the noninjured group because this score minimized false-positives. A score of 2 or more (out of 3) inappropriate horizontal changes were thought to indicate submaximal effort on the part of the subject. This approach and the appropriateness of the 33% cutoff score have not been tested in randomized controlled trials of injured subjects.

Extrapolating Static to Dynamic Performance as an Indicator of Evaluee Effort

Muscular strength underlies an evaluee's ability to generate static force and perform dynamic material handling activities. Based on this construct, Blankenship,[17] developer of the Blankenship System FCE model, believed there is a relationship between static force production and dynamic material handling performance. Based on his patient population, Blankenship[17] developed formulas to extrapolate static force production to dynamic lifting performance in order to identify expected and minimal levels of performance. The minimal performance result was termed a "validity" measure. For example, the static arm lift was used to project expected and validity dynamic lifting levels for the bilateral carry (80% and 60% of the average force produced, respectively). If an evaluee's dynamic carry performance failed to meet the validity level based on the static arm test, the validity criterion was not met and was part of the overall calculation of the "validity profile" developed by Blankenship. Brubaker et al[18] performed a single-blind randomized trial investigating the sensitivity and specificity of four of the Blankenship System FCE indicators of submaximal effort. They found 100% specificity of the participant's scores using the extrapolations for shoulder and overhead lifting and 78.6% sensitivity using the extrapolation of static to dynamic leg lift. The study subjects were not injured workers, although some subjects had musculoskeletal diseases and complaints. Further investigation using a population of subjects receiving worker's compensation is needed for further validation of this method.

Summary

Static testing provides a quick, relatively safe, and inexpensive method of strength assessment, but it should not be used in isolation to determine an evaluee's dynamic lifting ability because of its poor ability to predict dynamic performance. Horizontal strength change testing, heart rate response during static testing, the slope of the force curve, and extrapolation of static to dynamic performance seem to be potentially useful methods of determining an evaluee's effort level during FCE, but more research is required for these methods to be scientifically supported.

References

1. Caldwell LS, Chaffin DB, Dukes-Dobos FN, et al. A proposed standard procedure for static muscle strength testing. *Am Ind Hyg Assoc J.* 1974;35:201–206.
2. National Institute for Occupational Safety and Health. *Work Practices Guide for Manual Lifting.* Cincinnati, OH: National Institute for Occupational Safety and Health; 1981.
3. Hansson TH, Bigos SJ, Wortley MK, Spengler DM. The load on the lumbar spine during isometric strength testing. *Spine.* 1984;9:720–724.
4. Chaffin DB. Ergonomic guide for the assessment of human static strength. *Am Ind Hyg Assoc J.* 1975;30:505–510.
5. Lee GK, Chan CC, Hui-Chan CW. Consistency of performance on the functional capacity assessment: static strength and dynamic endurance. *Am J Phys Med Rehabil.* 2001;80:189–195.
6. Khalil TM, et al. Acceptable maximum effort (AME): a psychophysical measure of strength in back pain patients. *Spine.* 1987;12:372–376.
7. Chaffin DB, Herrin GD, Keyserling WM. Preemployment strength testing: an updated position. *J Occup Med.* 1978;20:403–408.
8. Gallagher S, Moore JS, Stobbe TJ. *Physical Strength Assessment in Ergonomics.* Fairfax, VA: American Industrial Hygiene Association; 1998.
9. Dempsey PG, Ayoub MM, Westfall PH. Evaluation of the ability of power to predict low frequency lifting capacity. *Ergonomics.* 1998;41:1222–1241.

10. Garg A, Mital A, Asfour SS. A comparison of isometric strength and dynamic lifting capability. *Ergonomics*. 1980;23:13–27.

11. Dakos M. The application of functional capacity evaluations in the provision of vocational expert services. *J Forensic Vocational Analysis*. 2004;7:105–117.

12. Matheson LN, Dakos M. Re-Visiting "How do you know he tried his best?"... The Coefficient of Variation As a Determinant of Consistent Effort. 2000. Available at: www.epicrehab.com/FreeResources/CV-and-Effort.pdf Accessed April 20, 2008.

13. Klimek E, Strait J. Volition in impairment rating: the validity of effort assessment. *Disability*. 1997;6:9–18.

14. Shechtman O, Sindhu BS, Davenport PW. Using the force-time curve to detect maximal grip strength effort. *J Hand Ther*. 2007;20:37–48.

15. Harber P, SooHoo K. Static ergonomic strength testing in evaluating occupational back pain. *J Occup Med*. 1984;26:877–884.

16. Berryhill BH, Osborne P, Staats TE, Brooks FW, Skarina JM. Horizontal strength changes: an ergonomic measure for determining validity of effort in impairment evaluations: a preliminary report. *J Disability*. 1993;3:143–148.

17. Blankenship K. *The Blankenship System Functional Capacity Evaluation: The Procedural Manual*. Macon, GA: American Therapeutics; 1994.

18. Brubaker PN, Fearon FJ, Smith SM, et al. Sensitivity and specificity of the Blankenship FCE system's indicators of submaximal effort. *J Orthop Sports Phys Ther*. 2007;37:161–168.

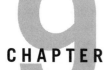

CHAPTER

Evaluating Movement and Positional Tolerance

Michael Coupland, CPsych, CRC, Margot Miller, PT, and Jill S. Galper, PT, M Ed

The ability of a person to perform repetitive movements and sustain positions is an important consideration when determining functional and work abilities. The evaluation of these abilities is included in functional capacity evaluations (FCEs). Workplace physical demands involve a complex interaction of physical motions (single and simultaneous), frequencies, strength demands, and positional tolerances, all within the context of a variety of environmental conditions. These motions were codified in the *Dictionary of Occupational Titles* (DOT) as physical demand conditions of jobs,[1] and the Canadian Classification and Dictionary of Occupations (CCDO)[2] adapted and revised them for Canadian use. The DOT and CCDO have been discontinued in favor of job cluster systems, the Occupational Information Network (O*NET) in the United States[3] and the National Occupational Classification[4] in Canada, but neither of these job cluster systems has developed physical demand conditions definitions of jobs. Therefore a "crosswalk" to the DOT and CCDO is necessary for analysis of the physical demands of each job.

In a general FCE, an evaluee's ability to repetitively perform or sustain a variety of activities is assessed by using standardized protocols that vary depending on the particular FCE model used. In a job-specific FCE, the test activities should simulate the specific job requirements. Job-specific testing is discussed in Chapter 14. In general and job-specific FCEs, the evaluee's abilities are assessed in the context of his or her injury or illness. The following activities, listed in the DOT,[1] are the activities most commonly evaluated during a general FCE (activities related to lifting and carrying are not listed; Chapter 6 discusses evaluation of dynamic lifting ability):

- Sitting: Remaining in the normal seated position
- Standing: Remaining on one's feet in an upright position at a work station without moving about
- Walking: Moving about on foot
- Climbing: Ascending or descending ladders, stairs, scaffolding, ramps, poles, and the like, using feet and legs and/or hands and arms. Body agility is emphasized. The DOT considers this factor important if the amount and kind of climbing required exceeds that required for ordinary locomotion.
- Balancing: Maintaining body equilibrium to prevent falling when walking, standing, crouching, or running on narrow, slippery, or erratically moving surfaces or maintaining body equilibrium when performing gymnastic feats. The DOT considers this factor important if the amount and kind of balancing exceeds that needed for ordinary locomotion and maintenance of body equilibrium.
- Stooping: Bending the body downward and forward by bending the spine at the waist. The DOT considers this factor important if it occurs to a considerable degree and requires full use of the lower extremities and back muscles.

- Kneeling: Bending legs at knees to come to rest on knee or knees
- Crouching: Bending the body downward and forward by bending legs and spine
- Reaching: Extending hand(s) in any direction
- Handling: Seizing, holding, grasping, turning, or otherwise working with hand or hands. Fingers are involved only to the extent that they are an extension of the hand.
- Fingering: Picking, pinching, or otherwise working primarily with fingers rather than with the whole hand or arm as in handling
- Feeling: Perceiving the attributes of objects, such as size, shape, temperature, and texture, by touching with skin, particularly that of fingertips
- Pushing: Exerting force on an object so that the object moves away from the force (includes slapping, striking, kicking, and treadle actions)
- Pulling: Exerting force on an object so that the object moves toward the force (includes jerking)

Based on an evaluee's performance during an FCE, each activity is assigned a frequency classification based on the definitions in the DOT. The frequency classifications are given in Table 9–1.[5]

TABLE 9–1	Definitions of Frequency Classifications of Job-Related Activities
Activity Frequency Title	**Activity Frequency**
Never	Not required
Occasional	Required 1%–33% of the workday
Frequent	Required 34%–66% of the workday
Constant	Required 67%–100% of the workday

In some FCE protocols, a range of repetitions is correlated with these frequency categories. For example, Blankenship,[6] originator of the Blankenship System FCE protocol, suggested the following:

- Occasional: up to 1 repetition every 15 minutes or up 32 repetitions per day
- Frequent: 1 repetition every 3 minutes or from 33 to 200 repetitions per day
- Constant: 1 repetition every 30 seconds or more than 200 repetitions per day

The material handling table in the WorkSTEPS (Austin, TX) FCE report lists a different range of repetitions for each frequency category described. These ranges are as follows: occasional, approximately 1 to 100 repetitions; frequent, approximately 100 to 500; and constant, 500 or more. Although these and similar classifications provide FCE evaluators with a framework for evaluating repetitive activity, there is no published research to validate them or the specific protocols used in these models to determine activity frequency. This lack of research also applies to many FCE models currently being used.

Environmental Factors and Functional Capacity Evaluation

Environmental factors can affect the extent to which a worker is able to tolerate a given activity and how much of a rest allowance the worker requires. These factors include temperature (extreme heat or cold), humidity, lighting, noise, vibration, dust, fumes, and poor ventilation. Although these factors are important to consider, they are not specifically assessed during an FCE unless the FCE is performed at the work site. Although the failure to replicate environmental conditions can be considered a limitation of FCE, one could argue that performing a general FCE in a controlled environment increases test safety and that an evaluee who is unable to perform within an "optimal" environment would probably function even less well in a less optimal environment. Later in this chapter, information is given about how Methods-Time Measurement (MTM) rest allowance standards, as adopted by the International Labor Organization, can account for "adverse" environmental conditions.

In addition to environmental factors, the test environment, meaning the surroundings where the FCE is being conducted, can vary and might impact evaluee performance. FCEs are performed in clinical settings, offices, at the work site, and, sometimes, in an evaluee's home.

Two studies about the impact of the FCE environment have been published. Reneman et al[7] studied the effect of three environmental conditions (normal, high noise, and high production) on the ecological validity of three static endurance tests used in the Isernhagen Work Systems FCE (now known as WorkWell Systems, Duluth, MN). The study concluded that the different conditions used did not influence the performance or perceived exertion of evaluees, but more research is needed. Innes and Straker[8] studied FCE protocols in clinical and work environments and noted that while there is usually more consistency and rigidity in the standard protocols compared with the work-site evaluations, many evaluators considered the work-site evaluation to have more validity because specific job-related activities were tested in the actual work environment. Chapter 21 provides further information on the FCE environment. The impact of test environment and environmental factors on evaluee performance in FCE needs further investigation.

Testing Methods

The methods used to assess an evaluee's positional tolerance and movement abilities vary (sometimes significantly) between FCE models, as does the availability of published research on these methods. The lack of research in this area underlies the difficulty FCE evaluators experience in generalizing the test results to an evaluee's 8-hour-per-day work ability and tolerance. There may be differences in an evaluee's predicted ability between models, although this factor has not been formally studied in regard to movement and positional tolerance. Further development of this area is needed because measurements must be reliable and valid in order for the measurement to be generalizable (the degree to which evidence of validity obtained in one situation can be generalized to another situation without further study of validity in the new situation). In addition to differences in testing methods, the operational definitions of test activities and positions used in an FCE protocol may vary between FCE models. For example, an overhead reach test in one model may require the evaluee's shoulders to be positioned at 90° with the hands positioned at crown height, whereas in another protocol, the upper extremities are fully elevated with the hands positioned above crown height.

This chapter discusses how movement and positional tolerances are assessed in an FCE. There are two general types of approaches to the assessment of an evaluee's repetitive movement abilities. The first approach determines the evaluee's abilities by asking the evaluee to repetitively perform an activity for a specified amount of time or number of repetitions. For purposes of discussion in this chapter, this approach is referred to as a "performance-based" approach. The second approach involves the use of the MTM approach. Approaches that use MTM are discussed in detail in this chapter and are followed by a discussion of the evaluation of positional tolerance.

Performance-based Assessment of Movement Abilities

Performance Parameters

In a performance-based approach, the evaluee is asked to perform a number of activities. The activities listed in the DOT are the activities typically assessed in a general FCE. In most FCEs using this approach, the evaluee is asked to perform a specified number of repetitive movements or to sustain a position for a specific period. The number of repetitions or time spent in a posture varies with the FCE protocol. The FCE evaluator considers quantitative and qualitative parameters and the evaluee's response to the activity when determining the evaluee's physical abilities.

Quantitative Parameters

Quantitative parameters relate to the "quantity" of the activity, such as time limits, distance moved, and number of repetitions. The quantitative criteria (also referred to as performance standards) for a movement or positional tolerance test should have operational definitions and be measurable. For example, an FCE protocol for kneeling should specifically define how the test is to be performed and for how long. The scoring criteria need to differentiate between "able to perform to full duration" and "unable to perform for any length of time" with identified frequencies in between. Based on the evaluee's performance, the protocol should define how the evaluator assigns an activity frequency (occasional, frequent, or constant) based on the evaluee's test result. It is difficult to obtain specific information about test procedures used in commercially available FCE models because the information is proprietary. (This difficulty is evident when reading the information provided by vendors of commercially available FCE models in the Appendix.) Comparison of different proprietary FCE protocols or of nonproprietary protocols with proprietary protocols is extremely difficult. The FCE protocol should have a method whereby the evaluator correlates performance on a specific test with the clinical examination results and the evaluee's performance during other activities requiring similar movements or postures. (This is referred to as "cross testing" in Chapter 16.) Some FCE evaluators label an evaluee's ability as "no activity limitation" or "no identified limitation" to indicate that neither the evaluee's symptoms nor clinical findings would limit performance of the activity. Data analysis and interpretation are discussed further in Chapter 16.

The test procedures used in an FCE protocol should have acceptable interrater and intrarater reliability and should be valid, meaning that the assigned frequency predicts the evaluee's 8-hour work ability. Unfortunately, there is a dearth of published research in peer-reviewed journals demonstrating reliability and validity of the methods used in many of the currently available FCE models. As stated by Reneman et al in their study of ecological validity published in 2001, "The performance standards of the three tests seem to be based on (a considerable amount of) experience, rather than on evidence. To our knowledge, no research is published to [support] the reliability and the validity of the tests that are the subject of this study."[7p228] Since publication of the study by Reneman et al,[7] two studies have been published that investigated reliability. Durand et al[9] studied the interrater reliability for 21 tasks used in the Physical Work Performance Evaluation (ErgoScience, Birmingham, AL). The results demonstrated "substantial" to "almost perfect" reliability for most of the items studied. Reneman et al[10] subsequently studied the ability of uninjured young (20–29 years old) subjects to sustain forward bend and elevated work postures, the relationship between the holding time in the postures and subject's perceived exertion, and the reliability of the testing procedures. Although the results indicated that generic formulas, curve estimations, and the subject's predictions could not reliably predict performance, the testing procedures were found to be reliable. Reneman et al[10] concluded that the determinations of ability are best identified through performance-based testing rather than reliance on the subject's belief or the use of generic formulas.

Many FCE evaluators use standardized protocols, such as the Purdue Pegboard Assembly and Minnesota Rate of Manipulation tests, to assess the fingering and handling abilities of evaluees. There are normative data available that classify performance based on the evaluee's demonstrated test speed or number of pieces completed. Although these scores provide information about the evaluee's *rate of performance,* the scores have not been shown to be valid predictors of an evaluee's ability to sustain activity. For example, the Purdue Pegboard Assembly test counts the number of pieces the evaluee assembles in 1 minute. The evaluee may repeat the test protocol three times. Although the Purdue Pegboard normative data then categorize performance speed, there are no published data that correlate the performance rate with sustained ability.

Although most FCEs describe frequency abilities as occasional, frequent, and constant, Osborne et al[5] questioned the need to assess an evaluee's ability beyond the frequent classification unless the FCE is job-specific. These authors stated that fewer than 1% of the occupations listed in the DOT require constant demand, so unless a specific job requires a constant level of frequency, there is no need for an FCE evaluator to test to a constant frequency level. In their view, an activity that exceeds occasional frequency requires endurance that cannot be assessed by having an evaluee perform a short bout of activity. A number of current FCE protocols use short activity bouts as the basis by which ability determination is made. For example, if an FCE protocol for a sustained kneeling test is a 5-minute test, an evaluee who kneels for 4 minutes could be considered to have "constant" ability because 4 minutes is within the 67% to 100% range of 5 minutes. Similarly, an evaluee who kneels for 2.5 minutes could be considered as having "frequent" ability because the demonstrated performance is within 34% to 66% of the total 5-minute duration. Finally, an evaluee who sustained kneeling for 30 seconds could be classified as having "occasional" ability because the performance is within 15% to 33% of the 5-minute task. The physiologic justification for the use of these extrapolations is unclear. Some FCE protocols repeat a test activity two or three times during the FCE process to determine if the evaluee's performance is stable or if performance declines over time. The FCE protocol should have specific scoring criteria for determining an evaluee's ability and make these criteria available to evaluees and referral sources who want to review and better understand their results.

To summarize, although quantitative parameters provide measurable information about an evaluee's performance, further study is needed to determine the reliability and validity of many of the current protocols and performance standards being used. The proprietary models claiming to base their performance standards on internal studies should subject those studies to peer review. Furthermore, standardization of terminology and definitions between FCE protocols is needed.

Quantitative parameters are only part of what evaluators consider in determining physical ability. Additional parameters are discussed in the following paragraphs.

Qualitative Parameters

Qualitative parameters are the factors observed by the evaluator during an activity and include the degree of muscle recruitment required for the task, movement quality (including motor control, coordination, use of external support, base of support, and pace), and the evaluee's posture. Qualitative scoring for a kneeling activity might include the evaluee's ability to sustain an upright posture and consider the number of deviations or difficulty the evaluee had while sustaining the posture during the test. The evaluee's transition in and out of the kneeling position is also considered. For example, what was the quality of the movement as the evaluee moved into kneeling or arose to standing? Was arm support required? Was the movement fluid and coordinated or performed slowly with difficulty? An FCE protocol should have scoring criteria that the evaluator uses to make ability determinations. In addition, the evaluator should correlate the observed performance with the clinical examination findings and other activities requiring similar movements during the FCE.

Evaluee-related Parameters

Evaluee-related parameters include the evaluee's physiologic response to the activity and symptom reports and behaviors. For example, an evaluator will note the evaluee's heart and respiratory rate during activity. A significantly increased heart rate after standing from a kneeling position or climbing a flight of stairs should be considered in determining the evaluee's ability to sustain activity. The evaluee's rating of perceived exertion using the 10- or 20-point Borg scale[11,12] is frequently used by evaluators, and some evaluators correlate the evaluee's rating of exertion with the heart rate. The evaluee's report of symptoms is also noted during and after an activity. Although the evaluee's report of symptoms and exertion is an important factor for consideration, it should not be relied on without correlation with observed performance and clinical examination findings because a number of published studies have demonstrated that a evaluee's perception of ability and pain correlate poorly with physical ability.[10,13,14] The impact of pain on data analysis is discussed further in Chapter 16.

Example: Repetitive Reaching Test

The following is an example of a fictitious repetitive reaching test using the performance-based method (as opposed to the MTM approach). The purpose of this example is to provide readers with a better understanding of how such a test might be performed during an FCE. The FCE protocol should define the test standard—how the test is to be performed and what the results mean in terms of the evaluee's ability to perform repetitive reaching. As noted earlier, most FCE models consider their methods proprietary and do not share this information with non-users. Once a test procedure is developed, it should be tested on healthy uninjured people without relevant disabilities and later on injured subjects, with further refinement (and validation) during the development phase. The following is an example of a performance-based model for repetitive reaching.

Activity Model Development: Repetitive Elevated Reaching
- Test purpose: To determine a patient's ability to perform repetitive elevated work with bilateral upper extremities. This activity primarily stresses the shoulders and cervical spine. (Because the activity involves fingering and handling, ie, picking up and moving bolts, this activity may be used as a cross-test for these activities. See Chapter 16 for discussion of cross-testing.)
- Define the test position.
    - Perform the reaching activity in a standing position. Elevated work is defined as having the hands at crown height, so the shoulders are at approximately 90° of elevation.

- A container with bolts is placed on the lower shelf of a shelving unit; position the shelf 29 inches from the floor.
- An empty container is placed on the top shelf of the shelving unit; position at the evaluee's crown height (top of head).
- Identify equipment or object weight, if appropriate.
  - Adjustable shelving unit with two shelves minimum
  - 50 No. 1 bolts
  - Stopwatch
  - Heart rate monitor
  - Two plastic containers, 6 × 24 × 12 inches (height, length, and width, respectively)
- Identify the test protocol.
  - Perform the bilateral reaching activity continuously for 5 minutes.
  - Transfer the bolts from the container on the lowest shelf to the container on the top shelf. Alternate your right and left hands. When the container on the top shelf is filled, begin removing the bolts and place them in the container on the bottom shelf. When the container on the lower shelf is filled, begin removing the bolts and place them in the container on the top shelf.
  - Continue the activity until the evaluator instructs you to stop.
- Identify duration of test and repetitions per minute or per cycle, if required.
  - The activity is performed for 5 minutes without interruption. The evaluator will alert you at the 2.5-minute mark.
  - Continue at a rate that allows you to continue for 5 minutes.
  - If at any time you feel it is not safe to continue the activity, alert the evaluator.
- Define performance standards (quantitative results).
  - Uninterrupted reaching performed at constant pace for 5 minutes
    - 35–67 reaches/min = frequent
    - 16–34 reaches/min = occasional
    - 1–15 reaches/min = rare
- Outline performance parameters (qualitative results)
  - Continuous bilateral reaching performed in a smooth, controlled manner for full duration of reaching activity
  - Minimal increase in heart rate and respirations during reaching
  - Normal scapulohumeral rhythm observed and appropriate recruitment of scapular muscles
  - Upright standing with neutral cervical posture maintained
- Document the evaluee's response to activity

- Report of pain or other symptoms: Does the report correlate with clinical examination findings and observations during the test?
- Report of fatigue: Does the report correlate with other similar activities, self-report, and examination findings?

The FCE evaluator would document the evaluee's ability to perform the reaching activity compared with the standard and identify limitations that interfere in reaching ability.

Use of Methods-Time Measurement (MTM) in Evaluating Movement

The MTM approach is a Predetermined Motion-Time Standards (PMTS) system. The PMTS systems were originally used by industrial engineers to determine the time needed to carry out manufacturing processes, establish estimates for production time and costs, and establish efficiency measures. The MTM system, the most widely developed and validated PMTS system in the world, was developed in the 1940s, published by Maynard et al[15] in 1948, and willed to the public domain in 1953, concurrent with the establishment of the MTM Association for Standards and Research. Since that time, the MTM system has continued to be validated in many work sites and production systems.[16] Further research has led to the development of personnel selection tests, disability evaluation measurement, treatment efficacy measurement, and rest allowance standards. By 1982, it was considered that there had been so much research published internationally "in such detail and such practicality" that the science had shifted from the basic science to the application level.[17]

The MTM Association coordinates worldwide development, training, and standardization practices.[18] The system identified standard motion groups, each with 2 to 175 classes, or cases, for a total of 460 fundamental motions. The standard motion groups that make MTM so relevant for testing work motions and positional tolerance are as follows:
- **Arm motions:** *Reach* and *move* (reaching with weight)
- **Hand motions:** *Turn, grasp, position, apply pressure, crank, disengage*
- **Body and foot motions:** *Walk, sidestep, turn body, sit, stand, bend and arise from bend, kneel and arise from kneel*
- **Simultaneous motions:** Coordinated use of any of these motions

The MTM Industrial Standard

MTM is a *criterion-referenced system*, rather than a population-based (normative) system. The concept of *normal* work is the basic premise of the MTM *Industrial Standard* (IS), which is the time it takes an average worker with average skill to perform a task throughout an average 8-hour day, with appropriate rest allowances, without undue stress or fatigue.[18] A *criterion-referenced data set* is one that establishes the level of ability of the domain being tested and establishes the criterion for the domain's entire population, not just the sample used for criterion referencing of the data set or criterion-referenced predictive validity studies. In this respect, the MTM system was designed as a criterion of "low-task" performance to account for variance among workers related to sex, age, and health status. The statistical "average" ability of the general workforce was demonstrated to be at 120% of the IS.[17]

A criterion-referenced example familiar to most readers of this text is the board certification examination. The items for the examination were solicited from a sample of current clinicians, often academicians. A cutoff point was established for passing the board examination, and the entire domain of clinicians was graded according to that pass-fail criterion for certification to meet minimum competency standards. Some examinees met only the minimum criterion, and some may have vastly exceeded the minimum criterion. However, all passing examinees received the same certification, despite their statistical variance in degree of competency. Clinicians who pass the examination are then considered *generalizable,* or competent within their scope of practice, in all types of patient environments.

Similarly, MTM-based testing compares an evaluee's results with the MTM IS criterion. The MTM evaluative process involves asking the evaluee to perform a number of tasks designed to evaluate positional tolerance and/or the ability to perform selected work motions or combinations of motions. The number and type of tasks chosen are dependent on the exact physical functions that the evaluator wants to assess and may change during testing to reflect evaluee performance (or nonperformance). Regardless of the tasks chosen, the MTM process, as applied in many FCEs, requires that evaluees complete a given task for several trials (often three), during which the amount of time it takes to do so is monitored. The evaluee's ability to work at an occasional, frequent, or constant level or not at all is based predominantly on the speed of task completions (albeit with adjustment factors; see "MTM Has Rest Allowances That Account for Constant Work"). Rest allowances reflect norms set in a number of studies of the relationship between the speed of task completion and the IS for that task. If an evaluee performs at a pace less than identified in the IS and there are no other variables accounting for low scores, the evaluator can attribute this performance to objective medical evidence of impairment or to poor effort. The issue of effort is of great significance in FCE testing, and the MTM system has a well-developed body of literature on the effort rating variance.

Reliability

The MTM system has demonstrated high internal consistency, with an 8% standard error of measurement at 95% confidence level (ie, if a person scores at 100% of the IS, the rater can assume the person would score from 92% to 108% of the IS 95% of the time). The original research found only 8% variance between workers within the same effort category (described later). Interobserver agreement studies were reported by Maynard et al.[15] The data demonstrated a high level of consistency and agreement. Reliability and validity studies performed at Cornell University and Western Michigan University reproduced these results.[16] Eady[19] in 1986 demonstrated reliability at 5% at a 95% confidence level for cycle times of approximately 1 minute. In a reliability study intended to validate MTM-2 and MTM-3, Knott and Sury[20] showed similar accuracy for cycle times between the MTM-1, MTM-2, and MTM-3 data sets for cycle times as low as 0.02 minutes. This research allows confidence that MTM-based tests can be performed reliably within the testing environment, given satisfactory evaluator training and test instructions.

Known reliability of tests has led to a body of research and literature hypothesizing that evaluee performance can be attributed to poor effort if the evaluee scores outside the aforementioned reliability variances. This hypothesis was tested with MTM-based tests and published in 1965 by Applewhite and Paulhe.[21] The investigators found that subjects instructed to give poor effort had a wider distribution of scores than subjects who gave average effort. The method of ascribing overall evaluee effort to the distribution of scores via use of a coefficient of variation (CV) has many weaknesses that are beyond the scope of this chapter (see Chapter 11). It should also be noted that impairment in the body area being tested will increase variability in the evaluee's results, so the CVs should not be considered indicators of evaluee effort in tests that involve body parts with clinical evidence of dysfunction.[22]

Validity

The IS is an achievable time for the majority of workers aged 18 to 65 years of both sexes in good health to perform the task. At least 95% of all workers can achieve the IS.[16] An important feature of MTM is that MTM motions are "universal" characteristics of work demanded by all jobs. Universal characteristics are more generalizable than "occupationals" (the characteristics required by a specific job) and "relationals" (the characteristics of a job relative to the environment). Generalizability theory, as first developed by Cronbach et al,[23,24] explicitly requires investigators to specify a universe of conditions over which they want to generalize. The extent to which different conditions are associated with different observations has implications for designing dependable observations. These principles of universality guided the development of the physical demand characteristics of the DOT and CCDO,[25] and the principles are embedded in the Uniform Guidelines on Employee Selection Procedures published by the US Department of Labor Equal Employment Opportunity Commission.[26]

The IS has continually been revalidated across many countries and work populations. The *Journal of Methods-Time Measurement* has continuously published articles since the mid-1950s. Additional studies have appeared in medical journals. For example, 65-year-old male clerical workers in Japan were given industrial tasks to perform and were able to meet or exceed the IS.[27] A Scandinavian study demonstrated that performance of repetitive tasks at the MTM IS by production workers did not elicit muscle fatigue.[28]

MTM and Predictive Validity of Personnel Selection

The MTM Association developed a series of personnel selection tests. A study found little difference between work performance predicted by the selections tests and actual work performance.[29–31] The MTM-based Purdue Elemental Motions test had greater predictive validity than did the Minnesota Rate of Manipulation test.[32]

MTM and the Predictive Validity With People With Disabilities

Evaluations based on MTM have been used with disability populations for more than 40 years. Farrell[32] compared the scores of rehabilitation clients on 14 MTM tests of basic motions of less than 30 seconds' duration with their workshop abilities and demonstrated that these short tests were predictive of the workshop abilities or attainable with treatment that addressed stamina or motivation. Bootle[33] reported good convergence of scores on PMTS testing with return to complex assembly, clerical, semiskilled, and skilled work outcomes within a worker rehabilitation sample. Hasselqvist[34] developed a Scandinavian system of evaluating work abilities for people with physical handicaps, and a derivative of the Scandinavian research has been referenced in a more recent study that demonstrated MTM testing to be a useful method for task analysis.[35] In Australia, Tichauer[36] used a battery of MTM-based tests and was able to correlate test results with the specific spinal cord lesion sites (eg, myotomes). The workability predetermined motion time system has been used in the Australian disability evaluation field.[37] In addition, from a legal defensibility position, Barnard[38] outlined the medicolegal strength of using a PMTS.

Chyatte and Birdsong[39-41] used MTM-based tests for evaluation of brain-damaged patients from a variety of causes beginning in 1968,[39] 1970,[40] and 1972.[41] They concluded from a study of 300 subjects that MTM-based tests showed meaningful change measurement with manual tasks, with and without moving weights. Todd et al[42] compared MTM-based evaluations of patients with cerebral palsy with the *AMA Guides*–derived impairment ratings. They concluded that the *AMA Guides*–derived impairment rating had little or no bearing on specific task function, whereas the MTM-based evaluation deals in specific task performance. The authors compared MTM-based assessment times with norm-based classifications of a work sample and found that the work sample overestimated work performance until the MTM criterion was added. Birdsong[43] reviewed the use of MTM-based evaluations as a monitoring and investigative technique at the Emory University School of Medicine, Atlanta, GA. The MTM approach has been used in evaluation of people with physical and mental handicaps and design of sheltered workshop tasks.[44,45] The MTM Association began a disability evaluation project in 1976 with United Kingdom, Scandinavian, and Dutch social services agencies for people with handicaps.[46-48] The tests were developed for people with mental handicaps in service delivery populations, including people with mental handicaps with "the possibility of adapt[ing] [the MTM-based test] to every individual candidate." This early work in the 1950s to 1970s established the relevance of the MTM data and its appropriateness for matching a worker to a job task and designing job accommodation and modification. Beginning in the late 1970s, MTM and other PMTS-based tests evolved into full sets of functional testing work samples and functional test batteries for work-injury populations. These include tests developed by the following companies: VALPAR Work Samples, Basic Motions of Work, Workability, Predictive Vocational Assessment, FWAP functional tests, MAST in England, Hanoun, BTE, ARCON/VerNova, and AssessAbility. Therefore, MTM-based tests have been widely used in work and incorporated into FCE systems by many commercial companies and academic organizations. Although most commercial testing companies with tests based on PMTSs have not published additional studies of reliability and validity, the basic scientific support for MTM is considerable. As noted in Chapter 21, further study of the reliability and validity of the MTM approach in determining a person's physical ability is, nevertheless, required.

MTM Has Rest Allowances That Account for Constant Work

The MTM time standards represent work under ideal conditions. Realistic performance requires some adjustment and/or allowance. The usual allowances are for personal time, fatigue, and minor unavoidable delay. The usual allowance for these variables is 15%. The International Labor Organization has published relaxation allowances for MTM data. Physiologic validation studies have been performed on these allowances with general agreement found with the International Labor Organization allowances.[49,50] Tests using the MTM approach with appropriate use of rest allowances have been generalizable to a wide variety of work settings, including manual labor, warehouse work, repetitive production tasks, fabrication, mail and package delivery and transportation, underground mining, sewing, health care, and insurance.[51-54] This robust evidence of generalizability allows an evaluator to predict return to most work settings where work is performed within normal and safe conditions. Where work conditions do not seem to be normal, safe higher scores are suggested as cutoff points for return to work. Return to piecework is often based on abilities at 120% of the IS, which is the pace at which piecework has been measured. Osborne et al[5] suggest that MTM-based tests refer to work pace and might not provide the data necessary to make accurate projections of an evaluee's ability to sustain frequent and constant work (ie, endurance) when testing for positional tolerance. This suggestion means that although FCE evaluators make frequency projections based on MTM-based tests, there is no clearly substantiated basis for doing so. Further research substantiating the validity of the application of the MTM method in FCEs is needed.

Effort Rating

According to the MTM approach, there is a range of scores possible within the context of normal effort, which is labeled as the MTM leveling system. The range of scores varies plus or minus 15% depending on effort, ranging from poor effort, poor to fair effort, fair effort, average effort, good effort, excellent effort, and excessive effort. See Table 9–2 for these operational definitions.

The elegance of this body of work on MTM leveling is that evaluators can consider all their evidence of patient-effort and opine about where, within the entire range of scores, is a score most feasible for a patient. For example, if the evaluator has concerns that a patient is giving "poor" effort, based on physical examination findings, inconsistency in testing, and heart rate and effort data, the evaluator may suggest that scores in the upper range would be feasible for the patient. On the other hand, if an evaluator has concerns that an evaluee is overexerting against his or her impairment, based on physical examination

TABLE 9–2	Effort* Rating in the Method–Time Management Approach
Type of Effort	**Description**
Poor	May take the form of a lackadaisical, dispirited attitude, accompanied by an obviously slow working pace; can also take the form of a great deal of unnecessary work undertaken with a frantic display of energy
Poor to fair	Between poor and fair efforts
Fair	Readily apparent that the patient is not putting forth the best effort but is not resorting to extreme time-killing practices characteristic of poor effort
Average	Patient works steadily and appears to take some interest in the work; level includes some characteristics of the good and fair effort levels; level can be maintained day after day without undue fatigue
Good	Patient works steadily at a pace that can be maintained day after day or week after week; motions have quickness or "snap"; patients conscientious about work and appear to be energetic and enthusiastic toward the job
Excellent	Patients work fast, take a keen interest in the work, and reduce false motions to a minimum as far as their skill permits; the level is difficult to maintain week in and week out, but possible for up all day and, perhaps, several days. A patient who usually performs at the good effort level may perform at the excellent level on some days when feeling particularly fit.
Excessive	Given by some workers who cannot work normally when they are being watched possibly owing to a tendency to show off or a reaction to being very nervous; pace cannot usually be maintained for more than an hour or two; can adversely affect a patient's skill level

Effort is defined as the will to work. Effort is related to the zest or energy with which a task is undertaken. Effort is controlled by the patient at all times.
Source: MTM Association

findings, inconsistency in testing, and heart rate and effort data, the evaluator may exercise caution and suggests that scores in the lower end would be more realistic. Although the reliability/validity of the leveling system has not been

CHAPTER 9

formally tested in the disability-systems' population, ie, using leveling to adjust scores has not been formally tested on individuals with disabilities, the leveling-system data have been accepted as an empirically derived range of scores within the universe of workers 18 to 65 years old and can be considered generalizable to a disability-systems' evaluee. Nonetheless, evaluator's cautious interpretation should be noted in the report. Further research is needed to support the validity of the leveling system within the framework of evaluating positional tolerance.

Non-credible Performance

On occasion, an evaluator may consider that even the corrected scores from any of the previously mentioned methods or MTM leveled scores underestimate an evaluee's capability. This judgment is usually made on the basis of a poor correlation between impairment (ie, lack of diagnostic confirmation of the impairment or physical examination findings inconsistent with a patient's testing performance) and the functional test results. There may also be side-by-side comparisons between tests that appear dissimilar yet stress identical muscle groups that lead the evaluator not to trust the veracity of the evaluee's effort. Repeated test trials may produce a CV that exceeds the cutoff score. Inconsistency of test-retest findings may demonstrate a statistical CV above the empirically derived standard for testing. The *AMA Guides to the Evaluation of Permanent Impairment,* Sixth Edition, gives very good guidance for this situation. In Table 2–1 in the *Guides 6th,* it states:

. . . . The physician must use all clinical knowledge, skill and abilities in determining whether the measurements, test results, or written historical information are consistent and concordant with the pathology being evaluated. If such findings, or an impairment estimate based on these findings, conflict with established medical principles, they cannot be used to justify an impairment rating.[55]

Case Examples Using the MTM Method

Case Example 1: A production worker has a well-documented right ankle fusion. The handling, bimanual handling, finger dexterity, and eye-hand-foot coordination testing is performed in a seated vs standing position. Test results show performance at 50% to 65% of the IS with a 1% to 7% CV (demonstrating consistency) when standing and 97% to 125% of the IS with a 3% to 7% CV (demonstrating consistency) when seated. Eye-hand-foot coordination is tested on the impaired vs unimpaired side while seated, and the testing confirms that any foot controls will need modification to allow left foot control. The evaluator concludes that the patient performed the evaluation in a valid manner and recommends (among other recommendations regarding lifting, walking, and carrying) a job accommodation of being permitted to sit for production work.

Case Example 2: A clerical worker has left shoulder pain and no objective evidence of impairment documented by diagnostic testing or medical examination. The results of seated right overhead reaching (on the unimpaired side) show performance at 75% of the IS with a 12% CV (demonstrating inconsistency) and results of seated left overhead reaching (suspect side) demonstrate 58% of the IS with a 22% CV (demonstrating inconsistency). The evaluator concludes the evaluee performed the evaluation in an unreliable and possibly self-limited manner and suggests that the evaluee is capable of performing at the upper level of the score range (leveling). The leveling is suggestive of constant right reaching overhead and frequent left reaching overhead, ie, leveling the score resulted in an increased estimate of the evaluee's ability. Alternatively, the physician may determine that the functional testing corroborates his or her clinical judgment that medical evidence seems insufficient to verify that impairment exists and return the evaluee to full duty.

Evaluating Positional Tolerance

There are few predictive and generalizable studies on work motions and positional tolerance. In regard to determining an evaluee's ability to sustain postures, FCE protocols vary in terms of which postures are evaluated, how tests are performed, and the parameters for scoring. With the exception of sitting, some protocols only routinely test to a frequent tolerance level because of the time required to assess constant ability (usually > 40 minutes per activity) and the belief that few occupations require constant work.[5] Quantitative, qualitative, and evaluee-related parameters are considered when identifying an evaluee's ability to sustain a given posture. Based on the percentage used in identifying frequency categories, some FCE protocols use the following quantitative parameters for determining an evaluee's positional tolerance:

■ Occasional tolerance, 1 to 20 minutes (33% of an hour)
■ Frequent tolerance, 21 to 40 minutes (35%–67% of an hour)
■ Constant tolerance, > 45 minutes (75% of an hour)

For example, if an evaluee demonstrates the ability to sit for 30 minutes, the ability is considered to be within the frequent level, as long as the evaluator did not observe significant signs of intolerance during the time the evaluee was sitting (eg, shifting in seat or leaning to one side) and the evaluee did not report significant discomfort. As noted with movement testing, there should be correlation between evaluee performance and symptom reports throughout the FCE and correlation of these reports with clinical examination findings. This correlation is critical for the FCE evaluator to distinguish between what an evaluee *can do* vs what an evaluee *is willing to do*. The FCE protocols should include details that specify how positional tolerances are evaluated. In a job-specific FCE, the test should replicate the specific job requirements. This replication is discussed in more detail in Chapter 14. As stated earlier, the predictive validity of these projections (values) has not been demonstrated in studies reported in the literature.

Summary

Determining an evaluee's movement abilities and positional tolerances is an important component of FCEs. FCEs use a performance-based approach or an MTM-based approach to determine an evaluee's abilities. FCE models differ in how tests are defined, performed, and interpreted and in the extent to which an evaluee's ability is estimated (ie, ability for occasional, frequent, or constant performance of an activity). More research is needed to validate the current testing and scoring methods used in the performance- and MTM-based approaches. Further investigation regarding "constant" activity is needed to determine when this level of testing in a general FCE is appropriate and relevant. At present, when requesting an FCE, the FCE evaluator should be asked about the level of testing routinely performed and the methods used to perform this testing, particularly if the requestor wants testing beyond the occasional level to clear an employee for a specific job-related task or tasks or wishes to determine an evaluee's maximum physical abilities.

References

1. US Department of Labor. *Selected Characteristics of Occupations as Defined in the Revised Dictionary of Occupational Titles.* Washington, DC: US Department of Labor; 1993. National Technical Information Service publication PB94–116282.
2. Manpower and Immigration Ministry. *Canadian Classification and Dictionary of Occupations.* Ottawa, Canada: Information Canada; 1971.
3. Occupational Information Network (O*NET) Web site. http://online.onetcenter.org/. Accessed May 24, 2008.
4. National Occupational Classification (NOC) in Canada. www5.hrsdc.gc.ca/NOC-CNP/app/index.aspx?lc=e. Accessed March 31, 2008.
5. Osborne P, Dakos M, Randolph DC. Functional testing for positional tolerance by frequency classification. *Disability.* August 2001:51–55.

6. Blankenship KL. *Industrial Rehabilitation I-A Seminar Series.* Macon, GA: American Therapeutics, Inc; 1990.

7. Reneman MF, Joling CL, Soer EL, Goeken LN. Functional capacity evaluation: ecological validity of three static endurance tests. *Work.* 2001;16:227–234.

8. Innes E, Straker L. Workplace assessments and functional capacity evaluations: current practices of therapists in Australia. *Work.* 2002;18:51–66.

9. Durand MJ, Loisel P, Poitras S, Mercier R, Stock SR, Lemaire J. The interrater reliability of a functional capacity evaluation: the physical work performance evaluation. *J Occup Rehabil.* 2004;14:119–129.

10. Reneman MF, Bults MM, Engbers LH, Mulders KK, Goeken LN. Measuring maximum holding times and perception of static elevated work and forward bending in healthy young adults. *J Occup Rehabil.* 2001;11:87–97.

11. Borg GA. Psychophysical bases of perceived exertion. *Med Sci Sports Exerc.* 1982;14:377–381.

12. Reneman MF, Fokkens AS, Dijkstra PU, Geertzen JHB, Groothoff JW. Testing lifting capacity: validity of determining effort level by means of observation. *Spine.* 2005;30:E40-E46.

13. Reneman MF, Jorritsma W, Schellekens JM, Goeken LN. Concurrent validity of questionnaire and performance-based disability measurements in patients with chronic nonspecific low back pain. *J Occup Rehabil.* 2002;12:119–129.

14. Gross DP, Battie MD. Construct validity of a kinesiophysical functional capacity evaluation administered within a worker's compensation environment. *J Occup Rehabil.* 2003;13:287–295.

15. Maynard HB, Stegemerton GJ, Schwab JL. *Methods–Time Measurement.* New York, NY: McGraw-Hill; 1948.

16. Karger DW, Bayha FH. *Engineered Work Measurement.* 4th ed. New York, NY: Industrial Press; 1987.

17. Karger DW, Hancock WM. *Advanced Work Measurement.* New York, NY: Industrial Press; 1982.

18. MTM Association for Standards and Research. *MTM-1 User Manual.* Des Plaines, IL: MTM Association for Standards and Research; 1972, 1990.

19. Eady K. Today's international MTM systems: decision criteria for their use. In: Shell RL, ed. *Work Measurement: Principles and Practice.* Norcross, GA: Industrial Engineering and Management Press; 1986:202–210.

20. Knott K, Sury RJ. Investigation into the minimum cycle time restrictions of MTM-2 and MTM-3. *Indust Eng Transactions.* 1986;18:392–397.

21. Applewhite PB, Paulhe GP, Thompson DA. Frequency distribution shape and work output. *Percept Mot Skills.* 1965;20:407–408.

22. Simonsen JC. Coefficient of variation as a measure of subject effort. *Arch Phys Med Rehabil.* 1995;76:516–520.

23. Cronbach LJ, Nageswari R, Gleser GC. Theory of generalizability: a liberation of reliability theory. *Br J Stat Psychol.* 1963;16:137–163.

24. Cronbach LJ, Gleser GC, Nanda H, Rajaratnam N. *The Dependability of Behavioral Measurements: Theory of Generalizability for Scores and Profiles.* New York, NY: John Wiley; 1972.

25. US Department of Labor. *The Revised Handbook for Analyzing Jobs.* Washington, DC: US Dept of Labor, Employment and Training Administration; 1991.

CHAPTER 9

26. Adoption of Questions and Answers to Clarify and Provide a Common Interpretation of the Uniform Guidelines on Employee Selection Procedures. www.eeoc.gov/policy/docs/qanda_clarify_procedures.html. Accessed March 31, 2008.

27. Yokomizo Y. Measurement of abilities of older workers. *Ergonomics.* 1985;28: 843–854.

28. Mathiassen SE, Winkel J. Physiological comparison of three interventions in light assembly work: reduced work pace, increased break allowance and shortened working days. *Int Arch Occup Environ Health.* 1996;68:94–108.

29. Anderson DS, Edstrom DP. MTM personnel selection tests: validation at a northwestern national life insurance company. *The Journal of Methods-Time Measurement.* July 1969;XV(3):pp 11–17.

30. Poock G K. Prediction of Elemental Motion Performance Using Personnel Selection Tests [dissertation].University of Michigan, 1967.

31. Drewes DW. Development and validation of synthetic dexterity tests based on elemental motion analysis. *J Appl Psychol.* 1961;45:179–185.

32. Farrell JM. The value of work study in occupational therapy. In: *Proceedings of the Fourth International Congress of the World Federation of Occupational Therapists.* London, England: Excerpta Medica; 1966:216–222.

33. Bootle EC. Graded movement assessment based on a predetermined time system. *Aust Occup Ther J.* 1976;23:130–144.

34. Hasselqvist O. The MTM method: with special reference to the physically handicapped. *Scand J Rehabil Med.* 1972;4:157–164.

35. Christmansson M. Repetitive and manual jobs: content and effects in terms of physical stress and work-related musculoskeletal disorders. *Int J Hum Factors Manufacturing.* 2007;4:281–292.

36. Tichauer ER. Industrial engineering in the rehabilitation of the handicapped. *J Industrial Engineering.* 1968;19:97–104.

37. Heyde GC. *Workability With Modapts: Mark III.* Sydney, Australia: Heyde Dynamics; 1990.

38. Barnard S. Modapts in the assessment of productivity for medico-legal purposes in Modapts for the 90's. Proceedings of the Preconference Workshop, 10th International Congress of the World Federation of Occupational Therapists and First International Modapts Conference Australian and New Zealand Modapts Association (ANZMA), Melbourne, Australia pp 1–26, ANZMA.

39. Chyatte SB, Birdsong JH. Assessment of brain damage with MTM. *The Journal of Methods-Time Measurement.* March/April 1968;XIII(2):15–18.

40. Birdsong JH, Chyatte SB. Further medical applications of methods-time measurement. *The Journal of Methods-Time Measurement.* 1970;15:19–27.

41. Chyatte SB, Birdsong JH. Methods–time measurement in assessment of motor performance. *Arch Phys Med Rehabil.* 1972;53:38–44.

42. Todd HC, Chyatte SB, Decker RS. Predetermined time standards: their application in workshop settings. *Arch Phys Med Rehabil.* 1979;60:222–226.

43. Birdsong JH. MTM and rehabilitation: a combination for potential profits. *The Journal of Methods-Time Measurement.* 1972;17:3–8.

44. Brickey M. MTM in a sheltered workshop. *The Journal of Methods-Time Measurement.* 1962;8:2–7.

45. McQuaid M, Winkler K. Using PMTS in handicapped workshops. *The Journal of Methods-Time Measurement.* March/April 1968;XIII:50–58.

46. Mink JA. MTM and the disabled. *The Journal of Methods-Time Measurement.* 1975;11:23–30.
47. Wilcock R. Some new dimensions on manual skills assessment and training in industry. *The Journal of Methods-Time Measurement.* 1980;7:20–27.
48. Wilcock R, Mink JA. The International MTM Directorate Rehabilitation Project. *The Journal of Methods-Time Measurement.* 1982;9:2–11.
49. International Labor Organization. *Introduction to Work Study.* 2nd ed. Geneva, Switzerland: ILO; 1969.
50. International Labor Organization. *Introduction to Work Study.* 3rd ed. Geneva, Switzerland: ILO; 1986.
51. Frievalds A, Goldberg JH. Specification of bases for variable relaxation allowances: standing, abnormal positions and use of muscular energy. *The Journal of Methods-Time Measurement.* 1969;14:2–7.
52. Frievalds A, Goldberg JH. Specification of bases for variable relaxation allowances: visual strain and low lighting. *The Journal of Methods-Time Measurement.* 1969;14:9–15.
53. Frievalds A, Goldberg JH. Specification of bases for variable relaxation allowances: environmental conditions. *The Journal of Methods-Time Measurement.* 1969;14:16–23.
54. Garg A, Saxena U. Maximum frequency acceptable to female workers for one-handed lifts in the horizontal plane. *Ergonomics.*1982:25:839–853.
55. Rondinelli R. *AMA Guides to Impairment Rating.* 6th ed. Chicago, IL: American Medical Association; 2007:20.

CHAPTER 10

Evaluating Aerobic Capacity

Harriët Wittink, PhD, and Tim Takken, MSc, PhD

Introduction to Aerobic Capacity

Aerobic testing in the workplace may serve two purposes: (1) to assess workers' health for health promotion and (2) to assess workers' capacity for work. In this chapter we address only the testing of workers' capacity for work. Physical fitness is essential for highly demanding and risky occupations, especially when public safety is involved. Physical fitness refers to the human ability to exert physical work. It is a multivariate concept that concerns not only aerobic capacity but also anaerobic capacity, muscular strength, endurance, flexibility, and coordination.[1]

In this chapter, we discuss how aerobic (cardiovascular) capacity relates to one's ability to perform work and how aerobic capacity can be assessed. Maximal aerobic capacity is also called maximal oxygen uptake ($\dot{V}O_2$max) or peak oxygen uptake ($\dot{V}O_2$peak). Expressed as an absolute rate in liters of oxygen per minute (L/min) or as a relative rate in milliliters of oxygen per kilogram of bodyweight per minute (mL/kg/min), it reflects the ability to perform external work and is determined by the performance of the cardiac muscle (O_2 delivery) and efficiency of the muscular system in extracting oxygen from blood for use in generating energy. The $\dot{V}O_2$peak directly affects the amount and intensity of physical activity a person is able to perform. Most physical activities are described in terms of their energy or metabolic cost.[2]

Physical activities are coded in metabolic equivalent (MET) intensity levels. One MET is considered a resting metabolic rate obtained during quiet sitting and equals an oxygen uptake of 3.5 mL/kg/min. The oxygen cost for physical activities ranges from 0.9 MET for sleeping to 18 MET for running at 10.9 mph.[2]

For occupational activities, the energy cost ranges from about 1.5 MET for sitting in a meeting to 17 MET for fast ax chopping in forestry. The higher a person's $\dot{V}O_2$max, the more energy is available to perform physical activities. For an individual person, a higher $\dot{V}O_2$max means that physical activity generates less fatigue or that the person is capable of performing at a higher level of energy demand, ie, "can do more."

Aerobic Capacity and Work Ability

If work demand exceeds a worker's capacity for sustained physical work, inevitably, fatigue will develop. A physiologic limit of 30% to 40% of $\dot{V}O_2$max is thought to be acceptable for an 8-hour work day,[3] although 50% of a worker's

$\dot{V}O_2$max has also been recommended.[4,5] Again, it follows that workers with higher levels of $\dot{V}O_2$peak have a higher capacity for sustained work or that these workers will experience their workload as less fatiguing than workers who have lower levels of $\dot{V}O_2$peak and do the same work. Workers who perform work above their capacity may become unduly fatigued or have insufficient time between their working days to sufficiently recover. Firefighters, for example, need to be highly aerobically fit to be able to perform their job duties. Oxygen uptake during fire suppression ranges from 60% to 80% of maximum with significant cardiopulmonary and thermoregulatory strain.[6] Based on this observation, 38 to 42 mL/kg/min has been most frequently cited as the desirable $\dot{V}O_2$max level for firefighters.[7] This measure indicates average fitness for healthy males younger than 50 years, but an average fit female of any age would not have this aerobic capacity because, on average, women have a 30% lower $\dot{V}O_2$max than do men. Firefighters with a $\dot{V}O_2$peak of less than 33.5 mL/kg/min have been found to be unlikely to safely perform expected work tasks for longer than a few minutes.[8] If the aerobic demand of work cannot be met, premature fatigue can put a person at risk for injury. It has been shown that inactive firefighters have a 90% greater risk of myocardial infarction than firefighters who are aerobically fit.[9]

In the US armed forces, women have more than twice the injury rate of men. For men and women, fewer push-ups, slower 3.2-km run times, lower peak $\dot{V}O_2$, and cigarette smoking were risk factors for time-loss injury. Among the men only, lower levels of physical activity before US Army Basic Combat Training and high and low levels of flexibility were also time-loss injury risk factors. Lower peak $\dot{V}O_2$ and cigarette smoking were independent risk factors for time-loss injury.[10]

Verstraten et al[11] reported an energetic workload of 35% $\dot{V}O_2$max for younger bricklayers (between 25 and 35 years of age) and 41% for older bricklayers (older than 45 years). This finding means that older bricklayers are slightly exceeding their physiologic limit at work. Meijer et al,[12] however, found that greater working heights (30 and 50 cm) for picking up the bricks and mortar significantly reduced oxygen uptake, up to 20%, especially when bricks were placed in the higher rows in the wall (±75-cm height of bricklaying) compared with a situation in which no adaptation was made in the storage height of bricks and mortar. Linden[13] demonstrated an inverse relationship between $\dot{V}O_2$max and absenteeism in customs officers. Gamble et al,[14] in a study on Belfast's ambulance men, showed that the physical demand of a simulated emergency task could be decreased from 81% to 71.4% of $\dot{V}O_2$max through aerobic and strength exercises.

There are several trends in Western society that negatively influence the average $\dot{V}O_2$max of the workforce that are of major concern; one of them is the aging workforce. It has been predicted that in 2025 there will be twice as many workers aged 50 years or older as aged 25 years or younger in the present 15 European Union (EU) member states. The work force of the entire European Union will attain its oldest age during the next 25 years. The International Labor Organization has estimated that by 2025, the proportion of people older than 55 years will be 32% in Europe, 30% in North America, 21% in Asia, and 17% in Latin America.[15] $\dot{V}O_2$max in absolute (L/min) and relative (mL/min/kg) terms shows a clear and linear decline with age among men and women, in part because of the decline of maximal heart rate combined with a reduction in cardiac stroke volume and the concomitant reduction in oxygen transport. In their longitudinal study, Fleg and coworkers[16] showed that the previously defined linear decline of aerobic capacity of 5% to 10% per decade is incorrect, particularly in the later decades of life. They found that the rate of decline in $\dot{V}O_2$max accelerated from 3% to 6% per 10 years in the 20s and 30s to more than 20% per 10 years in the 70s and beyond regardless of physical activity habits. The rate of decline for each decade was larger in men than in women from the 40s onward. The resultant reduction in $\dot{V}O_2$max may reduce the ability of a person to perform sustained work, and recommendations have been made to reduce the physical load of work according to the normal decline of physical capacity for workers older than 45 years.[15] It should be stressed that large individual variation exists and that an active 60-year-old can have more aerobic capacity than a sedentary 30-year-old. About 50% of the individual differences are probably due to genetic factors; the natural endowment can be further developed by physical training through exercise and/or habitual high levels of physical activity such as in physically demanding work.

Unfortunately, the literature reports fairly consistently that physically demanding work does not maintain or improve $\dot{V}O_2$max in aging workers.[17] Heavy manual work does not seem to sufficiently stress the cardiovascular system to produce a training effect in older workers,[18,19] although a positive association between heavy physical work and good cardiorespiratory fitness has been found in young males,[20] similar to Jonsson and Åstrand,[21] who stated that young men who sweat daily at work have better aerobic capacity than their nonperspiring counterparts. Karpansalo et al[22] report that heavy physical workload increases the risk of retirement on disability, especially owing to musculoskeletal disorders. The risk is especially increased among men with musculoskeletal or cardiovascular disease and poor cardiorespiratory fitness. Aerobic capacity thus matters a great deal when performing physically demanding work. Little evidence exists indicating that aerobic capacity matters when performing sedentary work.

Measuring Aerobic Capacity

The $\dot{V}O_2$peak* attained during a graded maximal exercise to volitional exhaustion is considered the single best indicator of aerobic exercise capacity by the World Health Organization.[23] $\dot{V}O_2$max is the reflection of the maximal oxygen flux through the mitochondria of the exercising muscle. Based on the Fick principle, $\dot{V}O_2$max is the product of cardiac output (heart rate × stroke volume) and the mixed arteriovenous oxygen difference.[24] Thus, $\dot{V}O_2$max is dependent on cardiac function and the ability of the muscles to extract (use) oxygen from the circulation. The "gold standard" for determining absolute $\dot{V}O_2$max in a person is by using a metabolic measurement system to analyze oxygen and carbon dioxide in expired air at regular intervals with a "plateauing" of $\dot{V}O_2$ during increasing workloads.[25] However, in many subjects, including children, patients, and athletes, a plateau in $\dot{V}O_2$ is not observed.[26-28] Several secondary parameters have therefore been established to determine $\dot{V}O_2$max without a $\dot{V}O_2$plateau. These parameters include a failure of the heart rate (HR) to increase with further increases in exercise intensity, a respiratory exchange ratio of more than 1.15, and a rating of perceived exertion of more than 17, which equals very hard or strenuous. Nevertheless, a healthy person would be able continue albeit he/she would have to really push him-/herself because it would feel very heavy and the person would be very tired (Borg 6–20 scale).[29]

Maximal HR may be predicted from age by using any of several published equations, such as 220 minus age; however, interindividual variability is quite high (Standard Deviation(SD), 10–12 beats/minute).[25,30] As a result, there is potential for considerable error in the use of methods that extrapolate submaximal test data to an age-predicted HRmax.[31] Tanaka et al[32] showed that the 220 minus age prediction method overestimates HRmax in young adults and progressively underestimates HRmax in adults older than 40 years. Based on a meta-analysis, confirmed by a laboratory study, they propose a regression equation of HRmax = 209 – 0.7 × age (SD 7–11 beats) for healthy, unmedicated, nonsmoking adults. A recent study confirmed a regression equation close to this (HRmax = 207 – 0.7 × age).[33] Because $\dot{V}O_2$max is strongly biased by body weight, it is usually expressed as $\dot{V}O_2$max per milliliter per minute per kilogram of body mass.[25,30] This procedure, however, underestimates the fitness of overweight and obese subjects.[34] Moreover, $\dot{V}O_2$max/kg of body mass also underestimates the $\dot{V}O_2$max of taller subjects.[35] Therefore, several other power equations have been suggested to raise $\dot{V}O_2$max in proportion

---

*Maximal exercise tests in patients are usually terminated when the subject, despite strong verbal encouragement from the experimenters, is unwilling or unable to continue. The appropriate term to use is therefore peak oxygen consumption ($\dot{V}O_2$peak), which represents the highest oxygen uptake during an exercise test to volitional exhaustion. Both terms are used interchangeably throughout this chapter.

to body mass raised to the power of $kg^{0.66}$, $kg^{0.75}$, and $kg^{0.87}$.[36-38] Adjusting body weight according to these formulas allows for a more accurate estimation of a person's $\dot{V}O_2max$ when expressed as $\dot{V}O_2max/mL/kg$.

The mode of exercise testing and the age and sex of the subject determine oxygen uptake with exercise testing. In general, the highest oxygen uptake is achieved with the type of exercise that uses the greatest amount of muscle mass. In healthy subjects, the highest $\dot{V}O_2max$ is obtained with treadmill testing owing to the quantity of the muscle mass involved, followed by bicycle testing. $\dot{V}O_2max$ achieved by bicycle testing is reported to be 5% to 15% lower than with treadmill testing in healthy subjects.[39,40] Åstrand and Rodahl[3] report a 5% to 7% difference in $\dot{V}O_2max$ between treadmill and bicycle testing in well-trained subject. Predicted $\dot{V}O_2max$ in mL/kg/min estimated from arm exercise testing is 60% to 70% of leg exercise in healthy subjects. The intra-arterial blood pressure during arm exercise is higher than in leg exercise at a given oxygen uptake or cardiac output, and the heart rate is also higher. The consequence is a heavier load on the heart. For completely untrained subjects, older subjects, or subjects whose cardiac status is unclear, this mode of exercise testing is not recommended. Healthy women reach 65% to 75% of male $\dot{V}O_2max$.[30] The lower oxygen uptake capacity in women may have to do with their lower hemoglobin concentration and higher body fat content. Per kilogram of lean body mass, $\dot{V}O_2max$ is not different between men and women.

Testing Protocols

In the early days of exercise physiology, it was quite common to use a discontinuous protocol.[25,41] In these protocols, exercise stages were performed on consecutive days until a subject reached his or her $\dot{V}O_2$plateau. These protocols were impractical in clinical and occupational settings because of the time constraints of the subject and laboratory personnel. Therefore, exercise protocols with a much shorter time between exercise stages (several minutes) were designed. The intervals between the exercise stages allowed physiologists to perform several measurements such as blood parameters and other invasive measurements, such muscle biopsies. Currently, most laboratories use continuous exercise protocols, and many different exercise protocols are available. Exercise stages vary from a couple of seconds in the so-called ramp protocols to 3 to 5 minutes if a steady state for most physiologic functions (HR and oxygen uptake). The use of computerized treadmills allows for smaller work increments at a higher frequency. These ramp protocols provide better hemodynamic and gas exchange responses during exercise than the protocols with longer exercise stages (ie, 3–5 minutes).[42,43] Determinations of, for example, the ventilatory anaerobic threshold are easier in protocols with a shorter stage duration. [43,44] Since Hill et al[45-47] described the concept of $\dot{V}O_2$max in 1924, many test protocols have been designed for testing or predicting $\dot{V}O_2$max. In the following section, we describe several exercise testing protocols, including maximal and submaximal exercise tests.

Maximal Exercise Tests

Treadmill Tests

A large number of treadmill protocols have been developed to measure $\dot{V}O_2$max. Pollock et al[48] suggested that $\dot{V}O_2$max could be estimated from exercise time determined by the use of standardized treadmill protocols. In their study, a correlation of $r = 0.88$ was found between exercise time on the Bruce protocol and $\dot{V}O_2$max. Longer walking and running times were associated with higher aerobic capacity.

The Bruce Protocol

The Bruce protocol is the most widely used treadmill protocol in clinical exercise testing.[49] This test was originally developed for cardiac patients by Bruce et al[50] in the 1960s. The test involves a change of speed and elevation every 3 minutes so that the incremental increases for each stage are relatively large for each stage (2–3 MET). Oxygen uptake values expressed in METs were derived from testing healthy subjects and were established for each minute of testing for the Bruce treadmill protocol.[51] In the modified version of the Bruce treadmill protocol, the speed stays constant for the first three stages, starting at 1.7 mph at 0% incline. After the third stage, the speed and grade increase every 3 minutes. McInnis et al[52] compared the modified Bruce and the Bruce protocols in patients with documented coronary artery disease and found that the physiologic responses at matched submaximal rates were similar.

In a sample of 75 patients with chronic low back pain (CLBP), the correlation of $\dot{V}O_2$peak with minutes walked using a symptom-limited, maximal, modified Bruce protocol was $R = 0.70$.[53] After adjustment for age and sex, the relationship was highly significant ($t = 7.49$; $P = .0001$), with more minutes walked on the treadmill resulting in higher peak $\dot{V}O_2$. Age had a significant inverse relationship with time walked ($t = -2.60$; $P = .01$), but sex had no effect ($t = -1.14$; $P = .26$). The relationship of time walked with predicted $\dot{V}O_2$max was also significant ($t = 1.99$; $P = .05$) when adjusted for age and sex, but less so than the relationship between time walked and $\dot{V}O_2$peak.

Disadvantages of the Bruce protocol are large interstage increments in work that can make estimation of $\dot{V}O_2$max less accurate and a fourth stage that can be run or walked, resulting in different oxygen costs.[54]

The Balke Protocol

In the 1950s, Balke[55] and Balke and Ware[56] described a treadmill protocol they used in exercise tests on Air Force personnel. In this protocol, the workload is increased by increasing the angle of the treadmill while the walking speed remains unchanged. Originally a speed of 5.3 km/h and a horizontal angle of the treadmill, with a 1° increase in angle every minute, was used.[55,56] Based on the endurance time or the final angle of the treadmill, an estimation of the $\dot{V}O_2$max could be made by using the following formula[56]:

$$\dot{V}O_2\text{max} = \text{Walking Speed (m/min)} \times \text{Body Mass (kg)} \times (0.73 \times \text{angle}/100) \times 1.8$$

In this formula, the angle is expressed as a percentage, and 1.8 is the factor of the oxygen uptake that is needed to generate 1 m/kg of work. Since the original study by Balke,[55] many modifications have been made[57,58] to limit the exercise time during the treadmill test. The optimal time for an aerobic capacity test is between 8 and 12 minutes, on average.[59]

The Ellestad Protocol

Another treadmill protocol is the Ellestad protocol. This protocol was developed by the American cardiologist Myrvin Ellestad.[60] Originally this test stopped when a subject achieved 95% of predicted peak heart rate. Later this "rule" was dropped and the test was stopped when the subject stopped because of volitional exhaustion. This test starts at a speed of 2.7 km/h with a 10% incline. The speed of the treadmill is increased every 2 or 3 minutes with large uneven steps in workload (1.2–2 km/h). Just as in the Bruce protocol, the first step of the protocol may be too demanding for elderly, unfit, and/or obese subjects.

Comparison of Protocols

Pollock et al[48] compared the Bruce, Balke, and Ellestad protocols in healthy men and found no significant differences in $\dot{V}O_2$max, HRmax, and maximal blood pressure. Prediction equations were established for all three protocols.[48,61–63]

Bicycle Ergometry Testing

Cycle ergometry is one of the oldest methods to measure the exercise capacity of a subject. The first cycle ergometer was developed in 1896 by the French medical student Elisée Bouny. Later, several other mechanically braked and electromagnetically braked cycle ergometers were developed in the United States[64] and Europe.[65]

Maximal Cycle Ergometer Protocols

In Europe, most maximal exercise tests are performed on the cycle ergometer, whereas in North America, the treadmill is more commonly used. This difference reflects the use of the bicycle as a mode of transportation in daily life in Europe. Cycle ergometry has some advantages over treadmill exercise testing: It is portable and less expensive than treadmill testing. Because the body is more stable during cycling and the bicycle is less noisy, blood pressure can be determined more easily and fewer movement artifacts are observed in electrocardiograms during exercise. Moreover, the workload and work efficiency can be precisely determined during cycle ergometry, whereas in treadmill exercise, only an estimation can be calculated. In addition, the $\dot{V}O_2$max can be easily predicted from the peak workload (Wpeak). As a rule of thumb, every watt costs about 10.3 mL O_2/minWpeak, which can be computed as follows when a nonramped protocol has been used.[66]

$$Wpeak = POf + (t/T \times D)$$

Where POf is the power output (W) of the last completed workload, t is the time (in seconds) that the last uncompleted workload was maintained, T is the duration (in seconds) of each completed workload, and D is the power output difference (watt) between consecutive workloads.

The disadvantage of bicycle protocols for American subjects is that many may not be accustomed to cycling and muscular fatigue may occur prematurely, preventing subjects from reaching their maximal capacity. $\dot{V}O_2$max is 10% to 15% lower in cycle vs treadmill testing in subjects not accustomed to cycling.

With computerized ergometers, it is possible to deviate from the conventional protocols in which the workload is increased every 1 to 5 minutes. By using an incremental or ramp approach, there is a smaller increase in workload per time unit, providing a more linear increase in workload, which facilitates the determination of the ventilatory anaerobic threshold.[28] Usually, the ventilatory anaerobic threshold occurs at an exercise intensity between 40% and 60% of $\dot{V}O_2$max. As mentioned previously, an exercise time of between 8 and 12 minutes gives the best quality and quantity of data during clinical exercise tests,[59] which implies that a ramp protocol should be individualized, based on the subject's fitness. For adults, the following method is applied. First, an estimation of $\dot{V}O_2$ during unloaded cycling is made by using the following formula:

$$\dot{V}O_2\text{unloaded (mL/min)} = 150 + (6 \times \text{weight})$$

Thereafter, an estimation of $\dot{V}O_2$max is made by using one of the following formulas:

$$\text{Men: } \dot{V}O_2\text{peak (mL/min)} = (\text{Length [cm]} - \text{Age [years]}) \times 20$$

$$\text{Women: } \dot{V}O_2\text{peak (mL/min)} = (\text{Length [cm]} - \text{Age [years]}) \times 14$$

The increment in workload per minute is calculated as follows:

$$(\dot{V}O_2\text{peak} - \dot{V}O_2\text{unloaded})/100$$

Several prediction equations for $\dot{V}O_2$max and other aerobic parameters such as minute ventilation and HR have been provided in the literature and are given in Table 10–1.

TABLE 10–1   Reference Values for Aerobic Exercise Testing Variables in Healthy Adults[67]

Variable	Equation
Wpeak (kpm/min)*	$20.4 \times \text{Height} - 8.74 \times \text{Age} - 288 \times \text{Sex} - 1909$
$\dot{V}O_2$max (L/min)	$0.0046 \times \text{Height} - 0.021 \times \text{Age} - 0.62 \times \text{Sex} - 4.31$
$\dot{V}O_2$max (mL/min; male)	$W \times (50.75 - 0.372 \times \text{Age})$
$\dot{V}O_2$max (mL/min; female)	$(W + 43) \times (22.78 - 0.17 \times \text{Age})$
HRmax (beats/min)	$202 - 0.72 \times \text{Age}$ $210 - 0.64 \times \text{Age}$
O_2pulse (mL/h)	$0.28 \times \text{Height} - 3.3 \times \text{Sex} - 26.7$ $\dot{V}O_2$max Predicted/HRmax Predicted

TABLE 10–1   Reference Values for Aerobic Exercise Testing Variables in Healthy Adults[67] (continued)

Variable	Equation
VEmax (L/min)	$26.3 \times VC - 34$
VEmax/MVV (%)	$\sim72 \pm 15$
AT (L/min)	$0.024 \times Height - 0.0074 \times age - 2.43$ Normal > 40% of $\dot{V}O_2$max Predicted **Note:** there are two methods to calculate AT

*Peak work load (Wpeak), 6 kpm/min = 1 watt; length, cm; weight (W), kg; sex, 0 = female, 1 = male.
Abbreviations: kpm indicates, kilopond-meter; $\dot{V}O_2$max, maximal oxygen uptake; HR, heart rate; VC, vital capacity; VE, minute ventilation; MVV, maximal voluntary ventilation; and AT, anaerobic threshold

Submaximal Aerobic Tests

It is important to understand that the most accurate way to measure $\dot{V}O_2$max in *one person* is through direct measurement of $\dot{V}O_2$max. In an occupational setting, this is neither practical nor feasible. A variety of submaximal tests have been developed for estimating aerobic capacity when direct measurement is not possible (see Noonan and Dean[68]). These tests usually involve running or walking for a given time or distance, such as the 12-minute walk-run test,[69] the shuttle test,[70] various step tests,[71,72] and the 2-km walk test.[73] Longer distances and shorter test times are associated with higher levels of aerobic fitness. Other tests estimate $\dot{V}O_2$max by submaximal testing and extrapolation to maximal HR by treadmill walking or bicycling against a predetermined load with measurement of HR.[74,75] These tests were primarily developed for testing aerobic capacity in healthy people and were validated by comparing actual measured $\dot{V}O_2$max with predicted $\dot{V}O_2$max or with test performance. Nomograms and prediction equations, derived from exercise testing in large samples of subjects, were developed to estimate $\dot{V}O_2$max in healthy populations. Even though they include corrections for age and sex, they reflect a *mean* aerobic fitness level for a particular sex at a particular age and, therefore, can never be as precise as direct measurement of oxygen uptake. Fear, excitement, and related emotional stress may cause a marked elevation of HR at submaximal work rates without $\dot{V}O_2$max or performance capacity being affected, which results in an underestimation of the person's actual aerobic fitness level when, for example, nomograms are used to extrapolate HR and the workload at maximal heart rates. It is usually recommended that the test load be sufficiently high to bring the HR up to or more than 150 beats per minute in younger subjects.[3] Motivation has a role, especially in timed or distance tests in which the subject can set his or her own pace. Aerobic fitness is more accurately predicted from a submaximal exercise test when the subject is well motivated.[69] Untrained persons often have underestimated predictions of their $\dot{V}O_2$max values.[3] These tests have a measurement error of about 10% to 20% of $\dot{V}O_2$max, which is often unacceptable in the occupational setting when subjects are being tested to determine fitness to perform the demands of their occupations.

Submaximal Cycle Ergometer Protocols

Three frequently reported submaximal bicycle ergometer exercise tests are the physical work capacity (PWC)150, PWC160, or PWC170[76–78]; the Åstrand-Ryhming bicycle ergometer test[69,79–,81]; and the Young Men's Christian Association (YMCA) bicycle test.

1. The PWC tests are performed on a stationary cycle ergometer. The subject is required to pedal continuously at a set pace (50 or 60 rpm). During the 9-minute protocol, the workload is increased twice (at 3 and 6 minutes), making three loads in all. The HR is measured during the last 15 seconds of each load, and the workload increases are regulated so that the HR achieved at the end of the test approaches 150, 160, or 170 beats/min. The workload corresponding to an HR of 150, 160, or 170 beats/min is then extrapolated. The higher this value, the more fit the person. Major criticisms of this method are that it does not account for the decline of maximal HR with age and does not take into account differences in resting HR. Efforts have been undertaken to develop a test that takes predicted maximal HR into account: the PWC75%[82] and the PWC65%.[83]

2. The Åstrand-Ryhming bicycle ergometer test[75] is a submaximal test from which aerobic fitness is measured. Subjects cycle at a measured exercise intensity (50 rpm) while the HR is continuously monitored until a steady state of HR is reached above a target level of 140 beats/min for subjects younger than 50 years and 120 beats/min for older subjects.[3] The workload is then correlated with the HR by using the Åstrand-Ryhming nomogram.[3,75] The obtained value is corrected for age and sex. The nomogram was derived from healthy Scandinavian subjects, which showed underestimated values in untrained persons by 10% to 15%.[3,75] Sanchez and Donoso[84] found an underestimation of 15.4% to 27.7% of predicted $\dot{V}O_2$max using the Åstrand-Ryhming nomogram in Chilean workers. Rowell et al[85] found that the nomogram method underestimated predicted $\dot{V}O_2$max by 26.8% (7.2%) in sedentary healthy subjects. Accuracy of prediction from the nomogram improved with higher levels of aerobic fitness. Differences in maximal and resting HRs also influence predicted $\dot{V}O_2$ in the Åstrand and Ryhming test[75] and, thus, its validity. Attempts have been

made to correct the Åstrand-Ryhming test for resting HR but, unfortunately, have been done only for young men.[86]

3. The YMCA bicycle test is a multistage protocol consisting of three or four consecutive 3-minute stages of continuous exercise.[87] Subjects cycle at a measured exercise intensity (50 rpm) at stage 1 starting at 25 watts (women and less fit men) or 50 watts (men and very fit women) while the HR is continuously monitored. Successive stages depend on HR during stage 1 until a steady state of HR is reached above a target level of 110 to 150 beats/min (the HR range at which the relationship between $\dot{V}O_2$ and workload is most linear). The HR measured during the last minute of each stage is plotted against workload. The line generated from the plotted points is extrapolated to the age-predicted HRmax. A perpendicular line is dropped to the x-axis to estimate the work rate this person would achieve if taken to maximal testing. The HR method using the YMCA $\dot{V}O_2$-HR relationship seems to be effective in predicting energy expenditure during physical activities at submaximal intensities but not at maximum efforts.[88] Although the YMCA test is widely used, the scientific evidence for this test is limited.

Submaximal Treadmill Test Protocols

Ebbeling and coworkers[89] described a submaximal treadmill test for healthy subjects between 20 and 59 years of age. In this test, subjects walk at a safe and comfortable walking speed between 3.2 and 7.2 km/h with an inclination of 0% for 4 minutes, after warm-up. After this stage, the HR should be between 50% and 70% of the predicted HRmax (using 220 – age), and the inclination is increased to 5%. Hereafter, the test is finished, and the cool down–recovery phase starts. The estimated $\dot{V}O_2$max from this test compares well with directly measured $\dot{V}O_2$max in subjects with a $\dot{V}O_2$max less than 60 mL/kg/min (nonelite athletes). However, more research is needed to establish the sensitivity to change of this test.[68] One of the weaknesses of this test is the use of submaximal HRs because many factors can influence HR (eg, medication, ambient temperature, and anxiety). The $\dot{V}O_2$max can be predicted by using the following formula:

$$\dot{V}O_2\text{max (mL/kg/min)} = 15.1 + 21.8 \times (\text{Speed [mph]}) - (0.327 \times \text{HR})$$
$$- (0.263 \times \text{Speed [mph]} \times \text{Age}) + (0.00504 \times \text{HR}$$
$$\times \text{Age}) + (5.98 \times \text{Sex [0, female; 1, male]}).$$

The Fire Department of New York stairmill protocol is used to measure aerobic capacity in firefighters in the United States and Canada. The protocol for this test (and a treadmill protocol) is available at www.swfd.org/iaff.pdf (accessed November 2007). This is a 3-minute, submaximal test. The worker is asked to walk at a constant rate of 60 steps per minute for 3 minutes at level 4, after a warm-up at level 3. The HR is measured during the final 15 seconds of the exercise and recorded. The following equations are used to establish $\dot{V}O_2$max:

$$\text{Males: } \dot{V}O_2\text{max} = 113.34 - 0.15 \times (\text{Weight}) - 0.32 \times (\text{Final HR}) - 0.54 \times (\text{Age})$$

$$\text{Females: } \dot{V}O_2\text{max} = 88.22 - 0.31 \times (\text{Final HR}) - 0.32 \times (\text{Age})$$

Shuttle Run Tests

The 20-m shuttle run test was derived from the Cooper test by the Leger et al[90] as a field test to predict $\dot{V}O_2$max. This test involves continuous running between two lines 20 m apart in time to recorded beeps. For this reason, the test is also often called the "beep" or "bleep" test. The time between recorded beeps decreases each minute (level). There are several versions of the test, but one commonly used version has an initial running velocity of 8.0 km/h, which increases by 0.5 km/h each minute. Recently, a square shuttle run test was developed, which seems to better estimate the $\dot{V}O_2$peak.[91]

Field Tests

Shuttle Walk-Run Tests

Because the first step of the shuttle test was too demanding for many clinical patients, modifications of the original shuttle test were made. These tests started at a much lower level of 1.8, 2, or 5 km/h instead of at 8 km/h.[92-94] Singh et al[92] developed a shuttle walking test for patients with pulmonary disease. This test started at 1.8 km/h, with an increase in walking velocity of 0.55 km/h each minute. Patients had to walk at these increasing speeds back and forth on a 10-m course until fatigue. Bradley et al[93] modified this test by adding several more demanding shuttles and allowing the patients to run during the test.

Verschuren et al[94] modified the original shuttle run protocol for subjects with mild cerebral palsy. Subjects started at a much lower speed, depending on functional ability, and the speed was increased at a much lower rate (0.2 km/h/min).

Walk Tests

Walk tests have become more and more popular to assess aerobic capacity in clinical settings. Since the introduction of the 15-minute walking test by Balke[95] in 1963, several investigators have used a walk test in research and clinical practice. Cooper[69] originally developed a 12-minute run test. In the years after publication of the test developed by Cooper,[69] many modifications have been made. One of these modifications is the 6-minute walk test[96] for patients. The 6-minute walk test provides a simple, relatively quick, inexpensive, and safe test.[97] The 6-minute walk test has been used for different kinds of measurements. It has replaced the symptom-limited cardiopulmonary exercise test[98] and has been used to evaluate the efficacy of a therapy or to establish a prognosis.[99,100]

Solway et al[101] identified the 6-minute walk test as the test of choice when using a functional walk test for clinical or research purposes. Most research on this test has been done in patients with cardiac or chronic obstructive pulmonary disease, but the 6-minute walk test might be the preferred method to determine the functional capacity of people with rheumatic disease.[102] Gibbons et al[103] reported that some familiarity with the test is required. Reliability is optimized when the administration of walk tests is standardized according to the guidelines of the American Thoracic Society[104] and one practice walk is performed. The guidelines of the American Thoracic Society also provide standardized encouragements during the test. The distance covered by the patients can be compared with several prediction equations obtained from data of healthy subjects (Table 10–2). From both distances, a percentage of predicted distance can be calculated by using the equations, several of which have been established. It is recommended to use the equation most comparable with the age group of the patients being tested.

TABLE 10–2   Prediction Equations for the 6-Minute Walk Test in Healthy Subjects

Author	Subject Age, y	Track Length, M	Prediction Equation (m)
Troosters et al[105]	50–85	50	Distance = 218 + (5.14 × Height [cm] – 5.32 × Age [y]) – (1.80 × Weight [kg]) + 51.31 × Sex [1, male; 0, female]
Gibbons et al[103]	20–80	20	Distance = 868.8 – (2.99 × Age) – 74.7 × Sex [male, 0; female, 1]
Enright and Sherrill[106]	40–80	30	Male: Distance = (7.57 × Height [cm]) – 5.02 × Age [y] – (1.76 × Weight [kg]) – 309 Female: Distance = (2.11 × Height [cm]) – 2.29 × Weight – (5.78 × Age) + 667

CHAPTER 10

Another test is the Pack Test. This is a work capacity test that consists of a 4.83-km (3-mile) hike over level terrain carrying a 20.5-kg (45-pound) pack used to assess job-related work capacity for wildland firefighters.[107] To qualify for arduous fire-line work, a worker must complete the pack test in 45 minutes or less. Jogging during the test is not permitted. Tests taken at altitude should be adjusted (Table 10–3).

TABLE 10–3   Correction for Altitude in the Pack Test Performance*

Altitude (ft) for 3-mi Test	Correction for the Pack Test (s)
4000	30
5000	45
6000	60
7000	75
8000	90

*Add the correction to the required test time.

The energy cost of the Pack Test is similar to fire-line work. Pack Test performance relates directly to muscular fitness. Because of the test distance, the Pack Test is an excellent indicator of a person's capacity to perform prolonged arduous work under adverse conditions and functional reserve to meet unforeseen emergencies.

Additional field tests for wildland firefighters were developed to qualify people for moderate and light duties (Table 10–4).

TABLE 10–4   Additional Field Tests to Assess Fitness in US Wildland Firefighters*

Fitness Requirement	Test	Description
Arduous (45 mL/kg/min), lift > 50 lb	Pack	3-mi hike with 45-lb pack in 45 min
Moderate (40 mL/kg/min), lift 25–50 lb	Field	2-mi hike with 25-lb pack in 30 min
Light (35 mL/kg/min), light lifting	Walk	1-mi hike in 16 min

*Source: "The Pack Test" Work Capacity Testing for Wildland Firefighters: Ensuring Wildland Firefighters Safety. USDA March 2002. Available at: www.fs.fed.us/fire/safety/wct/2002/PackTest_Info_Sheet.pdf

Step Tests

The first step test was developed in the Harvard Fatigue Laboratory during World War II by Brouha et al.[108] This test was developed as a simple field measure to assess exercise capacity, especially in the military setting.

During this so-called Harvard Step Test, subjects had to step up and down on a 20-in platform step at a rate of 30 steps per minute for 5 minutes or until exhaustion. For most subjects, it was a submaximal test. On completion of the test, the subject immediately sits down, and the total number of heartbeats is counted between 1 and 1.5 minutes after the subject finished the test. From this value, a fitness index is calculated, providing a poor, average, or good rating. The correlation between this test and directly measured $\dot{V}O_2$ is moderate to large ($r = 0.6$ to 0.8).[108] Several other step tests have been developed since 1943, including the Queens College Step Test, Home Step Test, Chester Step Test, and the Canadian Home Fitness Test. The advantages of these tests are the lack of equipment needed, low costs, and ease of administration (can be self-administered). Step tests have the disadvantage that anthropometric factors (eg, leg length and body mass) are often not considered in the score, although it is known that these factors have a role in test performance. Moreover, the reliability of the recovery HR is not always very high because of large day-to-day variability.[109] Step tests may not be suitable for people whose ability to balance is diminished because no handrail is used.[68] It is also difficult to monitor people while they are stepping, and several medications can alter the HR response (eg, beta blockers and methylphenidate). Further studies are needed to validate step tests for people with various diagnoses.

When to Test Aerobic Capacity

The US Department of Labor *Dictionary of Occupational Titles* (DOT) provides information about the work characteristics of most jobs in the United States in terms of the physical demands that these jobs place on the workers. In the DOT, the energy requirements of jobs are defined. The energy requirements range from 1.5 to 2.1 MET (5.3 to 7.4 mL/kg/min) for sedentary work to more than 7.5 METs (> 26.3 mL/kg/min) for very heavy work. Using a physiologic limit of 40% $\dot{V}O_2$max for an 8-hour working day[3] means that a sedentary worker should have an aerobic capacity of 3.8 to 5.3 MET (13.3 to 18.5 mL/kg/min) to perform work without undue fatigue. Average "fair" normative values for all age groups in men and women are well beyond this, suggesting that aerobic capacity testing is not necessary for all workers with sedentary jobs. Workers, however, who have had a prolonged period of immobilization or bed rest may have profound deconditioning and should be tested. Also, workers who have (or had) conditions or medical treatments that affect $\dot{V}O_2$max (eg, cardiopulmonary, central or peripheral neurologic problems, and chemotherapy) should be tested aerobically. Aerobic testing should be a standard part of physical capacity determination[110-113] to ensure that a worker is capable of meeting the energy requirement of the job when the physical demand level of the job is medium or high, especially for workers who are women older than 40 years or men older than 50 years. In these age groups, the energy requirement of the physical work demands begins to exceed "fair" aerobic capacity.

Choosing a Test

Care should be taken to ensure that the aerobic capacity tests used are appropriate for the job requirement to ensure validity of the test results. A job-specific functional capacity evaluation (FCE) will better simulate the work situation by providing higher validity for fitting the energy demands of the job to a person's aerobic capacity. Bicycle tests may be preferred for workers with gait or balance problems or when doing an exercise electrocardiogram. The protocol should be tailored to the person to yield a fatigue-limited exercise duration of approximately 10 minutes. Shorter durations may produce a nonlinear relationship between $\dot{V}O_2$ and work rate, whereas durations of more than 12 minutes may cause subjects to terminate exercise because of muscle fatigue or orthopedic problems.[114] It makes sense to choose a test that will not exacerbate a musculoskeletal problem. For example, a step test may not be the best test to assess aerobic capacity in a worker with knee problems. The test may be stopped prematurely owing to an increase of pain or symptoms, making interpretation of the test difficult. A modified version of a test may be chosen in a disabled population. In a sample of patients with CLBP, for example, 17% of the sample was unable to complete the initial stage of the Bruce protocol (walking at 1.7 mph at 10% grade).[115] For this population, the modified Bruce treadmill test may be a better option. Treadmill, bicycle, and upper extremity ergometry[116] exercise testing were compared in a small sample of 30 patients with CLBP. Significantly higher HRs, peak $\dot{V}O_2$, and predicted $\dot{V}O_2$max in mL/kg/min were achieved with the modified Bruce treadmill test than with the bicycle or upper extremity ergometry tests, despite pain.

Drawing Conclusions

When possible, it is recommended that $\dot{V}O_2$peak be measured directly in a maximal exercise test using a metabolic measurement system, especially in a population more likely to be limited by pain than by cardiac output. With enough data points, the $\dot{V}O_2$max can be estimated from the work rate achieved at a submaximal HR, but a significant potential for error exists owing to the 10- to 12-beat/min SD in the HRmax in healthy people. When people stop testing prematurely because of pain, the test result is more a reflection of what a person is willing and able to do than of aerobic capacity. The chosen protocol may have been too demanding or the worker insufficiently motivated or in too much pain to tolerate testing. Motivation always has a role in aerobic capacity testing, as is true for all FCE tests, and test results should be compared with other FCE test results. Did the worker perform badly on all tests that load the affected body part? It is, for example, unlikely that a worker who is able to come to the clinic, park the car, and walk at least 10 minutes to the testing site would be unable to walk for more than 2 minutes on a treadmill. Verbal encouragement is important during FCE testing to ensure that the subject is maximally motivated.

Various criteria for maximal effort during an exercise test have been proposed, with the most commonly used criteria for maximal effort as follows: the occurrence of a $\dot{V}O_2$plateau, a blood lactate concentration 3 minutes after the end of the test higher than 8 mmol/L, a respiratory exchange ratio of more than 1.1, an HRpeak within 10 beats of the age-predicted HRmax, a rating of perceived exertion on the 6–20 Borg scale[117] of 18 or more, a reduced pedal rate during cycling, and signs of subject exhaustion and/or intense effort.[114]

Summary

Aerobic capacity is an important part of an FCE and is indicated to determine whether a patient does or does not have the aerobic capacity to perform work or activities of daily living. There is a wealth of exercise test procedures for the direct and indirect evaluation of aerobic capacity. In this chapter, we have reviewed the most commonly used test procedures in the occupational and clinical settings. Exercise testing should be matched in a mode selection that is closest to the job activity.

References

1. Bouchard C, Shephard R. Physical activity, fitness and health: the model and key concepts: physical activity, fitness and health. International proceedings and consensus statement. Champaign, IL: Human Kinetics; 1994:77–88.

2. Ainsworth BE, Haskell WL, Whitt MC, et al. Compendium of physical activities: an update of activity codes and MET intensities. *Med Sci Sports Exerc.* 2000;32(9 suppl):S498-S504.

3. Åstrand P, Rodahl K. *Textbook of Work Physiology: Physiological Bases of Exercise.* 3rd ed. New York, NY: McGraw-Hill Book Co; 1986.

4. Ilmarinen J. Job design for the aged with regard to decline in their maximal aerobic capacity, part I: guidelines for the practitioner. *Int J Ind Ergon.* 1992; 10:53–77.

5. Ilmarinen J. Job design for the aged with regard to decline in their maximal aerobic capacity, part II: the scientific base for the guide. *Int J Ind Ergon.* 1992; 10:53–77.

6. Lemon PW, Hermiston RT. The human energy cost of fire fighting. *J Occup Med.* 1977;19:558–562.

7. Sothmann MS, Landy F, Saupe K. Age as a bona fide occupational qualification for firefighting: a review on the importance of measuring aerobic power. *J Occup Med.* 1992;34:26–33.

8. International Association of Fire Fighters. *Fire Service Joint Labor Management Wellness-Fitness Initiative.* 2nd ed. Washington, DC: IAFF; 1999.

9. Peate WF, Lundergan L, Johnson JJ. Fitness self-perception and VO_2max in firefighters. *J Occup Environ Med.* 2002;44:546–550.

10. Knapik JJ, Sharp MA, Canham-Chervak M, Hauret K, Patton JF, Jones BH. Risk factors for training-related injuries among men and women in basic combat training. *Med Sci Sports Exerc.* 2001;33:946–954.

11. Verstraten PJFD, Beekman IA, Binkhorst RA. The physiological stress and strain of bricklayers in construction industry [dissertation]. Department of Physiology, University of Nijmegen, The Netherlands, 1987.

12. Meijer MJF, Bulthuis BM, Brinkhorst RA. The load on bricklayers: the influence of work pace on physiological and perceived load on the bricklayer [dissertation]. Department of Physiology, University of Nijmegen, The Netherlands, 1988.

13. Linden V. Absence from work and physical fitness. *Br J Ind Med.* 1969;26:50–53.

14. Gamble RP, Boreham CA, Stevens AB. Effects of a 10-week exercise intervention programme on exercise and work capacities in Belfast's ambulance-men. *Occup Med (Lond).* 1993;43:85–89.

15. Ilmarinen JE. Aging workers. *Occup Environ Med.* 2001;58:546–552.

16. Fleg JL, Morrell CH, Bos AG, et al. Accelerated longitudinal decline of aerobic capacity in healthy older adults. *Circulation.* 2005;112:674–682.

17. Nygard CH, Luopajarvi T, Ilmarinen J. Musculoskeletal capacity and its changes among aging municipal employees in different work categories. *Scand J Work Environ Health.* 1991;17(suppl 1):110–117.

18. Ilmarinen J, Louhevaara V, Korhonen O, Nygard CH, Hakola T, Suvanto S. Changes in maximal cardiorespiratory capacity among aging municipal employees. *Scand J Work Environ Health.* 1991;17(suppl 1):99–109.

19. Savinainen M, Nygard CH, Ilmarinen J. A 16-year follow-up study of physical capacity in relation to perceived workload among ageing employees. *Ergonomics.* 2004;47:1087–1102.

20. Tammelin T, Nayha S, Rintamaki H. Cardiorespiratory fitness of males and females of northern Finland birth cohort of 1966 at age 31. *Int J Sports Med.* 2004;25:547–552.

21. Jonsson BG, Åstrand I. Physical work capacity in men and women aged 18 to 65. *Scand J Soc Med.* 1979;7:131–142.

22. Karpansalo M, Manninen P, Lakka TA, Kauhanen J, Rauramaa R, Salonen JT. Physical workload and risk of early retirement: prospective population-based study among middle-aged men. *J Occup Environ Med.* 2002;44:930–939.

23. Shephard RJ, Allen C, Benade AJ, et al. The maximum oxygen intake: an international reference standard of cardiorespiratory fitness. *Bull World Health Organ.* 1968;38:757–764.

24. Fick A. *Ueber die Messung des Blutquantums in den Herzventrikeln.* Wurzburg, Germany: Report of the XIV Session of the Physical-Medical Society, Würzburg; 1870: XVI.

25. Taylor HL, Buskirk E, Henschel A. Maximal oxygen intake as an objective measure of cardiorespiratory performance. *J Appl Physiol.* 1955;8:73–80.

26. Rowland TW. Does peak $\dot{V}O_2$ reflect $\dot{V}O_2$max in children? evidence from supramaximal testing. *Med Sci Sports Exerc.* 1993;25:689–693.

27. Lucia A, Rabadan M, Hoyos J, et al. Frequency of the $\dot{V}O_2$max plateau phenomenon in world-class cyclists. *Int J Sports Med.* 2006;27:984–992.

28. Wasserman K, Hansen JE, Sue DY, Casaburi R, Whipp BJ. *Principles of Exercise Testing and Interpretation.* 3rd ed. Baltimore, MD: Lippincott Williams & Wilkins; 1999.

29. Howley ET, Bassett DRJ, Welch HG. Criteria for maximal oxygen uptake: review and commentary. *Med Sci Sports Exerc.* 1995;27:1292–1301.

30. Åstrand PO. *Experimental Studies of Physical Work Capacity in Relation to Sex and Age.* Copenhagen, Denmark: Munkgaard; 1952.

31. American College of Sports Medicine. *ACSM's Guidelines for Exercise Testing and Prescription.* 6th ed. Philadelphia, PA: Lippincott Williams & Wilkins; 2000.

32. Tanaka H, Monahan KD, Seals DR. Age-predicted maximal heart rate revisited. *J Am Coll Cardiol.* 2001;37:153–156.

33. Gellish RL, Goslin BR, Olson RE, McDonald A, Russi GD, Moudgil VK. Longitudinal modeling of the relationship between age and maximal heart rate. *Med Sci Sports Exerc.* 2007;39:822–829.

34. Owens S, Gutin B. Exercise testing of the child with obesity. *Pediatr Cardiol.* 1999;20:79–83.

35. Tanner JM. Fallacy of per weight and per surface area standards and their relation to spurious correlation. *J Appl Physiol.* 1949;2:1–15.

36. Schmidt-Nielsen K. *Scaling: Why Is Animal Size So Important?* Cambridge, England: Cambridge University Press; 1984.

37. Kleiber M. Body size and metabolism. *Hilgardia.* 1932;6:315–353.

38. Weibel ER, Hoppeler H. Exercise-induced maximal metabolic rate scales with muscle aerobic capacity. *J Exp Biol.* 2005;208(pt 9):1635–1644.

39. Hermansen L, Saltin B. Oxygen uptake during maximal treadmill and bicycle exercise. *J Appl Physiol.* 1969;26:31–37.

CHAPTER 10

40. Hermansen L, Ekblom B, Saltin B. Cardiac output during submaximal and maximal treadmill and bicycle exercise. *J Appl Physiol.* 1970;29:82–86.

41. Mitchell JH, Blomqvist G. Maximal oxygen uptake. *N Engl J Med.* 1971;284:1018–1022.

42. Will PM, Walter JD. Exercise testing: improving performance with a ramped Bruce protocol. *Am Heart J.* 1999;138(6 pt 1):1033–1037.

43. Myers J, Buchanan N, Walsh D, et al. Comparison of the ramp versus standard exercise protocols. *J Am Coll Cardiol.* 1991;17:1334–1342.

44. Whipp BJ, Davis JA, Torres F, Wasserman K. A test to determine parameters of aerobic function during exercise. *J Appl Physiol.* 1981;50:217–221.

45. Hill AV, Long CNH, Lupton H. Muscular exercise, lactic acid and the supply and use of oxygen, part I. *Proc R Soc Biol.* 1924;96:438–475.

46. Hill AV, Long CNH, Lupton H. Muscular exercise, lactic acid and the supply and use of oxygen, part II. *Proc R Soc Biol.* 1924;96:438–475.

47. Hill AV, Long CNH, Lupton H. Muscular exercise, lactic acid and the supply and use of oxygen, part III. *Proc R Soc Biol.* 1924;96:438–475.

48. Pollock ML, Bohannon RL, Cooper KH, et al. A comparative analysis of four protocols for maximal treadmill stress testing. *Am Heart J.* 1976;92:39–46.

49. Bruce RA. Exercise testing for evaluation of ventricular function. *N Engl J Med.* 1977;296:671–675.

50. Bruce RA, Blackmon JR, Jones JW, Strait G. Exercise testing in adult normal subjects and cardiac patients. *Pediatrics.* 1963;32(suppl):742–756.

51. American College of Sports Medicine. *Guidelines for Exercise Testing and Prescription.* 4th ed. Philadelphia, PA: Lea and Febiger; 1991.

52. McInnis K, Balady G, Weiner D, Ryan T. Comparison of ischaemic and physiologic responses during exercise tests in men using the standard and modified Bruce protocols. *Am J Cardiol.* 1992;69:84–89.

53. Wittink H, Rogers W, Gascon C, Sukiennik A, Carr DB. Relative contribution of mental health and exercise-related pain increment to treadmill test intolerance in patients with chronic low back pain. *Spine.* 2001;26:2368–2374.

54. Fletcher GF, Balady GJ, Amsterdam EA, et al. Exercise standards for testing and training: a statement for healthcare professionals from the American Heart Association. *Circulation.* 2001;104:1694–1740.

55. Balke B. Optimum physical working capacity, its measurement and change as a result of the working fatigue [in German]. *Arbeitsphysiologie.* 1954;15:311–323.

56. Balke B, Ware RW. An experimental study of physical fitness of Air Force personnel. *U S Armed Forces Med J.* 1959;10:675–688.

57. Grumet J, Hizon J, Froelicher V. Special considerations in exercise testing: protocols, equipment, and testing athletes. *Prim Care.* 1994;21:459–474.

58. Rowland TW. Crusading for the Balke protocol. *Pediatr Exerc Sci.* 1999;11:189–192.

59. Buchfuhrer MJ, Hansen JE, Robinson TE, Sue DY, Wasserman K, Whipp BJ. Optimizing the exercise protocol for cardiopulmonary assessment. *J Appl Physiol.* 1983;55:1558–1564.

60. Ellestad M. *Stress Testing.* Oxford, UK: Oxford University Press; 2003.

61. Froehlicher V, Thompson A, Davis G, Triebwasser J. Prediction of maximal oxygen consumption: comparison of the Bruce and Balke treadmill protocols. *Chest.* 1975;68:331–336.

62. Foster C, Jackson AS, Pollock ML, et al. Generalized equations for predicting functional capacity from treadmill performance. *Am Heart J.* 1984;107:1229–1234.

63. Bruce R, Kusumi F, Hosmer D. Maximal oxygen intake and nomographic assessment of functional aerobic impairment in cardiovascular disease. *Am Heart J.* 1973;85:546–562.

64. Benedict FG, Cady WG. *A Bicycle Ergometer With an Electric Brake.* Washington, DC: Carnegie Institute of Washington; 1912. Publication no167.

65. Krogh A. A bicycle ergometer and respiration apparatus for the experimental study of muscular work. *Scand Arch Physiol.* 1913;33:375–380.

66. Kuipers H, Verstappen FT, Keizer HA, Geurten P, van Kranenburg G. Variability of aerobic performance in the laboratory and its physiologic correlates. *Int J Sports Med.* 1985;6:197–201.

67. ATS/ACCP Statement on cardiopulmonary exercise testing. *Am J Respir Crit Care Med.* 2003;167:211–277.

68. Noonan V, Dean E. Submaximal exercise testing: clinical application and interpretation. *Phys Ther.* 2000;80:782–807.

69. Cooper KH. A means of assessing maximal oxygen intake: correlation between field and treadmill testing. *JAMA.* 1968;203:201–204.

70. Siconolfi SF, Garber CE, Lasater TM, Carleton RA. A simple, valid step test for estimating maximal oxygen uptake in epidemiologic studies. *Am J Epidemiol.* 1985;121:382–390.

71. Leger LA, Lambert J. A maximal multistage 20-m shuttle run test to predict $\dot{V}O_2$max. *Eur J Appl Physiol Occup Physiol.* 1982;49:1–12.

72. Francis KT. Fitness assessment using step tests. *Compr Ther.* 1987;13:36–41.

73. Oja P, Laukkanen R, Pasanen M, Tyry T, Vuori I. A 2-km walking test for assessing the cardiorespiratory fitness of healthy adults. *Int J Sports Med.* 1991; 12:356–362.

74. Åstrand I. Aerobic work capacity in men and women with special reference to age. *Acta Physiol Scand.* 1960;49:1–92.

75. Åstrand PO, Ryhming I. A nomogram for calculation of aerobic capacity (physical fitness) from pulse rate during submaximal work. *J Appl Physiol.* 1954;7:218–221.

76. Sjostrand T. Changes in the respiratory organs of workmen at an ore smelting works. *Acta Med Scand.* 1947;196(suppl):S687–S699.

77. Cady L, Bischoff D, O'Connell E, Thomas P, Allan J. Strength and fitness and subsequent back injuries in firefighters. *J Occup Med.* 1979;21:269–272.

78. McQuade K, Turner J, Buchner DM. Physical fitness and chronic low back pain; an analysis of the relationship among fitness, functional limitations and depression. *Clin Orthop.* 1988;233:198–204.

79. Hurri H, Mellin G, Korhonen O, Harjula R, Harkapaa K, Luoma J. Aerobic capacity among chronic low-back-pain patients. *J Spinal Disord.* 1991;4:34–38.

80. Lindstrom I, Ohlund C, Eek C, et al. The effect of graded activity on patients with subacute low back pain: a randomized prospective clinical study with an operant-conditioning behavioral approach. *Phys Ther.* 1992;72:279–290.

81. Kellett KM, Kellett DA, Nordholm LA. Effects of an exercise program on sick leave due to back pain. *Phys Ther.* 1991;71:283–291.

82. Gore CJ, Booth ML, Bauman A, Owen N. Utility of pwc75% as an estimate of aerobic power in epidemiological and population-based studies. *Med Sci Sports Exerc.* 1999;31:348–351.

CHAPTER 10

83. Nielens H, Boisset V, Masquelier E. Fitness and perceived exertion in patients with fibromyalgia syndrome. *Clin J Pain.* 2000 Sep;16(3):209–213.

84. Sanchez J, Donoso H. Maximal oxygen uptake in Chilean workers of normal nutritional status. *Eur J Appl Physiol Occup Physiol.* 1988;57:26–32.

85. Rowell LB, Taylor HL, Wang Y. Limitations to prediction of maximal oxygen uptake. *J Appl Physiol.* 1964;19:919–927.

86. Legge BJ, Banister EW. The Åstrand-Ryhming nomogram revisited. *J Appl Physiol.* 1986;61:1203–1209.

87. Golding LA. YMCA *Fitness Testing and Assessment Manual.* Champaign, IL: Human Kinetics Publishers; 1989.

88. Garatachea N, Cavalcanti E, Garcia-Lopez D, Gonzalez-Gallego J, de Paz JA. Estimation of energy expenditure in healthy adults from the YMCA submaximal cycle ergometer test. *Eval Health Prof.* 2007;30:138–149.

89. Ebbeling CB, Ward A, Puleo EM, Widrick J, Rippe JM. Development of a single-stage submaximal treadmill walking test. *Med Sci Sports Exerc.* 1991;23:966–973.

90. Leger LA, Mercier D, Gadoury C, Lambert J. The multistage 20 metre shuttle run test for aerobic fitness. *J Sports Sci.* 1988;6:93–101.

91. Metsios GS, Flouris AD, Koutedakis Y, Nevill A. Criterion-related validity and test-retest reliability of the 20-m Square Shuttle Test. *J Sci Med Sport.* 2008; 11:214–217.

92. Singh SJ, Morgan MD, Scott S, Walters D, Hardman AE. Development of a shuttle walking test of disability in patients with chronic airways obstruction. *Thorax.* 1992;47:1019–1024.

93. Bradley J, Howard J, Wallace E, Elborn S. Validity of a modified shuttle test in adult cystic fibrosis. *Thorax.* 1999;54:437–439.

94. Verschuren O, Takken T, Ketelaar M, Gorter JW, Helders PJ. Reliability and validity of data for 2 newly developed shuttle run tests in children with cerebral palsy. *Phys Ther.* 2006;86:1107–1117.

95. Balke B. A simple field test for the assessment of physical fitness. *Report Civil Aeromedical Research Institute.* 1963;53:1–8.

96. Butland RJ, Pang J, Gross ER, Woodcock AA, Geddes DM. Two-, six-, and 12-minute walking tests in respiratory disease. *Br Med J Clin Res Ed.* 1982; 284:1607–1608.

97. Sadaria KS, Bohannon RW. The 6-minute walk test: a brief review of literature. *Clin Exerc Physiol.* 2001;3:127–132.

98. Nixon PA, Joswiak ML, Fricker FJ. A six-minute walk test for assessing exercise tolerance in severely ill children. *J Pediatr.* 1996;129:362–366.

99. Foley A, Halbert J, Hewitt T, Crotty M. Does hydrotherapy improve strength and physical function in patients with osteoarthritis: a randomised controlled trial comparing a gym based and a hydrotherapy based strengthening programme. *Ann Rheum Dis.* 2003;62:1162–1167.

100. Guimaraes GV, Bellotti G, Bacal F, Mocelin A, Bocchi EA. Can the cardiopulmonary 6-minute walk test reproduce the usual activities of patients with heart failure? *Arq Bras Cardiol.* 2002;78:553–560.

101. Solway S, Brooks D, Lacasse Y, Thomas S. A qualitative systematic overview of the measurement properties of functional walk tests used in the cardiorespiratory domain. *Chest.* 2001;119:256–270.

102. Minor MA, Kay DR. Arthritis. In: Durstine JL, ed. *ACSM's Exercise Management for Persons With Chronic Diseases and Disabilities*. Champaign, IL: Human Kinetics; 1997:149–154.

103. Gibbons WJ, Fruchter N, Sloan S, Levy RD. Reference values for a multiple repetition 6-minute walk test in healthy adults older than 20 years. *J Cardiopulm Rehabil*. 2001;21:87–93.

104. Crapo RO, Casaburi R, Coates AL, Enright PL, et al. ATS statement: guidelines for the six-minute walk test. *Am J Respir Crit Care Med*. 2002;166:111–117.

105. Troosters T, Gosselink R, Decramer M. Six minute walking distance in healthy elderly subjects. *Eur Respir J*. 1999;14:270–274.

106. Enright PL, Sherrill DL. Reference equations for the six-minute walk in healthy adults. *Am J Respir Crit Care Med*. 1998;158(5 pt 1):1384–1387.

107. USDA Fire and Aviation Management. Wildland Fire Safety. Fit to Work. Available at: www.fs.fed.us/fire/safety/fitness/fit_work/fit_pg5.html. Accessed October 13, 2008.

108. Brouha L, Health CW, Graybiel A. A Step Test. A simple method of measuring physical fitness for hard muscular work in adult men. *Rev Can Biol*. 1943;2:89–91.

109. Takken T, van der Net J, Helders PJ. The reliability of an aerobic and an anaerobic exercise tolerance test in patients with juvenile onset dermatomyositis. *J Rheumatol*. 2005;32:734–739.

110. Pohjonen T. Age-related physical fitness and the predictive values of fitness tests for work ability in home care work. *J Occup Environ Med*. 2001;43:723–730.

111. Bilzon JL, Allsopp AJ, Tipton MJ. Assessment of physical fitness for occupations encompassing load-carriage tasks. *Occup Med (Lond)*. 2001;51:357–361.

112. Bilzon JL, Scarpello EG, Smith CV, Ravenhill NA, Rayson MP. Characterization of the metabolic demands of simulated shipboard Royal Navy fire-fighting tasks. *Ergonomics*. 2001;44:766–780.

113. Colledge AL, Johns REJ, Thomas MH. Functional ability assessment: guidelines for the workplace. *J Occup Environ Med*. 1999;41:172–180.

114. Fleg JL, Pina IL, Balady GJ, et al. Assessment of functional capacity in clinical and research applications: an advisory from the Committee on Exercise, Rehabilitation, and Prevention, Council on Clinical Cardiology, American Heart Association. *Circulation*. 2000;102:1591–1597.

115. Wittink HM. Physical fitness, function and physical therapy in patients with pain: clinical measures of aerobic fitness and performance in patients with chronic low back pain. In: Max M, ed. Pain 1999; An Updated Review [refresher course syllabus]. Seattle, WA: IASP Press; 1999:137–145.

116. Wittink H, Michel TH, Kulich R, et al. Aerobic fitness testing in patients with chronic low back pain: which test is best? *Spine*. 2000;25:1704–1710.

117. Borg G. Psychophysical basis of perceived exertion. *Med Sci Sports Exerc*. 1982; 14:377–381.

CHAPTER 10

11

Assessing Evaluee Effort

Bhagwant S. Sindhu, PhD, OTR and Phyllis M. King, PhD OT, FAOTA

Functional capacity evaluations (FCEs) have been reported to accurately describe work-related functional ability only when a person exerts a "sincere,"* maximal voluntary effort.[1-4] Submaximal effort may be exerted by a person during functional evaluation and treatment for a variety of reasons, unintentional or intentional. Submaximal effort may be unintentional owing to injury-related factors such as pain, fear of pain, and fear of reinjury.[2,5-8] In contrast, intentional submaximal effort, which has been termed *insincere, low, less than maximal,* and *less than honest* effort, may be exerted by an injured worker to exaggerate disability.[3,9-14] *Disability exaggeration,* also called "symptom magnification" and "malingering," has been defined as "intentional production of false or grossly exaggerated physical or psychological symptoms, motivated by external incentives such as avoiding military duty, avoiding work, obtaining financial compensation, evading criminal prosecution, or obtaining drugs."[15] The probable prevalence of disability exaggeration in personal injury litigation, workers' compensation, and disability claims has been reported to be between 25% and 30%.[16-18] Disability exaggeration results in a significant financial burden on the society. Correctly identifying workers who intentionally exert submaximal effort during an FCE is one way of reducing this burden.

Maximal vs Submaximal Efforts

Physiologic differences between maximal and submaximal efforts exist at the level of the neuromuscular junction and in the sensory feedback system. A neurophysiologic model of maximal and submaximal efforts, based on the German literature of the 1950s and 1960s,[19,20] has been described by Kroemer and Marras.[11,21-24] According to Kroemer and Marras,[23] an executive program regulates muscular contraction based on a strength output profile. This program originates in the cerebral and cerebellar regions of the central nervous system (CNS) and regulates force output using two strategies—rate coding and recruitment coding—at the neuromuscular junction.[23] *Rate coding* is the speed or frequency of motor neuron firing, whereas *recruitment coding* refers to the sequence of motor unit activation. Maximal effort requires maximal motor neuron firing and maximal recruitment of motor units. In contrast, submaximal effort requires the motor cortex to mix and precisely control the frequency of motor neuron firing and recruitment of a certain number and type of motor units.[21,23,25-27] Maximal and submaximal efforts also require different levels of

---

*Use of the phrase "sincerity-of-effort" and similar terms and phrases reflects common language found in the literature and is not meant to reflect intent.

sensory feedback. Sensory afferent fibers assist in calibration and modulation of the magnitude of effort[28,29] by influencing the order of motor unit recruitment and frequency of motor unit firing.[23,30] Consequently, maximal effort is a lower order task requiring full use of motor units, which involves simple motor control (maximal motor unit recruitment and firing) and minimal sensory afferent feedback.[21,23,25-27] Because of minimal sensory feedback, maximal effort is also considered more consistent (or less variable).[12,21-27,31] In contrast, submaximal effort is a higher order task, which requires a more complex motor control strategy. Maintenance of submaximal effort requires extensive and complex sensory afferent feedback.[23,26,27] Submaximal effort is also considered less consistent (or more variable) because it involves constant corrections of motor signals by sensory afferent fibers.[12,21-27,31]

CHAPTER 11

Examining a Sincerity-of-Effort Test

Sincerity of effort has been described as a person's conscious motivation to perform optimally during evaluation and treatment.[6] For example, sincerity of effort during strength testing means that a person, while completing a strength trial, exerts maximal voluntary effort.[32] Different methods have been used to determine sincerity of effort.[6,33,34] Ability of a method to determine sincerity of effort can be examined on the basis of its reliability, validity, and the research methods used to determine its reliability and validity.

Reliability

It is essential to have a reliable and valid assessment tool to identify sincerity of effort. The reliability of a valid test needs to be examined before its use in a clinical setting.[35] A reliable assessment performs with predictable consistency under set conditions.[36] "Without reliability, we cannot have confidence in the data we collect, nor can we draw rational conclusions from those data," state Portney and Watkins.[36] Reliability of sincerity-of-effort tests has been commonly examined by using two approaches—test-retest reliability and interrater reliability. Test-retest reliability establishes the degree to which a sincerity-of-effort test reveals the same results with its repeated administrations.[36,37] Interrater reliability establishes the degree to which different raters using a sincerity-of-effort test can independently obtain similar results. Both types of reliabilities have been examined by calculating Pearson correlation coefficients and intraclass correlation coefficients (ICCs). The ICC has become the preferred index for analyzing reliability because it reflects correlation (correspondence) and agreement.

Correlation indicates how scores vary together, whereas *agreement* identifies any significant differences between scores.[36] The ICC reliability values range between 0.00 and 1.00. "Reliability coefficients of measurements used for decision making or diagnosis of individuals need to be higher, perhaps at least 0.9 to ensure valid interpretations of findings."[36(p65)] However, an index greater than 0.9 is a guideline and not an absolute standard.[36] An unreliable sincerity-of-effort test cannot be valid because an inconsistent instrument cannot produce meaningful measurements.[36] Furthermore, a reliable test may not necessarily be valid.[36]

Validity

A valid measurement instrument collects data in an accurate and relevant manner.[38] A sincerity-of-effort test is a diagnostic tool that screens for the presence or absence of submaximal effort. An ideal sincerity-of-effort test would accurately discriminate between maximal and submaximal effort. That is, an ideal test would always indicate a positive result, ie, submaximal effort, when a person exerts submaximal effort, whether it is a nearly maximal or an extremely low effort. Also, an ideal test would indicate a negative result, ie, maximal effort, when a person exerts his or her maximal effort. Therefore, the validity of a sincerity-of-effort test can be evaluated in terms of its ability to assess the presence and absence of submaximal effort.[36] While considering effort as a dichotomous variable, ie, maximal effort vs submaximal effort, a sincerity-of-effort test can have four possible outcomes, which can be summarized by using a 2 × 2 contingency table (Table 11–1).[36] The four outcomes can be divided into true and false values. A true value occurs when a test correctly identifies a person as exerting maximal or submaximal effort. A true-positive result means that a person is correctly identified as exerting submaximal effort. A true-negative result means that a person is correctly identified as exerting maximal effort. In contrast, a false value occurs when a test incorrectly identifies a person as exerting maximal or submaximal effort. A false-positive result means that a person is incorrectly identified as exerting submaximal effort. A false-negative result means that a person is incorrectly identified as exerting maximal effort (Table 11–1).[36] By using these true and false values, the validity of a sincerity-of-effort test can be identified by calculating the following: (1) the sensitivity and specificity values, (2) the overall error rate, and (3) the area under its receiver operating characteristic (ROC) curve.

TABLE 11–1   Summary of Outcomes of a Sincerity-of-Effort Test*†

		Effort		
		+ **(Submaximal Effort)**	**−** **(Maximal Effort)**	**Total**
Sincerity-of-effort test	+ (Positive)	a (True-positives)	b (False-positives)	a + b
	− (Negative)	c (False-negatives)	d (True-negatives)	c + d
	Total	a + c	b + d	N = a + b + c + d

*Sensitivity = a/(a + c) = True-Positives/Total Submaximal Effort; Specificity = d/(d + b) = True-Negatives/Total Maximal Effort

†Adapted from Portney LG, Watkins MP. Table 6.2. Summary of analysis for screening test results. Upper Saddle River, NJ: Prentice-Hall Inc; 2000.

CHAPTER 11

Sensitivity and Specificity Values

Sensitivity and specificity indicate the accuracy of a test, or closeness to a true value.[39] *Sensitivity* is the ability of a test to identify submaximal effort when a person actually exerts submaximal effort. Sensitivity is calculated by using the formula a/(a + c) (Table 11–1). *Specificity* is a test's ability to identify maximal effort when a person actually exerts maximal effort. Specificity is calculated by using the formula d/(d + b) (Table 11–1).[36] Sensitivity and specificity values range between 0.0 and 1.0. A valid sincerity-of-effort test, as any other diagnostic tool, has high sensitivity and high specificity values.[7,40] "What qualifies as 'high' depends on how serious the consequence of making an error will be, but most clinical tests should have values above 0.8 to be considered high," states McClure.[40] A sincerity-of-effort test with a low sensitivity value may misclassify a person exerting submaximal effort as exerting maximal effort. Consequently, a person intentionally exerting less-than-maximal effort may be mistakenly labeled as exerting sincere effort. Therefore, low sensitivity of a test meant to identify submaximal effort may lead to seemingly ineffective treatment, increased unnecessary procedures, and elevated disability and health care costs.[6,11,13,41–43] In contrast, a sincerity-of-effort test with low specificity may misclassify a person sincerely exerting maximal effort as intentionally exerting less than maximal effort. This error may lead to inappropriate diagnosis and treatment, reduced worker compensation settlement, withheld payments, and even loss of job.[6,11,13,41–43] A low sensitivity value of a sincerity-of-effort test has been argued as being better than a low specificity value because "it is considered more ethical to miss subjects giving a deliberately submaximal effort rather than to misclassify as feigning a subject giving a genuine maximal effort."[33(p1828)] Unfairly misclassifying a sincere person as a malingerer can be very damaging to the person because it may promote clinically unfair decisions.[11,13,44] Consequently, a clinically valid sincerity-of-effort test has high sensitivity and high specificity values, perhaps greater than 0.9, that allow it to avoid mistakes in classifying people as sincere or as exerting less-than-maximal effort.

Overall Error Rate

Sincerity-of-effort tests are usually based on variables that are continuous, such as grip strength and lifting capacity scores. Generally, a continuous variable must be converted to a dichotomous outcome to differentiate between maximal and submaximal efforts, that is, "a cutoff score must be established to demarcate a positive or negative test."[36] An optimal cutoff value has the best combination of sensitivity and specificity values. Sensitivity and specificity values change with the cutoff value because an inverse relationship exists between the two. That is, as sensitivity increases, the specificity decreases, and vice versa.[11,13,24,36] An optimal cutoff value can be identified as the cutoff with the lowest overall error rate, ie, the least amount of error in identifying maximal and submaximal efforts. For each cutoff value, true- and false- positive and negative values can be found to calculate sensitivity and specificity values and overall error rates.[11,13,24,38] The overall error rate can be calculated by using the formula, $(1 - \text{sensitivity}) + (1 - \text{specificity})$.[36]

Receiver Operating Characteristic Curve

Another way to evaluate how different cutoff values affect sensitivity and specificity is by plotting the ROC curve.[45] The ROC curve is a plot of true-positive rates (sensitivity) against false-positive rates $(1 - \text{specificity})$. The ROC curve can identify the optimal combination of sensitivity and specificity values.[45] The area under the ROC curve, or the area under the curve (AUC), is an index of separation of signal (true-positive) and noise (false-positive) distributions. The AUC is a measure of discriminability, ie, the ability of the test to discriminate between maximal and submaximal efforts. A higher AUC value indicates a more effective test,[45] with an ideal test having an AUC of 100%.[36]

Research Methods

In addition to reliability and validity, evaluation of a sincerity-of-effort test must include examining research methods, which include factors such as study design, type of study participants, and type of instructions. Two study designs that have been commonly used to examine sincerity-of-effort tests are between-subjects designs[2,3,5,46] and within-subjects designs.[4,47–49] Even though both designs include the same manipulated variable (maximal vs submaximal efforts), the two designs are not equivalent because they may not be answering the same question.[50] The reason they differ is that in the between-subjects design, each subject experiences maximal or submaximal effort, whereas in the within-subjects design, subjects experience one level of effort in the context of the other.[50] Researchers may favor one design over the other based on their strengths. A between-subjects design allows for legitimate generalization of results because each person exerts maximal or submaximal efforts.[51] Furthermore, selection bias can be eliminated by random assignment of subjects to study groups.[52] In contrast, a within-subjects design maximizes the use of resources because the same subjects exert maximal and submaximal efforts, ie, fewer subjects yield the same number of data points as in a between-subjects design.[50,53] Furthermore, a within-subjects design has increased statistical power to detect differences because scores are compared within each subject.[50,53] Therefore, the results from the two designs may be different and should be compared with caution.[50]

Many studies report the validity of a sincerity-of-effort test only among healthy people. However, the test needs to be validated on people being assessed with the test, ie, people with an injury or a specific medical condition. Healthy subjects have been included in validity studies because of ease of subject recruitment and absence of injury-related factors that may confound study results. In contrast, recruiting a homogeneous group of people with injuries poses challenges. Also, injury-related factors such as pain, fear of pain, and fear of reinjury may affect the ability of a participant with an injury to exert maximal voluntary effort.

The nature of instructions given for exerting submaximal effort also varies among studies on sincerity of effort. In some studies, submaximal effort has been exerted as a percentage of maximal effort, ie, 75%, 60%, 50%, or 25%.[2,3,5,46–48] In other studies, submaximal effort has been exerted by feigning weakness[4,7,49] or by imagining pain.[7,54–56] It has been suggested that instructions may be interpreted differently by subjects.[15] Furthermore, exerting submaximal effort as a percentage of maximal effort may identify a difference that is more pronounced than often observed in clinical practice.[4] However, only a few studies have examined the impact of different instructions on nature of effort. One study found greater reduction in range of cervical motion with imagined pain vs simulating a situation of financial gain.[55] Another study did not find differences between submaximal grip efforts exerted as 50% of maximal effort vs according to an imagined pain level.[56] Therefore, studies using different types of instructions should be compared with caution until more research is conducted on this topic.

Methods Used for Assessing Evaluee Effort

Methods used for detecting sincerity of effort may be divided into assessments that are widely used and assessments not widely used in the clinical setting.[24] The methods widely used in the clinic can be administered easily and in a relatively short time. Widely used methods also require minimal calculations and minimal equipment, for example, grip strength–based tests.[11–13,14,24,41,42,57,58] Some methods are not widely used in the clinic because they require a lengthy administration time, involve complicated calculations, and use expensive equipment, for example, FCEs and isokinetic tests.[49] Methods such as the horizontal strength change[59] have been developed to test sincerity of effort and, while promising, need to be further examined (see Chapter 8). Other methods can cause pain and discomfort, for example, tests involving supramaximal stimulation of muscles. In this section, first we describe some of the methods widely used for detecting sincerity of effort. Second, we examine the use of FCEs for determining sincerity of effort. Last, we describe some of the promising methods for determining sincerity of effort, which need to be further examined before routine use in the clinic.

Widely Used Methods

Clinicians use a variety of tests to detect submaximal effort, for example, the Waddell nonorganic signs, correlation between musculoskeletal evaluation and FCE findings, documentation of pain behavior, documentation of symptom magnification, and ratio of heart rate and pain intensity.[6] Table 11–2[60–67] identifies some of the methods most widely used by clinicians to evaluate sincerity of effort.[6] Although these methods are commonly used, evidence supporting the reliability and validity of measurements obtained by using these methods for the purpose of sincerity-of-effort determination is lacking.[6,8,11–13,14,24,41,42,57,58] Some of these methods are described next, which include tests used to determine level of effort exerted during grip strength testing (coefficient of variation, rapid exchange grip test, and five-rung grip test) and the Waddell nonorganic signs.

TABLE 11–2	Widely Used Methods of Determining Sincerity of Effort*
Waddell nonorganic signs[60]	
Coefficient of variation[61]	
Bell-shaped curve[62]	
Rapid-exchange grip[63]	
Correlation between musculoskeletal evaluation and functional capacity evaluation[64]	
Documentation of pain behavior[65]	
Documentation of symptom magnification[66]	
Heart rate–pain intensity ratio[67]	

*Reprinted from Lechner DE. The well-designed functional capacity evaluation: application in forensic vocational analysis. *Journal of Forensic Vocational Analysis*. 2004;7:89.

Coefficient of Variation (CV)

The CV is based on premise that submaximal exertion is more variable and less consistent than a maximal effort. The CV uses scores of at least three grip strength trials and is calculated by dividing the Standard Deviation (SD) by the mean value of the grip strength trials. The resulting value is multiplied by 100 to calculate a percentage. To distinguish between maximal and submaximal efforts, the CV is compared with a predetermined cutoff value. A CV value larger than the cutoff value is labeled as submaximal and insincere.[12,13,24] The cutoff values commonly used by clinicians range between 10% and 20%.

The CV is commonly used by clinicians because it is based on a standardized grip test, is simple to calculate, and differentiates between maximal and submaximal efforts as suggested by some studies.[24] However, the CV may not be an appropriate sincerity-of-effort test because some studies have indicated that it does not distinguish between maximal and submaximal efforts.[68,69] This finding could be because variability in repeated measures of maximal effort has been reported to range from 10% to 24%,[24,70,71] submaximal efforts of certain isometric tasks have been reported to be reproducible,[6] and variability between trials may increase because of psychological factors, such as fear of reinjury and pain.[43] For the CV to be a valid measure of sincerity of effort, the mean and SD of repeated grip strength trials should increase proportionally, ie, people with greater average grip strength should exhibit greater variability in grip strength trials.[24,43] However, an inverse relationship has been described between grip

CHAPTER 11

strength and its variability.[72] Also, means and SDs of grip strength do not change proportionally.[12,42] Finally, the CV is an invalid measure of sincerity of effort because it has been shown to have poor test-retest reliability[2] and low sensitivity and specificity values.[13]

Rapid-Exchange Grip (REG) Test

Lister[63] developed the REG test in 1983 to identify patients exerting submaximal effort. The REG test requires a person to quickly grip a dynamometer with alternating hands. The REG test involves comparing REG scores with those of static grip (SG) test scores. An SG test consists of slow, maximal grips and may be administered by using the five-rung (5R) test or the maximal static grip test. During a sincere, maximal effort, the REG score is expected to be less than the SG score, resulting in a negative REG test score. During an insincere, submaximal effort, the REG score is expected to be greater than the SG score, resulting in a positive REG test score.[73] The REG testing protocol varies with respect to hand switch rates (varying from 45 to 100 rpm), grip repetitions (three and five repetitions), type of SG score used for comparison (the 5R and the maximal static grip test), and patient positioning while testing and handling the dynamometer.[11,58,73] Clinicians tend to use the REG test because it is simple to administer, does not require special equipment, and requires a short administration time.[11,58,73] However, the REG test may not be an appropriate sincerity-of-effort test because literature provides contradictory evidence for its use.[73] Also, clinicians do not use a standard testing protocol,[11,58,73] and the use of different speeds of alternating grips[74] and different handle settings[11,58,73] play an important role in the effectiveness of the REG test. Furthermore, the sensitivity and specificity values of the REG test have not been found to be sufficiently high.[11,75]

Five-Rung Grip (5R) Test

The 5R test, also known as the 5-position grip test, involves maximally gripping the Jamar dynamometer at its five available handle settings. On graphing the scores, a maximal effort produces a skewed bell-shaped curve, whereas a submaximal effort produces a flat line. Four methods have been used to analyze the data from the 5R test: (1) visual analysis of grip strength curves,[62,76] (2) use of repeated-measure analysis of variance with two within-subject factors,[77–81] (3) normalization of grip strength scores,[82,83] and (4) SD of grip strength scores across all five trials.[84] Clinicians commonly use the 5R test because it is easy to administer and requires a short administration time.[14,41] However, the 5R test may not be an appropriate sincerity-of-effort test because it depends on the strength of the gripping hand. Hence, the test yields biased results when assessing sincerity of effort in people with upper extremity injuries[41] and cannot distinguish between injured maximal effort and uninjured submaximal effort.[14] Furthermore, conflicting evidence exists on its effectiveness as a sincerity-of-effort test.[80,81]

Nonorganic Signs

In the early 1980s, Waddell et al[60] first described nonorganic signs as clinical signs in patients with low back pain. They defined eight tests for these signs and grouped them into five types: (1) tenderness, (2) simulation tests, (3) distraction test, (4) regional disturbances, and (5) overreaction. Scoring positively on these tests suggested the person might benefit from psychological testing.

These signs were not intended to detect insincerity of effort but, unfortunately, became frequently used by clinicians in standardized evaluations to imply lack of sincerity of effort. Subsequent studies have been conducted on the reliability of nonorganic sign testing.[60,74,85–87] Limitations in generalization, statistical power, and research design of these studies warrant caution in interpreting the results. Numerous studies have been conducted to determine the validity of nonorganic signs for predicting treatment outcomes in people with low back pain.[60,88–97] Some studies supported the validity of nonorganic signs for predicting outcomes.[60,89–91] Other researchers questioned the predictive validity of nonorganic signs.[88–97] Often, contradictory findings were reported for the same study.[88–91,94] This disagreement highlights a lack of solid evidence in the literature to suggest nonorganic signs can be used to detect sincerity of effort. Until there is a stronger scientific basis for the use of nonorganic signs to determine sincerity of effort, it is suggested that nonorganic signs be strictly viewed as identifying people whose physical recovery may be affected by psychosocial factors.

Functional Capacity Evaluations

One of the most challenging and controversial aspects of an FCE involves determining the patient's sincerity of effort.[8] When FCEs were first developed, they did not contain methods for detecting sincerity of effort. However, given the eventual demand for this information by employers, attorneys, and case managers, methods were developed and incorporated into this testing. This information is then used to assess the "validity" of the evaluation. Clinicians are often asked to provide ratings of the level of effort. Although the therapist can compare performance during an FCE with other information such as reported impairments in activities of daily living, there are few data regarding the accuracy of these types of ratings.[98] Furthermore, limited evidence exists on using

CHAPTER 11

FCEs to detect sincerity of effort.* The methods examined can be categorized into dynamic tests,[49] lifting tasks,[2-4] and combined predictive ability methods.[5,46]

Dynamic Tests

The torque-velocity test of the BTE-Primus (BTE Technologies, Baltimore, MD) has been examined for its ability to discriminate between maximal and submaximal grip efforts and has been suggested not to be appropriate for use in the clinic.[49] It was hypothesized that the torque-velocity relationship of an isotonic grip would be linear during maximal vs submaximal efforts. The study included 32 healthy people who participated in one session each of maximal and submaximal efforts. In each session, four isotonic grip-strength tests were performed at loads of 20%, 30%, 40%, and 50% of isometric test scores. For maximal and submaximal efforts, torque values were plotted against velocity values at each of the four loads. The linearity of the relationship between torque and velocity was examined by calculating the intercept, slope, correlation coefficient (r), and coefficient of determination (r^2) for each plot. Paired t tests revealed significant differences between maximal and submaximal efforts for intercept and r^2 values. Maximal isotonic grip effort velocities were found to have high test-retest reliabilities (ICC $r = 0.737–0.901$). The ROC curve revealed that value of $r^2 = 0.80$ had the best combination of sensitivity (0.69) and specificity (0.72). Furthermore, the test misclassified 31% of submaximal effort and 28% of maximal effort, with an overall error of 59%. This high error rate suggests that the test may not have adequate sensitivity and specificity values to justify its use in the clinic.[49] However, this test should be further examined in simpler joints such as the elbow.[49] The reason is that a torque-velocity relationship is reproducible for a geometrically simple joint that involves few muscles[99] and, therefore, may be used to determine sincerity of effort.

Lifting Tasks

Jay et al[2] studied the validity of sincerity-of-effort tests included in the EPIC Lift Capacity (ELC). The ELC includes four methods of detecting sincerity of effort: (1) percentage increase in heart rate, (2) percentage increase in systolic blood pressure, (3) spinal or hand function sorts, and (4) subjective evaluation of the worker's physical exertion. According to the ELC protocol, a 10% or greater increase in systolic blood pressure or heart rate indicates sincere effort. The spinal and hand sorts are sets of drawings used to identify perception to perform daily living tasks and material handling tasks. A sort is rated as reliable or unreliable based on a person's responses (also see Chapter 5). The subjective

---

*Information regarding the purported reliability and validity of sincerity-of-effort-testing in many proprietary models are often unpublished.

evaluation involves an EPIC evaluator rating an evaluee's effort as reliable, questionable, or unreliable. As part of the subjective evaluation, the evaluator observes for behaviors considered to be associated with maximal effort, such as recruitment of accessory muscles and flexing or extending the spine in a whip-lash-type motion. For the study, 41 subjects with a previously diagnosed musculoskeletal condition were randomly assigned to one of two groups. The control group exerted maximal effort, and the experimental group exerted 50% of maximal effort. By using the predictive values reported by the authors,[2] excellent specificity (0.94) and good sensitivity (0.78) and overall error rate (0.28) were found. Multiple regression analysis revealed that the four methods explained 94.9% of variance in the evaluator's determination of effort level. Among the four methods, subjective evaluation accounted for the largest proportion of variance (92%). These findings suggest that subjective evaluation of a lifting task has the potential to identify sincerity of effort during a lifting task. However, it is not clear whether previously injured subjects included in this study had injury-related signs and symptoms at the time of participating in the study. Therefore, it seems that these results should be validated in a patient population.

The PILE lumbar lifting protocol, which is similar to the ELC, has also been examined for its ability to distinguish between maximal and submaximal efforts in an active workers' compensation population.[3] A total of 17 sincerity-of-effort tests were evaluated, which included functional lifting capacity, change in heart rate, change in pain intensity, tests involving hand grip (5R test, REG test, and CV), inconsistent range of motion to functional status, the Waddell nonorganic signs, overall visual and verbal pain behaviors, and comparing inconsistent self-perceived functional status with tested functional status. While a subject performed functional lifting, four competitive test behavior observations were also examined, which included: (1) biomechanical slowing, (2) accessory muscle use, (3) sliding the load over self or using the lower extremity to push or nudge the load, and (4) trembling or muscle fatigue.[3] For the study, 90 subjects with low back pain were randomly assigned to one of two groups. Subjects in the control group exerted maximal effort, and subjects in the experimental group exerted 60% of maximal effort. A test response was considered positive if it correctly predicted maximal effort. Also, maximal effort was believed to have been exerted if one or more competitive behaviors were observed. These competitive behaviors were found to be significantly different between maximal and submaximal efforts ($P = .029$). The tests that were found to be positive were as follows: (1) biomechanical competitive test behavior, (2) 5R test based on the visual method of analyzing the bell curve, (3) REG test (in comparison with increases >12 lb and in comparison with static squeezes), and (4) self-terminating the test. After reviewing all the available information, the FCE administrator was asked to give an overall opinion as to whether the participant was giving 100% effort or 60% effort. Based on the judgment of the administrator, the sensitivity was 0.65 and specificity was 0.84. Findings indicate that the PILE protocol may not be appropriate for detecting sincerity of effort. The predictive ability of the PILE may be improved by including tests that have high sensitivity and specificity values.[3]

Reneman et al[4] studied the validity of a method involving visual observation of a lifting task to detect sincerity of effort. The study included 15 healthy subjects and 16 people with chronic low back pain (CLBP) using a repeated measures design. Subjects completed the lifting test outlined in the Isernhagen Work System (IWS) FCE. The test involved lifting increasingly heavy weights in four to seven steps until reaching a maximum. Heart rate, duration of test, and self-rating of effort were recorded after each weight was lifted five times. Subjects rated their effort using the CR-10 scale (see Chapter 5), where ratings exceeding 10 were coded as representing maximal effort. For participants with CLBP, as a general safety precaution, the lifting task was terminated if a participant reached 85% of their age-related maximum heart rate. All lifts were recorded using a video camera. The recordings were evaluated by nine raters, who were physical or occupational therapists. The therapists rated the lifts using the CR-10 scale as well as according to the observational criteria of the IWS for the level of effort, which consisted of four categories—light, moderate, heavy, and maximal. Inter-rater reliability was identified as high for the CR-10 (ICC $r = 0.76$–0.78) and moderate for the IWS observational criteria (Kappa $= 0.50$–0.58). The validity of the observational criteria CR-10 as sincerity-of-effort tests at group level was identified by comparing the indices of effort of performances by participants to observer ratings of effort. Sensitivity was calculated as ability to identify maximal effort, and specificity was calculated as ability to identify submaximal effort, ie, the degree to which observers agreed with subjects when the latter described their effort as not yet at maximal. For healthy subjects, sensitivity values ranged between 0.43 and 0.53 and specificity values ranged between 0.85 and 0.90. For participants with CLBP, sensitivity values ranged from 0.05 to 0.07 and specificity values were 1.0. "Inadequate" sensitivity values in patients with CLBP were attributed to participants not reaching maximal effort.[4]

As noted previously, it is important for a sincerity-of-effort test to be able to identify maximal effort, as unfairly misclassifying persons as exerting what they believe to be maximal effort as not doing so can be very damaging when the discrepancy can have a negative impact on financial compensation, treatment of their condition, or psychological well being.[11,13,41,44] In this study, observers described effort as maximal only in those circumstances when the subjects exhibited physical signs indicating that they were unable to tolerate any increase in weight. Given this definition, the difference in sensitivity found when ratings of healthy subjects were compared to those of patients with low back pain was perhaps unsurprising, as one might expect those with back pain to be more hesitant to lift at a level that would result in this degree of physiologic strain. In other words, while effort may not have been "maximal," it may have represented the maximum weight that subjects believed that they could physically tolerate (although we do have no way of knowing this). Therefore, the visual observation test should be used with caution. Also, because only the lifting task was tested in healthy people *and* people with CLBP, generalizations to other tests or diagnoses *can* as of yet not be made.

Combined Predictive Ability Methods

Almost two decades ago, the Baltimore Therapeutic Equipment (BTE) work simulator and the Jamar hand dynamometer were used to examine the combined predictive ability of five sincerity-of-effort tests[46]: (1) the 5R test that assessed grip strength variability using the visual method,[90] (2) the CV of three grip strength trials, (3) the CV of ulnar deviation strength measured using BTE tool 302, (4) the CV of wrist extension strength measured using BTE tool 502, and (5) comparison of mean grip score measured using the Jamar dynamometer with mean grip score measured using BTE tool 162. In a within-subjects design, 40 healthy subjects were requested to exert maximal and 50% of maximal efforts. Data analysis included performing a binomial experiment to calculate the probability of passing four or more tests. For passing four or more tests, the sensitivity value was 93.9% and specificity value was 86.3%,[46] which would make this method valid for detecting sincerity of effort. However, this method has not been validated in a patient population. Furthermore, the combined ability of the five tests to detect submaximal effort was not cross-validated. According to Portney and Watkins,[38] the data obtained on an experimental sample usually differ from data obtained on subsequent samples. Consequently, the error components within the predictive equations will usually be greater on subsequent samples than they were on the original sample, which also reduce the accuracy of a test. Hence, predictive models obtained from validation studies should be cross-validated on another sample to determine if the test criteria can be generalized across samples.[36(p107)] Therefore, this method should be used with caution for determining sincerity of effort.

A recent study examined the combined ability of 19 methods that have been included in the Blankenship FCE for detecting sincerity of effort.[5] The Blankenship's 19 methods were based on grip effort force-time (F-T) curves, CV, extrapolation of static strength to dynamic strength, frequency of lift with regard to amount of weight lifted, and the rater's subjective report of the worker's behavior throughout the functional evaluation. The study included 49 subjects (31 injured and 18 healthy). The subjects were randomly assigned to one of two groups: 100% effort or 50% effort. The 19 tests together revealed a sensitivity value of 0.8 and a specificity value of 0.84, with an overall error rate of 0.36. The ROC curve indicated the best cutoff value to be 70% of positive test results, ie, the FCE report is considered valid when 14 of 19 tests (74%) indicate maximal effort. The area under the ROC curve was determined to be 88%. Based on high sensitivity and specificity values and a high AUC, the

Blankenship FCE seems to be a fairly good method for identifying sincerity of effort. However, this method should be used with caution because a small percentage of people exerting maximal effort may be incorrectly classified as exerting submaximal effort. Also, it seems that some of these tests may not be effective in detecting sincerity of effort because it takes 14 of 19 tests to achieve sensitivity and specificity values of 0.8. It may be that using fewer tests can reduce the burden on the assessor by decreasing the time and cost of assessment but still maintaining the predictive ability.

Promising Methods

Isokinetic Measurements   *Future research needed*

A method that has potential for discriminating between maximal and submaximal efforts involves isokinetic testing.[100] Isokinetic machines can change resistance and accommodate to muscular contraction, which may make it easier to detect discrepancies in effort.[100] Isokinetic testing has been examined in different body parts, including the hand,[101] elbow,[102] shoulder,[103–105] trunk,[47,106–109] knee,[110] and ankle.[111] The difference score (DEC) of isokinetic testing is a promising method for discriminating between maximal and submaximal efforts. The DEC involves calculating the ratio of eccentric and concentric strength at a slow speed and subtracting it from the ratio of eccentric and concentric strength at a fast speed.[101,102,104–108,110–113] The DEC has been examined in healthy people[55,101,102,104–107,110,111] and in people with trunk,[109] upper extremity, and lower extremity disorders.[113] Among healthy people, the DEC had sensitivity values between 0.68 and 0.88 and specificity values between 0.94 and 1.00.[104,111] The DEC cutoff values calculated in healthy people correctly identified 89% of patients with trunk disorders and 97% of patients with upper and lower extremity disorders as *exerting maximal effort* when they had actually exerted maximal effort.[108,113] Future research needs to compare maximal and submaximal efforts exerted by people with musculoskeletal disorders.

Motion Parameters

The analysis of motion parameters has been found to be a promising method for discriminating between maximal and submaximal efforts.[7,54,100,114] An excellent example is the trunk motion parameters examined by Marras et al[7] and Ferguson et al.[54] The premise of this method is that sincere motions have greater repeatability than insincere motions. The trunk motions examined were controlled and uncontrolled sagittal flexion and extension, uncontrolled axial twisting about the waist, and uncontrolled lateral flexion of the trunk. Controlled motions required subjects to restrict twisting movements within 2° of their tolerance, whereas uncontrolled motions did not specify tolerance.[7,54] By using a repeated-measures study design, Marras et al developed a predictive model by examining 216 trunk motion parameters for their discriminatory ability by including 100 subjects with low back disorders and 100 healthy subjects. The overall error of the model ranged between 8% and 25%, with sensitivity and specificity ranging between 0.75 and 0.92.[7] Subsequently, the reliability and validity of the predictive model were examined in healthy subjects using a randomized controlled study design. The model revealed excellent sensitivity (0.9) and specificity (1.0) values as well as test-retest and interrater reliability. Further validation of the model using clinical patients is necessary.[54]

Force-Time Curves

Another method that has potential for effectively discriminating between maximal and submaximal efforts involves examining various characteristics of F-T curves generated from isometric muscle contractions.[22,115–117] The F-T curves were first examined for their ability to distinguish between maximal and submaximal efforts in 1983 by Gilbert and Knowlton,[22] who randomly assigned 36 subjects to a "sincere" or a "faker" group. The sincere group performed maximal grip effort (MGE), and the faker group performed 75% of MGE. The resulting F-T curves were analyzed for the following characteristics: rate of force application (SLP), peak force, ratio of average force to peak force (DEV), and ratio of peak force to body weight (WTRATIO). The sum of z scores of all the variables correctly identified effort in 87.5% of the females and 80% of the males. The DEV was the only significant predictor of effort for females, whereas DEV, SLP, and WTRATIO were significant predictors for males.[22] However, the sensitivity and specificity values and the overall error rates have not been identified. In the early 1990s, Chengalur et al[115] and Smith et al[116] assessed the differences between maximal and submaximal efforts by using measures generated from the plateau phase of the F-T curve: ratio of average and peak force, CV, peak-average difference, and peak-average root difference. A predictive equation combined these measures to identify submaximal effort. The equation revealed the peak-average root difference to be the most important measure.[115,116] However, the peak-average root difference seems to be invalid because it represents a very small amount of variability requiring a multiplication factor of 10^8 and, thus, is subject to a significant round-off error.[44]

The slopes of the force-generation phase and the force-decay phase of the F-T curve have also been found to differentiate between maximal and submaximal grip efforts. The force-generation phase involves rapid or gradual development of force, and the force-decay phase involves a steady rate of force development that may decrease gradually over time, indicating onset of fatigue.[118–122] A study included 30 healthy subjects who participated in two sessions, in one session

CHAPTER 11

exerting maximal effort and in the other session exerting submaximal effort by feigning weakness. The slopes revealed excellent results, with sensitivity values ranging between 0.8 and 0.93 and specificity values ranging between 0.93 and 1.0. Also, the overall error rates ranged between 7% and 33%.[117] A second study including 40 people with upper extremity injuries revealed contrasting findings. Overall error rates were 55% to 60% for the slope of the force-generation phase. However, the patients formed a heterogeneous study sample, with various causes of disease, including acute and chronic musculoskeletal conditions. Therefore, future research should focus on examining slopes in homogeneous patient populations.[56]

Bilateral Test

Schapmire et al[48] examined a testing protocol for identifying sincerity of effort that involved simultaneous measurement of grip and pinch strength. The premise of this protocol is that for maximal effort, the strength scores would be consistent during bilateral testing of grip and pinch because it is a lower order task that requires less feedback when processed by the CNS. For submaximal effort, in contrast, the strength scores would be less consistent during bilateral testing because it is a higher order task that requires more feedback when processed by the CNS. The study included 100 healthy subjects. Each subject participated in two testing sessions 1 to 3 days apart. In one session, subjects exerted maximal effort and in the other session, 50% of maximal effort. In each session, a subject completed 66 strength trials, which consisted of performing isometric grip and pinch tests. The study protocol consisted of bilateral tests (simultaneous grip and pinch trials) and unilateral tests (grip or pinch trials) performed in a random sequence. This protocol identified noncompliance by using seven criteria that were based on CV and change scores. *Noncompliance*, defined as failing two of seven criteria, resulted in a sensitivity value of 99% and specificity value of 100%. Overall reliability of the testing protocol was calculated as $\phi = 0.99$.[48] Further validation of this protocol in a clinically relevant population is necessary.

Visual Target Grip Test

In a recent study, Shechtman et al[123] examined a method based on "tricking" a person into exerting maximal effort during grip strength testing. This method depends on visual feedback for replicating grip force. The premise of this method is that incorrect visual feedback tricks a person into exerting maximal grip effort. In a repeated-measures design, 30 healthy subjects exerted maximal and submaximal grip efforts in random order. For maximal and submaximal efforts, first a "target line" was set on an oscilloscope based on the subject's nonvisual grip force efforts. Next, the subject aimed to reach the target line while performing repeated gripping. Finally, the gain of the oscilloscope was secretly cut in half, requiring subjects to exert twice as much force to reach the same target line. Providing incorrect visual feedback caused a 53% increase in grip force during submaximal effort but only a 10% increase in grip force during maximal effort. At the percentage difference cutoff value of 55%, the test revealed a sensitivity value of 0.83 and a specificity value of 0.93. However, this test may not be safe enough for clinical use because it results in an increased grip force exertion during maximal and submaximal efforts, which could raise the potential for reinjury in persons with hand pathology.[123] To reduce the potential for reinjury, future research needs to examine gain values of the oscilloscope that require an increase in force exertion that are not as high as double the initial value.

CHAPTER 11

Factors Influencing Sincerity of Effort

Examination of various promising methods has been accompanied by mounting evidence suggesting that interpretation of these methods to suggest insincere effort is inappropriate. Evaluees with musculoskeletal disorders may exhibit less than full effort for reasons other than secondary gains: pain, fear of pain, depression, lack of understanding of procedures, and anxiety.

Pain

Pain behavior is a variable often measured and considered to influence performance on FCEs. Pain behavior is often monitored through visual observation and verbal cues, the presence of nonorganic clinical signs, reviewing the relation between change in heart rate and self-reported pain intensity, and discrepancies between self-reported functional limitations (see Chapter 5) and actual test results.[3] Unfortunately, none of these methods has been examined adequately. Studies reviewing the ability of these tests to differentiate between submaximal and maximal effort used small samples and included nonpatient volunteers or previously injured populations currently not receiving workers' compensation.[3] Research suggests that pain behavior may be influenced by a variety of factors: environmental,[124] verbal reinforcement,[125] and ethnicity.[126]

Pain behavior that is inconsistent with self-reports is often documented as suspicious. However, the literature addressing the correlation between observed behaviors and self-reports of pain intensity is contradictory.[127–130] These discrepancies point to the need for further evaluation of these associations. Pain behavior is believed to be only one aspect of the complex experience of pain.[131] By not including psychosocial and cognitive aspects, clinicians may be accused of an incomplete assessment. Informal, nonstandardized descriptions of pain during clinical practice are subject to considerable error and bias. During some FCEs, clinicians compare visual observations of signs of effort with the person's willingness to perform. If a person stops before what the clinician perceives could be maximum effort, the clinician cannot identify the reasons underlying this self-limiting behavior without further investigation. The person could be self-limiting owing to pain, fear of reinjury, anxiety, depression, fatigue, or other factors. Another common practice used by clinicians to determine sincerity of effort is to attempt to interpret a person's subjective comments during functional performance. This is only one source of information related to pain, and it leaves the clinician open to misinterpretation and bias.

Pain is often reported to be the cause of functional limitations. It is not clear if FCEs can validly measure physiologic capacity in people experiencing pain. It is difficult to assess the validity of pain complaints because pain is a private experience. Studies suggest there is little relationship between underlying pathophysiology and the experience of pain.[132,133] Pain is viewed as a multidimensional phenomenon that is influenced by many factors, such as affect, previous experience, and cultural beliefs, in addition to sensory input.[134] The correlation between these measures and sincerity of effort is unknown.

There have been some studies that have attempted to evaluate the impact of pain on function. In a study conducted by Hart,[135] the reported function (ie, perception of the level of activity the person believed he or she was capable of performing) was poorly or not related to reports of pain, supporting the results of other studies on the impact of symptoms on actual performance.[136-143] Patients also perceived their level of function as unrelated to their reports of pain. Moffroid et al[138] reported little correlation between self-reporting of inactivity and the results of physical testing. Linton[139] reported no significant correlation between self-report of pain intensity and actual activity levels, and Rainville et al[140] confirmed that pain measures did not generally correlate with measured levels of activity. Other authors have reported poor relationships between a person's report of pain and actual performance when using pain drawings and observed functional tasks.[60,136,137,140,141] Hart[135] found a lack of a relation between perception and reported function and implied independence of the constructs of perceived pain and perceived performance.

Psychosocial Factors

There is a paucity of studies that have directly examined the relationship between psychosocial factors and FCE results.[98] Although it is beneficial to test and examine an overriding hypothesis about the relationship between psychosocial factors and FCE results, such a hypothesis does not exist. Many of the relationships between psychosocial factors and function are complex, and multiple mechanisms have been proposed to explain these relationships. Some researchers suggest that a biopsychosocial perspective must be taken when dealing with determining sincerity of effort.[142] This approach considers three broad categories of measures—physical, psychological/self-report, and overt behavior/function. However, these three categories may not always display high concordance with one another. This is not unique to the area of pain and function. For example, the psychology literature noted that self-report, overt behavior, and physiological indices of behavior in general sometimes show low correlations among one another.[142] Therefore, unlike a construct that is based on overt behavioral or physiologic index, direct overlap cannot be automatically expected when self-report measure is used as the primary index for pain. A summary of research on psychosocial factors and function is given in Table 11–3.[98] This information supports the notion that certain psychosocial factors influence functional activity and FCE measures. Commonly used questionnaires that evaluate self-reported function and pain are described in Chapter 5.

CHAPTER 11

TABLE 11–3	Summary of Results of Studies on Psychosocial Factors and Functions*		
Variable	Nature of Relationship	Related to Self-reported Function	Related to Functional Activity
Anxiety/pain-related fear	Poorer function	Strong evidence	Strong evidence
Depression	Poorer function	Strong evidence	Weak evidence
Catastrophizing	Poorer function	Strong evidence	Weak evidence
Posttraumatic stress disorder	Poorer function	Strong evidence	No evidence
Self-efficacy	Better function	Strong evidence	Strong evidence
Job dissatisfaction/ job stress	Poorer function	Moderate evidence	No evidence
Illness behavior/ nonorganic signs	Poorer function	Some evidence	Strong evidence
Secondary gain	Poorer function	Some evidence	Weak evidence

*Reprinted from: Geisser ME, Robinson ME, Miller QI, Bade SM. Psychosocial factors and functional capacity evaluation amoung persons with chronic pain. *J Occupational Rehabilitation.* 2003;13:270.

Heart Rate and Pain Intensity

Some FCEs compare ratings of pain intensity on a visual analogue scale or verbal ratings with the individual's heart rate. The premise is that as pain increases, so should heart rate. If an increase in heart rate is not demonstrated as the person expresses an increase in pain, the person is viewed as consciously trying to exaggerate the pain. This notion originated with a study conducted by Borg et al[67] in 1981. They found a positive correlation between the heart rate and pain intensity of patients with angina pectoris while exercising with a specific bicycle ergometry protocol. However, the physiologic relationship among chest pain, heart rate, and workload is not the same as the relationship among musculoskeletal pain disorders, heart rate, and workload. Therefore, extrapolation of the findings of the study by Borg et al[67] to musculoskeletal dysfunction is inappropriate.

Only one study has addressed the physiologic response to pain in patients with chronic pain.[143] In this study, physiologic responses to repeated painful stimuli in persons with and without back pain were measured. Both groups demonstrated an increase in skin conductance fluctuations and respiratory rates, but they did not demonstrate increases in heart rate. No correlation was found between the responses to painful stimuli and the heart and respiratory rates. In summary, using autonomically mediated physiologic measures to validate self-report measures of pain is a practice used by some clinicians to obtain objective measures of pain. However, preliminary research suggests the relationship among pain intensity, physiologic responses, and pain perception is complex and poorly understood.[143–146]

Clinical Examination

Sometimes, lack of a correlation between measures of impairment determined during musculoskeletal evaluations and functional measures is used as evidence to suggest the patient is demonstrating less-than-maximum effort. However, research suggests that impairment is not directly correlated with function.[147–149]

Detecting deception or lack of sincerity of effort during the clinical examination requires a thorough knowledge of what is expected for the condition in question and the capacity to observe or elicit what is expected and what is not. Inappropriate signs should not exclude the presence of physical pathology but should raise questions about psychological factors that may be influencing the behavior.

Conclusions

Health care providers can fall into a number of "assumption traps" when attempting to assess sincerity of effort. Research has shown that a lack of sincerity-of-effort cannot be reliably identified by facial expression testing, questionnaires, sensory testing, physiologic measurements, or clinical examination. No approach for detecting sincerity-of-effort has been directly correlated with outcome.[6] No single test or test factor serves as the absolute means to discredit the performance of a tested person.

Many studies assessing the reliability and validity of tests determining sincerity-of-effort have involved healthy subjects or subjects with disease or injury who are asked to produce submaximal effort. This methodology is problematic. First, the generalizability is limited owing to the absence of application of these methods to people with real motivational issues to perform at submaximal effort. Second, many studies have used "normal" and "normal with the request to fake" groups as control groups. If this design is used, one cannot accurately suggest that the observed group differences are due to the effects of malingering. Another theoretical problem with sincerity-of-effort research is the type of instruction given. Some studies advised subjects to give a percentage of maximal effort (ie, 75%, 50%, and 25%), whereas other studies requested a faked effort. These differences in instruction are open to different interpretations by subjects.[15]

Other studies discuss interpersonal contextual influences on sincerity-of-effort.[132] The clinician's presence and how questions are presented may affect the patient's emotional reactions and attitude during testing that impacts behavioral performance on an FCE. One study using simulation research indicated that clinicians perceived people as more honest if they reported self-damaging information, and people who presented more positive or self-serving information were viewed as malingering. In this case, perception of the examiner may influence decisions about malingering that are based primarily on observation of the patient.[132]

Interview methods for detection of sincerity-of-effort also remain understudied.[132] Few studies control for many of the factors (besides the factors under evaluation) that affect actual effort. For this reason, many advocate for more objective measures of level of effort. At best, when obvious function-to-function discrepancies, gross inconsistencies in functional performance, or attempts to feign maximal effort are observed during an FCE, the clinician can report this behavior. However, underlying motivation is not necessarily ascertained. If self-limiting behavior predominates during an FCE, further psychological, psychosocial, or environmental evaluation may be helpful in fully understanding what is contributing to this behavior.

Some basic questions remain. Do we need to measure sincerity-of-effort? If so, what method is most accurate? Is it a legitimate task for the physician or clinician to determine a person's sincerity-of-effort? The majority of clinicians and physicians have no special expertise in this assessment. Further discussion is warranted, and more rigorous research is required to answer these fundamental questions. Until there is more definitive scientific evidence supporting a reliable, valid, and predictive means of determining an evaluee's level of effort, evaluators are cautioned about making level-of-effort decisions that are based on methods with known scientific limitations, especially when they are made based solely on one method. Such decisions leave practitioners open to error and bias and, as noted previously, can have a profound effect on an evaluee's future. The best a practitioner can do at this time is to obtain subjective information via client-interview and objective data using multiple methods of testing. Triangulation of such data will provide information on consistency in effort. Inconsistencies in the information gathered from FCEs should prompt the evaluator (or individual ordering the FCE) to further investigate other factors that may be contributing to the evaluee's performance.

References

1. Baker JC. Burden of proof in detection of submaximal effort. *Work.* 1998; 10:63–70.
2. Jay MA, Lamb JM, Watson RL, et al. Sensitivity and specificity of the indicators of sincere effort of the EPIC lift capacity test on a previously injured population. *Spine.* 2000;25:1405–1412.
3. Lemstra M, Olszynski WP, Enright W. The sensitivity and specificity of functional capacity evaluations in determining maximal effort: a randomized trial. *Spine.* 2004;29:953–959.
4. Reneman MF, Fokkens AS, Dijkstra PU, Geertzen JH, Groothoff JW. Testing lifting capacity: validity of determining effort level by means of observation. *Spine.* 2005;30:E40–E46.
5. Brubaker PN, Fearon FJ, Smith SM, et al. Sensitivity and specificity of the Blankenship FCE system's indicators of submaximal effort. *J Orthop Sports Phys Ther.* 2007;37:161–168.
6. Lechner DE, Bradbury SF, Bradley LA. Detecting sincerity of effort: a summary of methods and approaches. *Phys Ther.* 1998;78:867–888.
7. Marras WS, Lewis KE, Ferguson SA, Parnianpour M. Impairment magnification during dynamic trunk motions. *Spine.* 2000;25:587–595.
8. Lechner DE. The well-designed functional capacity evaluation: application in forensic vocational analysis. *J Forensic Vocational Anal.* 2004;7:83–96.

9. Mitterhauser MD, Muse VL, Dellon AL, Jetzer TC. Detection of submaximal effort with computer-assisted grip strength measurements. *J Occup Environ Med.* 1997;39:1220–1227.

10. Tredgett M, Davis TR. Rapid repeat testing of grip strength for detection of faked hand weakness. *J Hand Surg [Br].* 2000;25B:372–375.

11. Shechtman O, Taylor C. The use of the rapid exchange grip test in detecting sincerity of effort, part ii: validity of the test. *J Hand Ther.* 2000;13:203–210.

12. Shechtman O. The coefficient of variation as a measure of sincerity of effort of grip strength, part i: the statistical principle. *J Hand Ther.* 2001;14:180–187.

13. Shechtman O. The coefficient of variation as a measure of sincerity of effort of grip strength, part ii: sensitivity and specificity. *J Hand Ther.* 2001;14:188–194.

14. Shechtman O, Gutierrez Z, Kokendofer E. Analysis of the statistical methods used to detect submaximal effort with the five-rung grip strength test. *J Hand Ther.* 2005;18:10–18.

15. Fishbain DA, Cutler RB, Rosomoff HL, Rosomoff RS. Chronic pain disability exaggeration/malingering and submaximal effort research. *Clin J Pain.* 1999;15:244–274.

16. Mittenberg W, Patton C, Canyock EM, Condit DC. Base rates of malingering and symptom exaggeration. *J Clin Exp Neuropsychol.* 2002;24:1094–1102.

17. Green P, Rohling ML, Lees-Haley PR, Allen LM. Effort has a greater effect on test scores than severe brain injury in compensation claimants. *Brain Inj.* 2001; 15:1045–1060.

18. Lees-Haley PR. MMPI-2 base rates for 492 personal injury plaintiffs: implications and challenges for forensic assessment. *J Clin Psychol.* 1997;53:745–755.

19. Beck W, Hettinger T. Is the evaluation of strength measurement in expert testimony reasonable [in German]? *Monatsschr Unfallheilkd Versicherungsmed.* Apr 1956;59(4):116–118.

20. Rohmert W, Sieber W. Untersuchungen über die Bewertung von Kraftmessungen bei der medizinischen Begutachtung. *Med Sachverstaend.* 1960;56:174–1977.

21. Astrand PO, Rodahl K, eds. *Textbook of Work Physiology.* 2nd ed. New York, NY: McGraw-Hill; 1977.

22. Gilbert JC, Knowlton RG. Simple method to determine sincerity of effort during a maximal isometric test of grip strength. *Am J Phys Med.* Jun 1983;62:135–144.

23. Kroemer KH, Marras WS. Towards an objective assessment of the "maximal voluntary contraction" component in routine muscle strength measurements. *Eur J Appl Physiol Occup Physiol.* 1980;45:1–9.

24. Shechtman O. Using the coefficient of variation to detect sincerity of effort of grip strength: a literature review. *J Hand Ther.* 2000;13:25–32.

25. Edgerton VR. Mammalian muscle-fiber types and their adaptability. *Am Zoologist.* 1978;18:113–125.

26. Milner-Brown HS, Stein RB, Yemm R. Changes in firing rate of human motor units during linearly changing voluntary contractions. *J Physiol.* 1973;230: 371–390.

27. Milner-Brown HS, Stein RB, Yemm R. The orderly recruitment of human motor units during voluntary isometric contractions. *J Physiol.* 1973;230:359–370.

CHAPTER 11

28. Kilbreath SL, Refshauge K, Gandevia SC. Differential control of the digits of the human hand: evidence from digital anaesthesia and weight matching. *Exp Brain Res.* 1997;117:507–511.

29. Lafargue G, Paillard J, Lamarre Y, Sirigu A. Production and perception of grip force without proprioception: is there a sense of effort in deafferented subjects? *Eur J Neurosci.* 2003;17:2741–2749.

30. Grimby L, Hannerz J. Recruitment order of motor units on voluntary contraction: changes induced by proprioceptive afferent activity. *J Neurol Neurosurg Psychiatry.* 1968;31:565–573.

31. Niemeyer LO. The issue of abnormal illness behavior in work hardening. In: Niemeyer LO, Jacobs K, eds. *Work Hardening: State of the Art.* Thorofare, NJ: Slack; 1989.

32. Hamilton Fairfax A, Balnave R, Adams R. Review of sincerity of effort testing. *Saf Sci.* 1997;25:237–245.

33. Hamilton Fairfax A, Balnave R, Adams RD. Variability of grip strength during isometric contraction. *Ergonomics.* 1995;38:1819–1830.

34. King PM. Analysis of approaches to detection of sincerity of effort through grip strength measurement. *Work.* 1998;10:9–13.

35. Johnston MV, Keith RA, Hinderer SR. Measurement standards for interdisciplinary medical rehabilitation. *Arch Phys Med Rehabil.* 1992;73:S3–S23.

36. Portney LG, Watkins MP. *Foundations of Clinical Research: Applications to Practice.* 2nd ed. Norwalk, CT: Appleton & Lange; 2000.

37. Streiner DL, Norman GR. Reliability. In: *Health Measurement Scales: A Practical Guide to Their Development and Use.* 2nd ed. Oxford, England: Oxford University Press; 1995:104–127.

38. Portney LG, Watkins MP. *Foundations of Clinical Research: Applications to Practice.* Norwalk, CT: Appleton & Lange; 1993.

39. Asal NR, Neas BR, Beebe L. *Principles of Epidemiology.* Oklahoma City, OK: University of Oklahoma Health Science Center; 2003.

40. McClure P. Sensitivity and specificity. *J Hand Ther.* 2001;14:219–220.

41. Gutierrez Z, Shechtman O. Effectiveness of the five-handle position grip strength test in detecting sincerity of effort in men and women. *Am J Phys Med Rehabil.* 2003;82:847–855.

42. Shechtman O. Is the coefficient of variation a valid measure for detecting sincerity of effort of grip strength? *Work.* 1999;13:163–169.

43. Robinson ME, Geisser ME, Hanson CS, O'Connor PD. Detecting submaximal efforts in grip strength testing with the coefficient of variation. *J Occup Rehabil.* 1993;3:45–50.

44. Shechtman O, Sindhu BS, Davenport PW. Using the force-time curve to detect maximal grip strength effort. *J Hand Ther.* 2007;20:37–48.

45. McNicol D. *A Primer of Signal Detection Theory.* London, UK: Lawrence Erlbaum Associates; 2005.

46. King JW, Berryhill BH. Assessing maximum effort in upper-extremity functional testing. *Work.* 1991;1:65–76.

47. Hazard RG, Reid S, Fenwick J, Reeves V. Isokinetic trunk and lifting strength measurements: variability as an indicator of effort. *Spine.* 1988;13:54–57.
48. Schapmire D, St James JD, Townsend R, Stewart T, Delheimer S, Focht D. Simultaneous bilateral testing: validation of a new protocol to detect insincere effort during grip and pinch strength testing. *J Hand Ther.* 2002; 15:242–250.
49. Shechtman O, Hope LM, Sindhu BS. Evaluation of the torque-velocity test of the BTE-Primus as a measure of sincerity of effort of grip strength. *J Hand Ther.* 2007;20:326–335.
50. Maxwell SE, Delaney HD. One-way within subjects designs: univariate approach. In: Maxwell SE, Delaney HD, eds. *Designing Experiments and Analyzing Data: A Model Comparison Perspective.* Mahwah, NJ: Lawrence Erlbaum Associates; 2000:455–494.
51. Poulton EC. Range effects in experiments on people. *Am J Psychol.* 1975;88:3–32.
52. Lachin JM, Matts JP, Wei LJ. Randomization in clinical trials: conclusions and recommendations. *Control Clin Trials.* 1988;9:365–374.
53. Minke A. Conducting repeated measures analyses: experimental design considerations. Paper presented at: Southwest Educational Research Association; January 23–25, 1997; Austin, TX.
54. Ferguson SA, Gallagher S, Marras WS. Validity and reliability of sincerity test for dynamic trunk motions. *Disabil Rehabil.* 2003;25:236–241.
55. Dvir Z, Penso-Zabludowski E. The effects of protocol and test situation on maximal vs submaximal cervical motion: medicolegal implications. *Int J Legal Med.* 2003;117:350–355.
56. Sindhu BS. *Effect of Upper Extremity Injury on Grip Strength Effort* [dissertation]. Gainesville: University of Florida; 2007.
57. Shechtman O, Anton SD, Kanasky WF Jr, Robinson ME. The use of the coefficient of variation in detecting sincerity of effort: a meta-analysis. *Work.* 2006; 26:335–341.
58. Shechtman O, Taylor C. How do therapists administer the rapid exchange grip test? a survey. *J Hand Ther.* 2002;15:53–61.
59. Berryhill BH, Osborne P, Staats TE, Brooks FW, Skarina JM. Horizontal strength changes: an ergometric measure for determining validity of effort in impairment evaluations: a preliminary report. *J Disabil.* 1993;3:143–148.
60. Waddell G, McCulloch JA, Kummel E, Venner RM. Nonorganic physical signs in low-back pain. *Spine.* 1980;5:117–125.
61. Simonsen JC. Coefficient of variation as a measure of subject effort. *Arch Phys Med Rehabil.* 1995;76:516–520.
62. Stokes HM. The seriously uninjured hand: weakness of grip. *J Occup Med.* 1983; 25:683–684.
63. Lister G. *The Hand: Diagnosis and Indications.* 2nd ed. New York, NY: Churchill Livingstone; 1984.
64. Isernhagen SJ. *Isernhagen Work Systems Functional Capacity Evaluation.* Duluth, MN: Isernhagen Work Systems; 1996.

65. Solomon PE. Measurement of pain behaviour. *Physiother Canada.* 1996;48:52–58.

66. Matheson LN. Use of the BTE work simulator screen for symptom magnification syndrome. *Ind Rehabil Q.* 1989;2:5–31.

67. Borg G, Holmgren A, Lindblad I. Quantitative evaluation of chest pain. *Acta Med Scand Suppl.* 1981;644:43–45.

68. Ashford RF, Nagelburg S, Adkins R. Sensitivity of the Jamar dynamometer in detecting submaximal grip effort. *J Hand Surg [Am].* 1996;21A:402–405.

69. Robinson ME, MacMillan M, O'Connor P, Fuller A, Cassisi JE. Reproducibility of maximal versus submaximal efforts in an isometric lumbar extension task. *J Spinal Disord.* 1991;4:444–448.

70. Bechtol CO. Grip test; the use of a dynamometer with adjustable handle spacings. *J Bone Joint Surg Am.* 1954;36-A(4):820–824; passim.

71. Young VL, Pin P, Kraemer BA, Gould RB, Nemergut L, Pellowski M. Fluctuation in grip and pinch strength among normal subjects. *J Hand Surg [Am].* 1989;14:125–129.

72. Krombholz H. On the association of effort and force of handgrip. *Percept Mot Skills.* 1985;60:161–162.

73. Taylor C, Shechtman O. The use of the rapid exchange grip test in detecting sincerity of effort, part i: administration of the test. *J Hand Ther.* 2000;13:195–202.

74. Spratt KF, Lehmann TR, Weinstein JN, Sayre HA. A new approach to the low-back physical examination: behavioral assessment of mechanical signs. *Spine.* 1990;15:96–102.

75. Joughin K, Gulati P, Mackinnon SE, et al. An evaluation of rapid exchange and simultaneous grip tests. *J Hand Surg [Am].* 1993;18:245–252.

76. Hildreth DH, Breidenbach WC, Lister GD, Hodges AD. Detection of submaximal effort by use of the rapid exchange grip. *J Hand Surg [Am].* 1989;14:742–745.

77. Hoffmaster E, Lech R, Niebuhr BR. Consistency of sincere and feigned grip exertions with repeated testing. *J Occup Med.* 1993;35:788–794.

78. Niebuhr BR. Detecting submaximal grip exertions of variable effort by electromyography. *Electromyogr Clin Neurophysiol.* 1996;36:113–120.

79. Niebuhr BR, Marion R, Hasson SM. Electromyographic analysis of effort in grip strength assessment. *Electromyogr Clin Neurophysiol.* 1993;33:149–156.

80. Niebuhr BR, Marion R. Detecting sincerity of effort when measuring grip strength. *Am J Phys Med.* 1987;66:16–24.

81. Niebuhr BR, Marion R. Voluntary control of submaximal grip strength. *Am J Phys Med Rehabil.* 1990;69:96–101.

82. Goldman S, Cahalan T, An K. The injured upper extremity and the Jamar five-handle position grip test. *Am J Phys Med Rehabil.* 1991;70:306–308.

83. Tredgett M, Pimble LJ, Davis TR. The detection of feigned hand weakness using the five position grip strength. *J Hand Surg [Br].* 1999;24B:426–428.

84. Stokes HM, Landrieu KW, Domangue B, Kunen S. Identification of low-effort patients through dynamometry. *J Hand Surg [Am].* 1995;20A:1047–1056.

85. Waddell G, Main CJ, Morris EW, et al. Normality and reliability in the clinical assessment of backache. *Br Med J (Clin Res Ed).* 1982;284:1519–1523.

86. Korbon GA, DeGood DE, Schroeder ME, Schwartz DP, Shutty MS Jr. The development of a somatic amplification rating scale for low-back pain. *Spine.* 1987;12:787–791.

87. McCombe PF, Fairbank JC, Cockersole BC, Pynsent PB. 1989 Volvo Award in Clinical Sciences: reproducibility of physical signs in low-back pain. *Spine.* 1989;14:908–918.
88. Lehmann TR, Russell DW, Spratt KF. The impact of patients with nonorganic physical findings on a controlled trial of transcutaneous electrical nerve stimulation and electroacupuncture. *Spine.* 1983;8:625–634.
89. Doxey NC, Dzioba RB, Mitson GL, Lacroix JM. Predictors of outcome in back surgery candidates. *J Clin Psychol.* 1988;44:611–622.
90. Dzioba RB, Doxey NC. A prospective investigation into the orthopaedic and psychologic predictors of outcome of first lumbar surgery following industrial injury. *Spine.* 1984;9:614–623.
91. Karas R, McIntosh G, Hall H, Wilson L, Melles T. The relationship between nonorganic signs and centralization of symptoms in the prediction of return to work for patients with low back pain. *Phys Ther.* 1997;77:354–360.
92. Waddell G, Main CJ, Morris EW, Di Paola M, Gray IC. Chronic low-back pain, psychologic distress, and illness behavior. *Spine.* 1984;9:209–213.
93. Waddell G, Morris EW, Di Paola MP, Bircher M, Finlayson D. A concept of illness tested as an improved basis for surgical decisions in low-back disorders. *Spine.* 1986;11:712–719.
94. Lancourt J, Kettelhut M. Predicting return to work for lower back pain patients receiving worker's compensation. *Spine.* 1992;17:629–640.
95. Bradish CF, Lloyd GJ, Aldam CH, et al. Do nonorganic signs help to predict the return to activity of patients with low-back pain? *Spine.* 1988;13:557–560.
96. Chan CW, Goldman S, Ilstrup DM, Kunselman AR, O'Neill PI. The pain drawing and Waddell's nonorganic physical signs in chronic low-back pain. *Spine.* 1993;18:1717–1722.
97. Lacroix JM, Powell J, Lloyd GJ, Doxey NC, Mitson GL, Aldam CF. Low-back pain: factors of value in predicting outcome. *Spine.* 1990;15:495–499.
98. Geisser ME, Robinson ME, Miller QL, Bade SM. Psychosocial factors and functional capacity evaluation among persons with chronic pain. *J Occup Rehabil.* 2003;13:259–276.
99. Wilkie DR. The relation between force and velocity in human muscle. *J Physiol.* 1949;110:249–280.
100. Robinson ME, Dannecker EA. Critical issues in the use of muscle testing for the determination of sincerity of effort. *Clin J Pain.* 2004;20:392–398.
101. Dvir Z. Identification of feigned grip effort using isokinetic dynamometry. *Clin Biomech (Bristol, Avon).* 1999;14:522–527.
102. Dvir Z. An isokinetic study of submaximal effort in elbow flexion. *Percept Mot Skills.* 1997;84(3 pt 2):1431–1438.
103. Fishbain DA, Abdel-Moty E, Cutler RB, Rosomoff HL, Steele-Rosomoff R. Detection of a "faked" strength task effort in volunteers using a computerized exercise testing system. *Am J Phys Med Rehabil.* 1999;78:222–227.
104. Dvir Z, Steinfeld-Cohen Y, Peretz C. Identification of feigned shoulder flexion weakness in normal subjects. *Am J Phys Med Rehabil.* 2002;81:187–193.
105. Chaler J, Dvir Z, Diaz U, et al. Identification of feigned maximal shoulder external rotation effort. *Clin Rehabil.* 2007;21:241–247.

CHAPTER 11

106. Dvir Z. Differentiation of submaximal from maximal trunk extension effort: an isokinetic study using a new testing protocol. *Spine.* 1997;22:2672–2676.

107. Dvir Z, Keating J. Identifying feigned isokinetic trunk extension effort in normal subjects: an efficiency study of the DEC. *Spine.* 2001;26:1046–1051.

108. Dvir Z, Keating JL. Trunk extension effort in patients with chronic low back dysfunction. *Spine.* 2003;28:685–692.

109. Hazard RG, Reeves V, Fenwick JW. Lifting capacity: indices of subject effort. *Spine.* 1992;17:1065–1070.

110. Dvir Z, David G. Suboptimal muscular performance: measuring isokinetic strength of knee extensors with new testing protocol. *Arch Phys Med Rehabil.* 1996;77:578–581.

111. Olmo J, Jato S, Benito J, Martin I, Dvir Z. Identification of feigned ankle plantar and dorsiflexors weakness in normal subjects [published online ahead of print March 27, 2008]. *J Electromyogr Kinesiol.* doi:10.1056.

112. Dvir Z, Gal-Eshel N, Shamir B, Pevzner E, Peretz C, Knoller N. Simulated pain and cervical motion in patients with chronic disorders of the cervical spine. *Pain Res Manag.* Autumn 2004;9:131–136.

113. Dvir Z. Clinical application of the DEC variables in assessing maximality of muscular effort: report of 34 patients. *Am J Phys Med Rehabil.* 2002;81:921–928.

114. Dvir Z, Prushansky T, Peretz C. Maximal versus feigned active cervical motion in healthy patients: the coefficient of variation as an indicator for sincerity of effort. *Spine.* 2001;26:1680–1688.

115. Chengalur SN, Smith GA, Nelson RC, Sadoff AM. Assessing sincerity of effort in maximal grip strength tests. *Am J Phys Med Rehabil.* 1990;69:148–153.

116. Smith GA, Nelson RC, Sadoff SJ, Sadoff AM. Assessing sincerity of effort in maximal grip strength tests. *Am J Phys Med Rehabil.* 1989;68:73–80.

117. Shechtman O, Sindhu B. Using the force-time curve to detect submaximal effort. *J Hand Ther.* 2005;18:461–462.

118. Sanjak M, Konopacki R, Capasso R, et al. Dissociation between mechanical and myoelectrical manifestation of muscle fatigue in amyotrophic lateral sclerosis. *Amyotroph Lateral Scler Other Motor Neuron Disord.* 2004;5:26–32.

119. Kamimura T, Ikuta Y. Evaluation of grip strength with a sustained maximal isometric contraction for 6 and 10 seconds. *J Rehabil Med.* 2001;33:225–229.

120. Househam E, McAuley J, Charles T, Lightfoot T, Swash M. Analysis of force profile during a maximum voluntary isometric contraction task. *Muscle Nerve.* 2004;29:401–408.

121. Hakkinen A, Malkia E, Hakkinen K, Jappinen I, Laitinen L, Hannonen P. Effects of detraining subsequent to strength training on neuromuscular function in patients with inflammatory arthritis. *Br J Rheumatol.* 1997;36:1075–1081.

122. Helliwell P, Howe A, Wright V. Functional assessment of the hand: reproducibility, acceptability, and utility of a new system for measuring strength. *Ann Rheum Dis.* 1987;46:203–208.

123. Shechtman O, Sindhu BS, Davenport PW. Using the "Visual Target Grip Test" to identify the level of effort during grip strength. Paper presented at: ASHT 30th Annual Meeting; October 4–7, 2007, 2007; Phoenix, AZ.

124. Cinciripini PM, Floreen A. An assessment of chronic pain behavior in a structured interview. *J Psychosom Res.* 1983;27:117–123.

125. Gairnes D, Pasina J. Comparison of verbal reinforcement and feedback in the operant treatment of disability due to chronic low back pain. *Behav Ther.* 1977;8:621–630.

126. Tursky B, Sternbach RA. Further physiological correlates of ethnic differences in responses to shock. *Psychophysiology.* 1967;4:67–74.

127. Richard JS, Nepomuceno C, Riles M, Suer Z. Assessing pain behavior: the UAB Pain Behavior Scale. *Pain.* 1982;14:393–398.

128. Dirks JF, Wunder J, Kinsman R, McElhinny J, Jones NF. A pain rating scale and a pain behavior checklist for clinical use: development, norms, and the consistency score. *Psychother Psychosom.* 1993;59:41–49.

129. Keefe FJ, Block AR. Development of an observation method for assessing pain behavior in chronic low back pain patients. *Behav Ther.* 1982;13:363–375.

130. McDaniel LK, Anderson KO, Bradley LA, et al. Development of an observation method for assessing pain behavior in rheumatoid arthritis patients. *Pain.* 1986;24:165–184.

131. Feuerstein M, Beattie PF. Biobehavioral factors affecting pain and disability in low back pain: mechanisms and assessment. *Phys Ther.* 1995;75:267–280.

132. Nachemson AL. Advances in low-back pain. *Clin Orthop.* 1985;200:266–278.

133. Robinson JP. Disability evaluation in painful conditions. In: Turk DC, Melzack R, eds. *Handbook of Pain Assessment.* New York, NY: Guilford Press; 2001:248–272.

134. Melzack R, Wall PD. *The Challenge of Pain.* New York, NY: Basic Books; 1982.

135. Hart DL. Relation between three measures of function in patients with chronic work-related pain syndromes. *J Rehabil Outcomes Meas.* 1998;2:1–14.

136. Fordyce WE, Lansky D, Calsyn DA, Shelton JL, Stolov WC, Rock DL. Pain measurement and pain behavior. *Pain.* 1984;18:53–69.

137. Fordyce W, McMahon R, Rainwater G, et al. Pain complaint: exercise performance relationship in chronic pain. *Pain.* 1981;10:311–321.

138. Moffroid M, Reid S, Henry SM, Haugh LD, Ricamato A. Some endurance measures in persons with chronic low back pain. *J Orthop Sports Phys Ther.* 1994; 20:81–87.

139. Linton SJ. The relationship between activity and chronic back pain. *Pain.* 1985; 21:289–294.

140. Rainville J, Ahern DK, Phalen L, Childs LA, Sutherland R. The association of pain with physical activities in chronic low back pain. *Spine.* 1992;17:1060–1064.

141. Waddell G. 1987 Volvo Award in Clinical Sciences: a new clinical model for the treatment of low-back pain. *Spine.* 1987;127:632–644.

142. Gatchel RJ. Psychosocial factors that can influence the self-assessment of function. *J Occup Rehabil.* 2004;14:197–206.

143. Peters ML, Schmidt AJ. Psychophysiological responses to repeated acute pain stimulation in chronic low back pain patients. *J Psychosom Res.* 1991;35:59–74.

144. Moltner A, Holzl R, Strian F. Heart rate changes as an autonomic component of the pain response. *Pain.* 1990;43:81–89.

145. Kregel KC, Seals DR, Callister R. Sympathetic nervous system activity during skin cooling in humans: relationship to stimulus intensity and pain sensation. *J Physiol.* 1992;454:359–371.

146. Coghill RC, Talbot JD, Evans AC, et al. Distributed processing of pain and vibration by the human brain. *J Neurosci.* 1994;14:4095–4108.

CHAPTER 11

147. Yelin EH, Henke CJ, Epstein WV. Work disability among persons with musculoskeletal conditions. *Arthritis Rheum.* 1986;29:1322–1333.

148. Althouse HL. Preplacement screening: revealing a true profile of musculoskeletal abilities. *Occup Health Saf.* 1980;49:25–30.

149. Jette AM. Concepts of health and methodological issues in functional status assessment. In: Granger CV, Gresham GE, eds. *Functional Assessment in Rehabilitation.* Baltimore, MD: Williams & Wilkins; 1984:46–64.

CHAPTER 12

Upper Extremity Functional Testing

Cynthia T. Kwasniewski, MS, OTR/L, CHT and Elaine Labovitz, OTR/L, CHT

A Difference in Emphasis

Although general and upper extremity (UE) functional capacity evaluations (FCEs) provide similar information, the emphasis placed on various aspects of the evaluation is different. For example, a general FCE provides specific sitting and standing tolerances, whereas a UE FCE usually includes examination of sensation, edema, and dexterity by using standardized tests, but only comments on standing or sitting unless there is a complaint or reported limitation. Some information, including the reason for referral, medical history, work history, job demands, specific injury history, reported functional abilities, and limitations and symptoms, is addressed in all FCEs. Although lifting, carrying, pushing, and pulling are assessed in both types of FCEs, there may be increased emphasis on handle types and hand and wrist positioning during tasks in a UE FCE.[1] Furthermore, it is inappropriate and counterproductive to assess only isolated joint motion without considering the overall physical functional requirements. Although these functions are not always formally evaluated, neck, back, and lower extremity function should be addressed in UE FCEs to determine an evaluee's ability to meet the critical demands of the job.

Because there is such a variance in UE diagnosis and related impairments, set rigid formats are generally not appropriate,[2] although there are areas that should be addressed in every test. This chapter addresses the test components specific to UE FCEs. Table 12–1 at the end of the chapter provides information (norms, validity, reliability) for a number of commonly used standardized tests. All UE FCEs should include assessment of sensation, pain, edema, range of motion, coordination and dexterity, muscle strength, grip and pinch strength, lifting, carrying, pushing and pulling, reaching, and any specific job tasks. The FCE evaluator bases decisions about which tests to include on the evaluee's diagnosis and performance during the FCE and on the referral questions. For example, a job-specific test will include evaluation of specific job demands, provided a detailed job analysis was provided (refer to Chapter 14, Job-Specific Functional Testing for Injury Management, for more information). The number of tests used in a UE FCE depends on what information is needed. Table 12–1 at the end of the chapter is a good resource to identify appropriate tests for individual situations. In addition, the case studies at end of the chapter give examples of specific test selection in a UE FCE.

Shoulder and Elbow Assessments

The ability of the shoulder and elbow to position the hand in space is critical to UE function. Problems involving the shoulder and elbow should be clearly documented in each test. Evaluees with shoulder and elbow injuries without distal arm (wrist and/or hand) involvement can be assessed with a general FCE or a UE FCE, based on the evaluator's discretion. In the UE FCE, assessment of range of motion, muscle strength, pain, and sensation includes the entire UE. Lifting and carrying, pushing and pulling, and reaching require activity of the shoulder *and* elbow. Most of the coordination and dexterity tests involve the elbow, and many also require shoulder function. Components of the Valpar (Valpar International Corporation, Tuscon, AZ), a commercially available testing method, such as Whole Body Range of Motion, incorporate shoulder and elbow mobility, and many job-specific tasks require shoulder and elbow function. Consequently, when shoulder and/or elbow involvement is accompanied by wrist and/or hand injury, a UE FCE should be performed.

Upper Extremity–Specific Components

Sensibility

Sensibility refers to the ability to feel or perceive a stimulus. Good sensibility of the hand is essential to good functional use. Even if the results of all other assessments are normal, loss of sensation can have a significant impact on a person's ability to use the hands in functional activities, including work. A comprehensive review of sensory physiology is beyond the scope of this chapter, but additional information is available.[3] There are multiple types of sensation and, therefore, multiple measures of sensory function. Each type of sensation fulfills a role in function; however, not all types need to be measured in every FCE. Although every UE FCE should include sensory screening, a good history and interview are critical to defining the need for specific tests. For example, in a person with a fracture and no history or complaints of nerve involvement, a Semmes-Weinstein mini-kit would be adequate unless the findings were abnormal. For an evaluee who has had a nerve repair or has nonspecific sensory complaints, more detailed testing, such as a full Semmes-Weinstein Test, is indicated. With the exception of the O'Riain Wrinkle Test and the Ninhydrin Test, all sensory testing is subjective.[4]

Semmes-Weinstein Monofilament Test

The Semmes-Weinstein Monofilament Test is a light touch–deep pressure threshold test that is based on the work of von Frey.[5] von Frey sorted horsehairs by thickness and stiffness and determined specific milligrams of pressure at which they would bend. He standardized the hairs and used them to test the amount of pressure a person first perceived as touch. This was a pressure test and was combined with tests for pain, touch, and temperature in a complete sensory battery.

In 1960, Semmes and Weinstein[6] developed a set of nylon monofilaments set in Lucite rods based on von Frey's test. See Figure 12–1. These filaments were laboratory-calibrated to exert specific pressure, which is the product of the length and diameter of each filament. The maximum pressure exerted is the point at which the filament bends. The amount of pressure applied is a product of the filament rather than the individual examiner. This is the only handheld test that controls for application force and vibration.[7] Sensation is classified into one of five categories based on the filament size perceived. For accuracy, filaments must be standardized at the factory and be straight before testing, and the humidity must be controlled. The test must also be administered in a standardized manner.[8,9,10(p76)] The Semmes-Weinstein Test measures constant pressure. Studies have questioned its correlation to functional sensation.[10(p76),11]

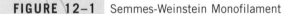

FIGURE 12–1   Semmes-Weinstein Monofilament

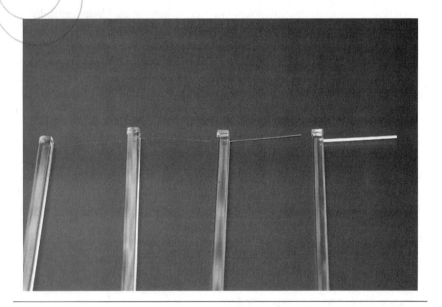

The original Semmes-Weinstein had 20 filaments and was designed to test all areas in a detailed manner. A five-filament mini-kit was designed[12] with six specific testing spots. It uses the filaments from each of the sensory loss categories and tests areas that are specific to each of the three sensory nerves of the hand. It is an excellent screening device and appropriate for use in an FCE. However, the full test should be performed in cases in which there is nerve involvement without full or near full recovery or in situations in which sensation seems to be impaired.[10(p77)]

The Weinstein Enhanced Sensory Test (WEST) The WEST is a variation of the Semmes-Weinstein Test. It has five monofilaments representing progressive levels of sensibility packaged into a single tool. Administration is similar to that of the brief Semmes-Weinstein, and the tests are often used interchangeably. Testing has determined that the respective filaments provide the same threshold results as the Semmes-Weinstein test.[13] However, the WEST measures force in milligrams and, because of its design, has its own validity studies.[14]

Two-Point Discrimination

The Static Two-Point, also known as the Weber Static Two-Point Discrimination Test,[10(p79),15] is a measure of innervation density. There are standards for performing the test, including instrumentation. The test should be performed using a Disk-Criminator (Disk-Criminator, Baltimore, MD), Boley Gauge (Boley Gauge, Research Design Inc. Houston, TX), or dull-pointed calipers. This test is also affected by variations in application of force by the examiner.[16] Testing has revealed poor reproducibility of the application of force and the addition of vibration from the examiner's hand even in the most careful application.[17] In the past, a paper clip was used but is no longer recommended because, in the manufacturing process, a burr can be created on the ends of the paper clip, which is not uniform and affects the sensory input during testing and, thus, the reliability of the test.

Moving Two-Point Discrimination The Moving Two-Point Discrimination Test[10(pp79–80),18] measures tactile gnosis (the ability to identify shapes and textures without vision) and has been found to correlate with hand function.[3,19] The tools used are the same as for the Weber Static Test, but the test is administered by moving the point(s) distally to proximally parallel to the long axis of the finger. In addition to the issues of inconsistent reproducibility of the application of force and of vibration found in static two-point testing, force measurements have been shown to vary with the topography as the points move across the skin.[17] It can be difficult to isolate testing to a single nerve. Only the fingertips are tested. There are no normative data for other areas.

Sharp-Dull

This test is not as frequently used as in the past. Its advantage was that it was portable and easy for anyone to do. Traditionally, a safety pin was used. Pain is considered a good indicator for protective sensation. Evaluees are asked to discriminate between sharp and dull stimuli. Problems with the test include the variability of pressure applied even within a single test, lack of validity and reliability studies, and the reaction of evaluees when they are told a pin or needle is used for assessment. A pin is no longer recommended when this test is performed because of infection concerns. A single-use sterile needle is the preferred tool.[10(p73)]

Vibration Testing

Vibration testing measures touch threshold and is used for placement in a sensory retraining program.[10(p77)] It is usually measured with tuning forks at 30 and 256 cps. There are some other options such as vibrometers,[10(p78),20] but these are more commonly used in research. There are standards for measuring vibration using tuning forks, but the standards do not eliminate the variable of hand pressure used by the tester, which is problematic in many sensory tests.[17] This problem also occurs in computerized forms of evaluation in which handheld devices are used.[16] "Normal" is based on comparison with the contralateral extremity, which makes the test inappropriate for patients with bilateral involvement.

Temperature

Although not a component of every UE FCE, hot-cold discrimination testing[10(p75)] can be important to evaluate in evaluees who are exposed to significant temperature changes, for example, chefs, ironworkers, and people working with dry ice. This test does not measure intolerance, which should be addressed elsewhere if that is an issue. It measures the ability to perceive temperature differences. The inability to perceive temperature could be a safety issue in many jobs.

Moberg Pick-up Test

This test measures the ability to distinguish various objects by using tactile feedback. It is primarily an assessment of median nerve function. Discrimination is a part of most jobs but becomes critical for employees such as mechanics and assembly-line workers whose vision may be obstructed during work.[10(p81),21]

Other Tests

The O'Riain Wrinkle Test This test measures sympathetic nerve function.[10(p74)] It can be an indicator of early sensory return, but its true use is in assessing sensory function in persons who cannot provide reliable feedback, such as young children and people with cognitive impairment. Results can be affected by nerve regeneration and may be useful only in recent, complete nerve injuries. Unlike most other sensory tests, it requires no subjective input from the testee. The evaluee's hand is placed in water that is 104°F for 30 minutes, and the amount of finger wrinkling is assessed and graded on a 0 to 3 scale, with 3 considered normal, compared with the other hand.

The Ninhydrin Test   The Ninhydrin Test[8,10(pp73–74)] measures sudomotor and sympathetic nerve function. Like the O'Riain Wrinkle Test, it requires no input from the testee and is appropriate for children and adults with cognitive impairment. The hand is cleaned thoroughly and wiped with alcohol or acetone. After a 30-minute period during which the hand has no contact with any surface, the fingertips are pressed against a good quality bond paper. The fingers are held in place for 15 seconds and traced with a pencil. The paper is then sprayed with Ninhydrin spray reagent and heated in an oven for 5 to 10 minutes at 200°F. Areas where sweat is detected will turn purple. However, the scoring, which is the same as for the wrinkle test, is subjective. The test is appropriate only for acute complete nerve lesions, and sudomotor function may return over time without sensory return. Results correlate with return of protective sensation but have not been found to relate to functional sensation. Because FCEs are not indicated during the acute period in which these tests are best used, these tests are not routinely seen in UE FCEs.

Volumetrics

Volumeters are used to measure volume based on the Archimedes' Principle. The volume of an irregular object, such as a hand, can be measured by submerging it in water and measuring the amount of water displaced. See Figure 12–2. Repeated measurements over time allow the status to be monitored. Volumetric measures are commonly performed at the beginning and end of a UE FCE. Even if there is no edema initially, volume is routinely measured before and after evaluation as an indicator of the evaluee's response to the evaluation. Volumeters are commercially available, and there are standardized procedures for measurement, set up, and patient preparation.[10(p14)] Volumeters have been found to be accurate within 1%.[22] Farrell et al[23] studied interrater and intrarater reliability using two standardized protocols and found both to be high with both protocols (Intraclass correlation coefficients (ICC) = 0.99). They used the manufacturer's directions for one group and a modified version of the American Society of Hand Therapists recommended protocol for the other. In addition, van Velze et al[24] found left nondominant hands to be 3.4% smaller than right dominant hands

---

FIGURE 12–2 | Volumeter

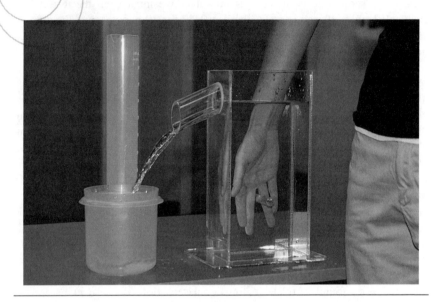

---

in laborers. Changes for left-hand–dominant people were observed to be smaller, but the sample was not large enough to draw conclusions in the study. Changes in volume of 10 ml or greater or 2% should be considered significant.[10]

Edema can also be measured by using a tape measure, which is done when swelling is beyond the range of the volumeter, for example, at the elbow, or very localized, for example, a single finger. There are standards for measurement at distances from landmarks, and these should be clearly noted in the report. For edema of a finger, a finger circumference gauge allows measurements to be made in a standard manner at the proximal and distal interphalangeal joints. Comparisons are made with the contralateral side and/or with previous measurements.

Dexterity and Coordination

Box and Block Test

Unilateral and gross manual dexterity is measured by using the Box and Block Test. It is frequently used in rehabilitation and research involving children and adults and is suitable for persons with low intelligence and/or limited manual dexterity. It is quick and easy to administer and can be homemade.[10(p92),25,26]

Purdue Pegboard

The Purdue Pegboard measures dexterity involving the gross movement of the hands, fingers, and arms and fingertip dexterity. This test has been used in the selection and/or return to work of employees in industrial jobs requiring assembly, packing, and operation of machines. Five separate scores can be obtained: (1) right hand, (2) left hand, (3) both hands, (4) right and left and both hands, and (5) assembly.[27]

Nine-Hole Peg Test

This test is a simple, timed test of fine motor coordination. Patients are scored on the time it takes to place and remove nine pegs in a board.[28–32] See Figure 12–3.

| FIGURE 12–3 | Nine-Hole Peg Board |

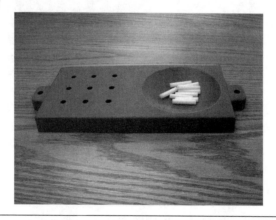

Jebsen Taylor Hand Function Test

This test evaluates a broad range of everyday hand functions. The Jebsen Taylor test can be administered to patients with a variety of diagnoses such as hemiplegia, rheumatoid arthritis, traumatic quadriplegia, brain injury, and UE injuries.[33]

Minnesota Rate of Manipulation Test (MRMT)

The MRMT is designed to measure manual dexterity or the speed of gross arm and hand movements during rapid eye-hand coordination tasks. See Figure 12–4. It is scored by totaling the number of seconds it takes to complete two, three,

| **FIGURE 12–4** | Minnesota Rate of Manipulation Test |

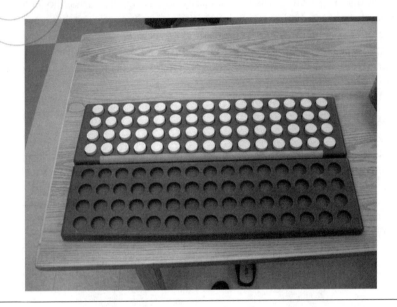

or four test trials. Each subtest has its own set of normative data. This test may be administered individually or in groups. Separate procedures are provided for administering the MRMT Displacing Test and Turning Test to the blind[*][34].

Bennett Hand Dexterity Test

The Bennett Hand Dexterity Test involves moving nuts, bolts, and washers from the left side of a box and mounting them on the right side. It measures skill in the use of ordinary tools such as wrenches and screwdrivers and is applicable in assembly, mechanical, and industrial positions that require similar tool use. It can also be used as an observational tool for assessing sequencing, planning, and spatial orientation skills. It has been used for prevocational and vocational students, injured workers, physically handicapped trainees, people who are mentally or emotionally handicapped, and people who are mentally retarded.[35]

---

[*]Because the MRMT is a standardized test, the authors have retained the usage of the term *blind* in adherence to the MRMT language.

Crawford Small Parts Dexterity Test

This test evaluates eye-hand coordination and fine motor dexterity. It is used to help predict success in jobs requiring intricate wiring of devices, electronic parts manufacturing, and engraving or adjustment of meters, clocks, watches, and other instruments. It also has percentage rankings for patients with physical disabilities and people with mental retardation.[36,37]

O'Connor Finger Dexterity Test

This dexterity test can be used to assess rapid manipulation of objects, especially small parts. It assesses fine motor skills.[38]

O'Connor Tweezer Dexterity Test

The O'Connor Tweezer Dexterity test assesses fine motor coordination and eye-hand coordination. It is similar to the O'Connor Finger Dexterity Test but requires the use of tweezers. A high score indicates an aptitude for work involving precision and steadiness in the use of small hand tools such as needed by surgeons, biological laboratory workers, watch repairers, and stamp collectors.[39]

Roeder Manipulative Aptitude Test

This test measures speed and dexterity in arm, hand, and finger movements. It is designed for students and for testing people for employment and/or upgrading of job and trade when dexterity is a main requirement. It can be used to assess performance in jobs that require assembly and disassembly of apparatus and precision placement and fitting of parts such as would be done by mechanics, repair persons, electricians, machinists, and drafts persons.[40]

Rosenbusch Test of Finger Dexterity

This dexterity test measures fine dexterity, specifically the speed of interdigital manipulation of objects by each hand separately. It is the only standardized test that focuses on the ability to simultaneously hold, manipulate, and place small objects.[2]

Stromberg Dexterity Test

The Stromberg test is a fast means of measuring finger dexterity for positions such as laundry worker, assembler, and welder. It can also be used for vocational evaluation and training programs. It is used for assessing speed and accuracy in the coordination of arm and hand movements.[41,42]

Grooved Pegboard Test

This test is a manipulative dexterity test consisting of 25 holes with randomly positioned slots. This test requires complex visual coordination because the pegs have a key along one side that must be rotated to match the hole before they are inserted. This test can be used in student laboratories and screening procedures in industry and in evaluation of lateralized brain damage.[43]

Apfel 19-Item Pick-Up Test

This test involves measurement of the time it takes a patient to transfer 19 standardized items from a specific position on a felt mat to an adjacent box. The items include a small square block (2 × 2 × ⅜ in), a roll of cloth bandage tape, a large rectangular block of redwood (16½ × 3½ × ½ in), a 2-in metal ring, an eraser (2¾ × ¾ × ⅛ in), a clothespin, a paper clip, a wing nut, a thimble, a stamp, a penny, a pencil, a rubber band, a wooden spool of thread (1½-in diameter), a safety pin, a toilet paper tube, a ping-pong ball (dented on one side for stability), a bolt (2 in long × 3⁄16 in diameter), and a matchbox (2 × ½ in). This test can be used for functional evaluation of the UE. It can be used in a wide age range and is portable and simple to administer.[44]

Strength

Grip and Pinch

Grip strength is determined by using a Jamar or similar gauge. See Figure 12–5. The gauge and normative data[45–47] used should be identified in the report. Norms are not transferable from different gauges or between manual and computer gauges. There are standardized positions for measuring grip strength,[10(pp42–43)] which are not always consistent from instrument to instrument. All instruments must be accurately calibrated and rechecked regularly to maintain accuracy. There are multiple protocols for measuring grip strength.

Grip strength measurements can serve two purposes in FCEs. Measurements can be used to determine grip strength for function or as an indicator of maximal voluntary effort. Grip strength protocols include single-trial and three-trial testing. Traditionally, three-trial testing using the mean force of three trials[10(p43)] has been the "gold standard" in measuring grip. However, recent research by Coldham

---

FIGURE 12–5   Jamar Grip Gauge

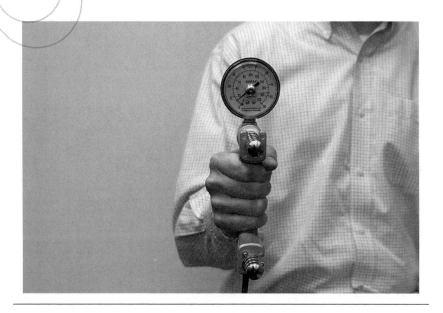

---

et al[48] compared the reliability between a one-repetition grip test with the mean and maximum force of three-repetition grip test protocols on symptomatic and asymptomatic subjects in a repeated-measures, crossover design study. Their results suggested that performing a one-repetition grip strength trial is as reliable and less painful for symptomatic subjects than the best of or the mean of three-repetition trials. Further research is needed to identify the most effective protocol for grip assessment.

Pinch strength measurements may be determined by using manual and computerized gauges. The "gold standard" for manual gauges is the B&L pinch gauge. See Figure 12–6. Positioning is not as standardized for pinch as for grip. When comparing pinch results with normative data, the position used when the normative data were obtained should be carefully duplicated. There is some evidence that pinch scores are transferable from instrument to instrument,[49] but this must be done with care. As with dynamometers, pinch gauges need to be calibrated and regularly rechecked.

Although pinch and grip strength assessments with force gauges are considered reliable and valid, they are dependent on patient compliance, so evaluee effort

---

FIGURE 12-6   Pinch Gauge

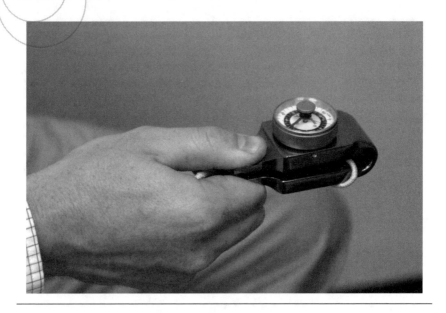

---

must be considered. Published normative data may not always be reliable owing to instrument calibration. Therefore, the American Society of Hand Therapists recommends contralateral comparison.[10(p44)] In addition, questions have arisen about measurement error and the amount of change needed in subsequent testing to detect true strength changes.[50] Five-level (Bell-Shaped Curve) and rapid-exchange tests are used to assess maximum voluntary effort and are addressed in the section "Assessing Evaluee Effort and Consistency."

Manual Muscle Testing

The UE FCE may assess the impact of injury and/or disease involving any part of the UE, but even if only the hand or a finger is involved, it is not uncommon to find weakness more proximal in the extremity due to disuse. Manual muscle testing (MMT) is a procedure to evaluate muscle strength and is included in most FCEs. In a UE FCE, MMT may include more detailed testing of intrinsic hand muscles. The MMT should be performed in the standard manner described by Kendall and McCreary[51] or Daniels and Worthington[52] with any variance in technique noted.

Commercially Available Tests

Valpar

Valpar Component Work Samples (VCWSs) were designed for use in the vocational evaluation field.[53] There are 21 individual work samples that have been identified as well suited for allied health uses. Each sample simulates different work factors that are required by different jobs. Most of the Valpar assessments provide Methods-Time Measurement (MTM) and norm-referenced information. Chapter 9 provides a detailed description of the MTM approach. A brief description of 20 samples follows. The VCWS 14, Integrated Peer Performance, is not included because it is given to three to five people simultaneously and would not be appropriate for a UE extremity FCE.

VCWS 1, Small Tools (Mechanical), helps assess the ability to work with small tools and parts in small, confined spaces, with work totally or partially blocked from view. It involves reaching, handling, fingering, feeling, near acuity, depth perception, and accommodation. It assesses motor coordination and finger and manual dexterity.

VCWS 2, Size Discrimination, simulates light work activities and involves reading, fingering, feeling, near acuity, depth perception, and accommodation and assesses size discrimination and manual and finger dexterity.

VCWS 3, Numerical Sorting, involves sorting, categorizing, and filing by numbered arrangement and using numbers and numerical series. It assesses clerical aptitude, motor coordination and finger and manual dexterity.

VCWS 4, Upper Extremity Range of Motion, is commonly used in allied health settings for assessment and treatment. It involves picking up nuts and reaching through a hole in the work sample box and placing the nut on the proper size screw. This sample assesses UE range of motion, endurance, reaching, fingering, feeling, near acuity, depth perception, accommodation, and color vision. It assesses motor coordination and finger and manual dexterity.

VCWS 5, Clerical Comprehension and Aptitude, requires answering telephones, sorting mail, alphabetical filing, bookkeeping, and typing. It involves reaching, handling, fingering, feeling, talking, hearing, and seeing and assesses motor coordination, finger and manual dexterity, and form perception.

VCWS 6, Independent Problem Solving, requires comparison of colored geometric shapes, presented on a series of cards, with the master key mounted on the work sample. It involves reading, handling, near acuity, accommodation, and color vision and assesses form perception, clerical perception, motor coordination, finger and manual dexterity, and color discrimination.

VCWS 7, Multi-Level Sorting, requires making rapid sorting decisions while performing work tasks that require physical manipulation and visual discrimination of objects (plastic chips) with different colors, letters, numbers, and combinations of these and placement of them in the correct slots. It involves reaching, fingering, near acuity, depth perception, accommodation, color vision, and field of vision and assesses motor coordination, finger and manual dexterity, form perception, and color discrimination.

VCWS 8, Simulated Assembly, requires the assembly of a three-part object (pin, spacer, and cap) in an assembly line manner as a motorized wheel spins. This test simulates repetitive assembly work and requires bimanual use of both UEs. It requires reaching, handling, fingering, feeling, near acuity, depth perception, accommodation, and field of vision and assesses motor coordination and finger and manual dexterity.

VCWS 9, Whole Body Range of Motion, requires the transfer of three colored shapes, one at a time, by screwing and unscrewing nuts from the board. The transfers occur from four levels. The levels include shoulder height to overhead, overhead to waist level, waist level to knee level, and knee level back to shoulder level. The test requires handling, fingering, feeling, near visual acuity, and depth perception. It assesses whole body range of motion, agility, and stamina through gross body movements of the trunk, arms, hands, legs, and fingers; finger and manual dexterity; motor coordination; and form perception. The test permits examination of the effects of kneeling, bending, stooping, repeated crouching, and overhead reaching on various work-related tasks. See Figure 12–7.

VCWS 10, Tri-Level Measurement, requires various inspections and measurements from very simple to very precise. It uses various measuring devices to decide whether 50 parts have been machined to various specifications. It requires reaching, handling, fingering, feeling, and sight and assesses finger and manual dexterity, form perception, spatial aptitude, general learning ability, clerical perception, and motor coordination.

FIGURE 12-7   VCWS 9

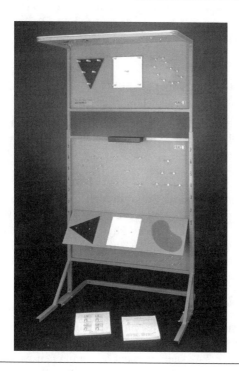

VCWS 11, Eye-Hand-Foot Coordination, assesses the ability to move the eyes, hands, and feet in coordination. It requires reaching, handling, fingering, feeling, and seeing and assesses eye-hand-foot coordination, motor coordination, finger dexterity, general learning ability, and spatial aptitude.

VCWS 12, Soldering and Inspection (Electronic), assesses the ability to acquire and apply the skills necessary to perform soldering tasks of varying complexity. This test requires reaching, handling, fingering, feeling, and seeing and assesses motor coordination, manual dexterity, general learning ability, spatial aptitude, form perception, and finger dexterity.

VCWS 15, Electrical Circuitry and Print Reading, assesses skills related to understanding and working with electrical circuits. It involves the use of a variety of tools to test electrical circuits for circuit continuity and to repair circuits. It requires patients to read electrical schematic prints and install wires, diodes, and resistors. The test requires reaching, handling, fingering, feeling, near acuity, depth perception, accommodation, and color vision and assesses spatial aptitude, form perception, motor coordination, and finger and manual dexterity.

VCWS 16, Drafting, assesses the ability to read blueprints and work in the drafting trades. Tasks require reaching, handling, fingering, feeling, and sight and assess spatial aptitude, general learning ability, verbal aptitude, form perception, motor coordination, manual and finger dexterity, clerical perception, and numerical skills.

VCWS 19, Dynamic Physical Capabilities, is designed to simulate the work tasks of a shipping clerk. It assesses sedentary to very heavy strength levels as outlined by the Department of Labor's Physical Demands.[53] It involves climbing, balancing, lifting, carrying, reaching, pushing and pulling, and variations in whole body positions. It also has the ability to evaluate the patient's work endurance and pace or rate of work completion.

VCWS 201, Physical Capabilities and Mobility Screening Evaluation, was designed to be a nonmedical screening of the 17 physical demand factors of the Department of Labor.[53] As such, it is not as comprehensive as VCWS 19; however, it screens climbing, balancing, stooping, kneeling, crouching, crawling, walking, standing, lifting, reaching, handling, fingering, feeling, pushing, pulling, seeing, and talking. It also screens the following non–Department of Labor physical factors: hand grip, palm press, horizontal press, vertical press, walking (heel-toe), walking (toes), walking (heels), and squatting-walking backward.

VCWS 202, Mechanical Assembly/Alignment and Hammering, contains four short independent exercises. The first, assembly, requires the patient to use wrenches to assemble two halves of a hard rubber block using bolts, springs, washers, and nuts. The second, alignment/driving, requires the patient to drive several bars through holes in the rubber block, using a rubber mallet, punch, wrench, and ball-peen hammer. The third task, disassembly, involves taking apart parts and putting them into proper containers. In the fourth task, hammering, the patient uses a claw hammer and inkpad to rapidly tap small targets on three hammering sheets. The test requires reaching, handling, fingering, feeling, and seeing and assesses motor coordination, finger and manual dexterity, and upper extremity strength.

VCWS 203, Mechanical Reasoning and Machine Tending, involves five exercises that require reaching, handling, fingering, feeling, and seeing and assesses motor coordination, finger and manual dexterity, and general learning ability.

VCWS 204, Fine Finger Dexterity, assesses the ability to perform work tasks that require a high level of finger dexterity in the dominant and nondominant hands. It requires reaching, handling, fingering, feeling, near acuity, depth perception, and visual accommodation and requires motor coordination and manual and finger dexterity.

VCWS 205, Independent Perceptual Screening (Spatial Aptitude), requires visualization of geometric forms and comprehension of two-dimensional representations of three-dimensional objects. It requires the completion of three tasks with vision occluded. It involves reaching, handling, fingering, feeling, and seeing and assesses spatial and general learning ability, form perception, motor coordination, and finger and manual dexterity.

CHAPTER 12

Baltimore Therapeutic Equipment Work Simulator

The Baltimore Therapeutic Equipment Work Simulator (BTE) is a magnet-based computerized work simulator. See Figure 12–8. By using multiple tool inserts, it allows for a wide variety of task simulations and is used in treatment and evaluation. Strength can be assessed isometrically or dynamically. Since its introduction in 1981, there have been multiple improvements in the system, and currently, four different units are commonly used as tools in FCEs: the W10, the W20, the Simulator II, and the Primus. In addition, BTE has developed a comprehensive functional testing system, the ER Functional Testing System, which can be used as a stand-alone FCE but is not UE-specific. See the Appendix for a description of this FCE model.

The W10 and the W20 are similar units (W20 allows for a greater variance in exercise head height). Both are older units that can be modified by adding the Quest, a computer link that facilitates data collection and reporting. The Simulator II is an updated version of the W20. The BTE Primus was introduced in 1994 and has different tools and measurements but similar issues with reliability and validity. All have been shown to be reliable in the static mode,[54,55] which is used in determining consistency of effort, but have wide variations in resistance when used in the dynamic mode,[56] the mode used in treatment and in

FIGURE 12–8	Baltimore Therapeutic Equipment Work Stimulator (BTE)

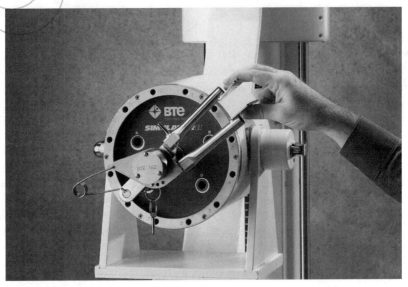

Courtesy of BTE Technologies, Inc. (www.btetech.com)

job simulation during FCEs. This variability occurs within machines and even within individual sessions, limiting its value in job simulation in which specific resistance levels need to be tested and potentially creating a risk for patients who may not be able to tolerate wide variances in resistance.

Dexter Hand Evaluation and Treatment System

The Dexter Hand Evaluation and Treatment System is a computerized evaluation system designed to collect data using attachment tools and accept data input such as from sensory tests and volumetrics. It gives the evaluator the ability to produce data analysis and customer reports. Algorithms of the American Medical Association's *Guides to the Evaluation of Permanent Impairment, Fifth Edition* are integrated into the system, enabling analysis and automated report generation. Attachment tools include computerized goniometers and dynamometers.

Brown et al[57] studied the concurrent validity of these components by comparing them with the gold standards of manual goniometry, Jamar dynamometers, and B&L pinch gauges. Bellace et al[58] compared the dynamometer component with the Jamar. They found the measurement statistically similar and, therefore, reliable.

Assessing Evaluee Effort and Consistency

The UE FCE identifies a person's ability to perform physical functional activities with the UEs. Important considerations are the client's level of effort and consistency of performance.[2] Assessment of effort and consistency of performance is done as part of a total assessment to help set appropriate capacity parameters. Tests that address the level and consistency of evaluee patient effort (described in Chapter 11) assess whether a person performed with maximum voluntary effort. There can be many reasons for submaximal effort, including fear of reinjury or pain, pain, fatigue, the effects of the impairment, and even the reliability of the measure being used in the particular situation.[2] In a literature review, Innes[59] found that "no single method of determining sincerity of effort can be recommended . . . extreme caution should be used when interpreting the results."

Many tests can be used to determine a client's level of performance in a UE FCE. One common combination is the King Protocol,[60] which combines five specific measures, ie, repeated grip measures at one position on the Jamar, the five-position grip test on the Jamar, static testing with tools 302 and 502 on the BTE, and comparison of right-left differences on the Jamar vs tool 162 on the BTE. The use of multiple measures enhances the ability to identify submaximal effort. King and Berryhill[60] used healthy subjects for their testing. By using probability measures, they found that a cutoff point of passing four of five tests yielded few false-positive (.0606p) and false-negative (.1363p) results in their test group. This protocol is highly dependent on the use of coefficients of variation (CVs) to determine sincerity of effort. The use of CVs has been criticized.[61–64] See Chapter 11 for a more detailed discussion of testing using healthy subjects.

Bell-Shaped Curve (Five-Level Grip Test)

According to Stokes et al,[65] grip assessment using the five positions of the dynamometer should produce a bell-shaped curve when exerting maximal voluntary effort. This test is used to measure evaluee effort. Multiple studies have been performed to assess the validity of this protocol and have produced conflicting results.[66–68] People with UE injuries and people with a weak grip may not produce a bell-shaped curve even when performing with maximum effort.

Rapid-Exchange Grip Test

The Rapid-Exchange Grip Test was originally proposed by Hildreth et al[69] as a method to identify submaximal performance. The test involves the evaluee rapidly producing maximum grip force with the gauge moved quickly between both hands. The test is based on the premise that exerting submaximal effort requires planning and that the rapid exchange of the gauge between hands during the test does not allow the evaluee the time to control effort. Rapid-Exchange results are compared with "static tests maximal." If the rapid-exchange results are higher than the maximal effort grip results, the test is considered a positive result or indicative of submaximal effort. Hildreth et al[69] did not specify the static grip test used, positioning during testing, or the rate of exchange, and subsequent studies have used different standards. The lack of a standardized protocol concerning administration and comparison testing limits the usefulness of this test. Shechtman and Taylor[70] found that the same person could be seen as giving maximal or submaximal effort depending on the test protocol used. Taylor and Shechtman[71] proposed a standard protocol for the Rapid-Exchange test but still found the test was not sufficiently sensitive or specific to reliably detect submaximal effort.[72] These tests were also discussed in Chapter 11.

Recent Protocols

In 2002, Schapmire et al[73] proposed the Simultaneous Bilateral Testing Protocol, which assesses multiple trials of unilateral and bilateral simultaneous grip and pinch testing. This testing involved the use of the CV and the bell-shaped curve and was tested only on asymptomatic people. Shechtman[74] developed the Visual Target Grip Test. This instrument uses incorrect visual feedback to "trick" the person into exerting maximal grip strength. Grip strength and electromyographic results of the "trick" measurement are compared with nontrick trials. This test is in the preliminary phase but may have future value in assessing maximal effort.

In addition to the tools used as part of the King Validity Protocol, various BTE tools have been identified for use in testing for submaximal effort.[62] Regardless of the specific tool, the CV is used, thus creating the same issues identified in the preceding paragraphs.

Job Task Simulation

In a job-specific UE FCE, the protocol includes evaluation of the evaluee's ability to perform the fine motor and UE activities that are required for his or her specific job. Some simulations can involve specific standardized components such as the Valpar or BTE. Information about an evaluee's ability can also be obtained from results of standardized coordination and dexterity tests. However, often a nonstandardized assessment that simulates an evaluee's specific job demands is necessary. This simulation may involve writing, typing, sorting, assembly, tool use, or any number of tasks. For the simulation, the evaluator must create a situation in which the evaluee is asked to duplicate specific work tasks and the evaluee's performance is evaluated for endurance, tolerance, and accuracy. Performance is then compared with identified job expectations.

UE Testing in Non-Upper Extremity Functional Capacity Evaluations

Individual components of UE FCEs may be used in a general FCE to assess evaluee effort and consistency, simulate a specific job component, measure coordination and dexterity in an FCE that is being done to determine appropriate job or training placement, assess dexterity as part of a general functional skills assessment, or as a means of providing activity for the client to perform while assessing sitting or standing tolerance. See Table 12–1 at the end of the chapter.

Assessing Effort and Consistency

Upper extremity tests, which have norms and CVs, are used as indicators of consistent maximal effort for evaluees with non-UE injuries. Issues such as pain, fear of reinjury, and fatigue and weakness may or may not be factors and need to be assessed during the interpretation of test results. The issues addressed for UE FCEs concerning the validity and reliability of measuring consistency of effort in this manner are the same. Chapter 11 provides further discussion.

Job Simulation

Any of the standardized coordination and dexterity tests can be used for specific job simulation as long as they closely match the actual work requirements. The various Valpar tests provide a wide variety of possible simulations and were designed to measure skills for job placement. In addition, the BTE has a variety of tools and can be adjusted to mimic various work situations.

Placement

When looking at job placement or training as opposed to return to a previous job, there is a need for a broader span of information. While comprehensive aptitude and interest testing is beyond the scope of an FCE, determining physical skills is essential. For example, a manual laborer with a back injury who cannot return to a previous job may be considering placement in a job that requires fine motor dexterity but minimal lifting. Consequently, in addition to addressing sitting and standing tolerance, an FCE performed to assess job placement or vocational rehabilitation must address the extent to which an evaluee has physical skills other than those referable to the initial occupation. Although it is not possible to screen for all possible options, a general assessment of manual dexterity and motor manipulation ability will be warranted in many such situations.

Sitting and Standing Tolerance

Sitting and/or standing tolerance is a critical component of an FCE and needs to be measured. This measurement is often done as part of a standardized evaluation system. However, there are times when specific postures or lengths of time need to be assessed. Ideally, this testing would be done using the station and tools required on the job, but this is not always feasible. The UE FCE components can be used to provide a simulated task while posture and tolerance are evaluated. In these cases, the component is not an evaluation measure but a prop and need not be used in a standardized manner. Evaluees can also be asked to complete psychometric testing during this time, especially if there is a need to assess sitting tolerance.

Case Studies

The following case studies are presented to illustrate how an FCE evaluator might use specific upper extremity tests in different clinical circumstances.

Case Study 1

A 35-year-old assembly worker sustained lacerations of the flexor digitorum profundus (extrinsic flexor muscle of the fingers at the distal interphalangeal joints), flexor digitorum superficialis (extrinsic flexor muscle of the fingers at the proximal interphalangeal joints), and median nerve in Zone 5 (forearm). He has completed traditional therapy and has been referred for an FCE to assess his ability to return to work. As part of the evaluation, the following assessment would be appropriate:

- Complete Semmes-Weinstein to assess sensibility return in the median nerve distribution
- Moberg Pick-up Test to assess fine motor function following median nerve injury
- VCWS 8, Simulated Assembly, to assess potential performance in his assembly job

- Intrinsic MMT and grip and pinch strengths to assess the strength of muscles innervated by the median nerve
- The MRMT and Nine-Hole Peg Test to assess dexterity and fine motor coordination, which involves sensory and motor function of the median nerve

Case Study 2

A right-handed 40-year-old construction worker sustained a distal radius fracture to his right arm. He developed a frozen shoulder during immobilization. He has completed traditional therapy and has been referred for an FCE. Case-specific key components of the evaluation would include the following:

- Upper extremity range of motion, MMT, and grip and pinch strengths to identify residual limitations
- Unilateral and bilateral lifts to various heights from floor to overhead; carry and push and pull
- VCWS 9, Whole Body Range of Motion
- VCWS 202, Mechanical Assembly/Alignment and Hammering
- Bennett Hand Tool Dexterity

These tests simulate functions required to perform his job. Residual limitations from a distal radius fracture, frozen shoulder, or both can limit the results of the assessment.

Case Study 3

A 30-year-old factory worker whose job involves picking and packing small bottles of pharmaceutical products has a clinical diagnosis of carpal tunnel syndrome, but the results of electrodiagnostic or electromyography and nerve conduction velocity tests (EMG/NCV) and magnetic resonance imaging (MRI) are negative. She complains of intermittent numbness and tingling, as well as pain, in the affected hand and has had no resolution of symptoms with conservative management including therapy, splints, rest, and cortisone injections. She has been referred for an FCE. She reports no numbness, tingling, or pain at the beginning of the evaluation.

Following obtaining a history and review of the job description, the assessment takes place in the following order: volumeter, range of motion, manual muscle testing, complete Semmes-Weinstein Monofilament Test, initial grip and pinch strengths, Nine-Hole Peg Test, and MRMT. At this point in the evaluation, she reports a slight aching in her wrist and hand but no sensory changes. With the Dynamic Lift and Carry and VCWS 7, Multi-Level Sorting, her sensory and pain symptom reports increase. Repeated Semmes-Weinstein Monofilament Test, grip and pinch strength, and volumetry would be performed to assess the effect of activity. Measurable changes would be an indication for further assessment of her condition, and she would be referred back to the referring physician with a report of findings.

CHAPTER 12

CHAPTER 12

TABLE 12–1   Upper Extremity Test

Test	Measures	Age Range	Norms	Test/Retest	Interrater	Validity
Apfel 19(44)	Handling		Yes	Yes	Yes	Yes
Bennett(35)	Finger dexterity, tool usage		Yes	Yes	No	Yes
Box and block(25,26)	Unilateral gross manual dexterity	20–75+		Yes	Yes	Yes
BTE-Dynamic(56)	Strength, endurance		No	No	No	No
BTE-Static(54,55)	Isometric strength		No	Yes	Yes	Yes
Circumferential measure(10)	Edema		No	No	No	Yes
Crawford(36,37)	Eye-hand coordination, fine motor dexterity, tool usage		Yes	No	No	Yes
Dexter(57,58)	ROM, grip, pinch		Yes	Yes	Yes	
Grip strength(45,46,47)	Grip strength	6–75+	Yes	Yes	Yes	Yes
Grooved pegboard(43)	Finger dexterity		Yes	No	No	No
Jamar bell-shaped curve(67)	Consistency of effort		Yes	No	No	No
Jebsen(10,33)	Seven test items to be representative of various hand tasks, finger dexterity, tool usage, ADLs		Yes	Yes		Yes
King protocol(59)	Consistency of effort		Yes	No	Yes	No

TABLE 12–1 Upper Extremity Test (continued)

Test	Measures	Age Range	Norms	Test/Retest	Interrater	Validity
Minnesota rate of manipulation(34)	Finger dexterity		Yes	Yes	No	No
MMT(51,52)	Muscle strength		Yes	Varies	Varies	Yes
Moberg pick up(10,12)	Finger dexterity, tool usage, sensibility		No	No	No	No
Moving two-point(18,74)	Tactile gnosis		Yes	No	No	No
Nine-hole peg test(30,31)	Finger dexterity	4–75+	Yes	Yes	Yes	Yes
Ninhydrin(10)	Sudomotor function		No	Yes	Yes	Yes
O'Connor finger(38)	Finger and fine motor dexterity		Yes	Yes	No	No
O'Connor tweezer(39)	Fine motor and eye-hand coordination		Yes	Yes	No	No
O'Riain wrinkle test(10)	Sympathetic nerve function		No	No	No	No
Pinch strength(46,49)	Tip, three jaw, and lateral pinch	6–75+	Yes	Yes	Yes	Yes
Purdue pegboard(27,28,29)	Gross movements of hands, fingers, and arms; fingertip dexterity; job simulation	14–60+	Yes	Yes	No	Yes
Rapid exchange(70,71)	Consistency of effort		Yes	No	No	No

CHAPTER 12

TABLE 12–1 Upper Extremity Test (continued)

Test	Measures	Age Range	Norms	Test/Retest	Interrater	Validity
Roeder(40)	Upper extremity speed and dexterity		Yes	Yes	Yes	Yes
Rosenbusch(42)	Finger dexterity		Yes	Yes	Yes	No
Semmes-Weinstein(6,7)	Sensibility		Yes	Yes	Yes	Yes
Sharp/dull(10)	Pain perception		No	No	No	No
Stromberg(41)	Finger dexterity		Yes	No	No	Yes
Temperature(10)	Temperature		No	No	No	No
Three-trial jamar(10,48)	Consistency of effort		Yes	No	No	No
Two-point discrimination(20)	Innervation density		Yes	No	No	No
Valpar(53)	Varies, *see individual tests*		Yes	No	No	Yes
Vibration(10)	Vibration		No	No	No	No
Volumeter(22,23,24)	Volume-edema		No	Yes	Yes	Yes
West(14)	Sensibility		Yes	Yes	Yes	Yes

References

1. Schultz-Johnson K. Upper extremity factors in the evaluation of lifting. *J Hand Ther.* 1990;3:72–85.
2. Johnson KS. Upper extremity functional capacity evaluation. In: Mackin EJ, Callahan AD, Skirven TM, Schneider LH, Osterman AL, eds. *Rehabilitation of the Hand and Upper Extremity.* 5th ed. Philadelphia, PA: Mosby; 2002.
3. Dellon AL. *Evaluation of Sensibility and Re-education of Sensation of the Hand.* Baltimore, MD: Williams & Wilkins; 1981.
4. Callahan AD. Sensibility assessment for nerve lesions-in-continuity and nerve lacerations. In: Mackin EJ, Callahan AD, Skirven TM, Schneider LH, Osterman AL, eds. *Rehabilitation of the Hand and Upper Extremity.* 5th ed. Philadelphia, PA: Mosby; 2002.
5. Von Frey M. The distribution of afferent nerves in the skin. *JAMA.* 1906;47:645–648.
6. Weinstein S. Tactile sensitivity of the phalanges. *Percept Mot Skills.* 1962;14:351–354.
7. Bell-Krotoski JA, Fess EE, Fiqarola JH, Hiltz D. Threshold detection and Semmes-Weinstein Monofilaments. *J Hand Ther.* 1993;6:155–162.
8. Von Prince K, Butler B Jr. Measuring sensory function of the hand in peripheral nerve injuries. *Am J Occup Ther.* 1967;21:385–395.
9. Werner JL, Omer GE Jr. Evaluating cutaneous pressure sensation of the hand. *Am J Occup Ther.* 1970;24:347–356.
10. Casanova JS, ed. *Clinical Assessment Recommendations.* 2nd ed. Chicago, IL: American Society of Hand Therapists; 1992.
11. Moberg E. The unsolved problem: testing functional value of hand sensibility. *J Hand Ther.* 1991;4:105–110.
12. Bell-Krotoski J. "Pocket filaments" and specifications for the Semmes-Weinstein Monofilaments. *J Hand Ther.* 1990;3:26–31.
13. Weinstein S. Fifty years of somatosensory research: from Semmes-Weinstein Monofilaments to the Weinstein Enhanced Sensory Test. *J Hand Ther.* 1993;6:11–22.
14. Schulz LA, Bohannon RW, Morgan WJ. Normal digital tip values for the Weinstein Enhanced Sensory Test. *J Hand Ther.* 1998;11:200–205.
15. Louis DS, Greene TL, Jacobson KE, Rasmussen C, Kolowich P, Goldstein SA. Evaluation of normal values for stationary and moving two-point discrimination in the hand. *J Hand Surg (Am).* 1984;9A:552–555.
16. Bell-Krotoski J, Weinstein S, Weinstein C. Testing sensibility, including touch pressure, two-point discrimination, point localization, and vibration. *J Hand Ther.* 1993;6:114–123.
17. Bell-Kotoski JA, Buford WL. The force/time relationship of clinically used sensory testing instruments. *J Hand Ther.* 1997;10:297–309.
18. Dellon AL. The moving two-point discrimination test: clinical evaluation of the quickly adapting fiber receptor system. *J Hand Surg (Am).* 1978;3:474–481.
19. Dellon AL, Kallman CH. Evaluation of functional sensation in the hand. *J Hand Surg (Am).* 1983;6:865–870.
20. Szabo RM, Gelberman RH, Williamson RV, Dellon AL, Yaru NC, Dimmick MP. Vibratory sensory testing in acute peripheral nerve compression. *J Hand Surg (Am).* 1984;9A:104–109.

CHAPTER 12

21. Ng CL, Ho DD, Chow SP. The Moberg Pick Up Test: results of testing with a standard protocol. *J Hand Ther.* 1999;12:309–312.

22. Waylett-Rendall J, Seilby DS. A study of a commercially available volumeter. *J Hand Ther.* 1991;4:10–13.

23. Farrell K, Johnson A, Duncan H, Offenbacker T. The intertester and intratester reliability of hand volumetrics. *J Hand Ther.* 2003;16:292–299.

24. van Velze CA, Kluever I, vander Merwe CA, Mennen U. The difference in volume of dominant and nondominant hands. *J Hand Ther.* 1991;4:6–10.

25. Desrosiers J, Bravo G, Hebert R, Dutil E, Mercier L. Validation of the box and block test as a measure of dexterity of elderly people: reliability, validity and norms studies. *Arch Phys Med Rehabil.* 1994;75:751–755.

26. Mathiowetz V, Volland G, Kashman N, Weber K. Adult norms for the box and block test of manual dexterity. *Am J Occup Ther.* 1985;39:386–391.

27. Tiffin J. *Purdue Pegboard Examiner Manual.* Yonkers, NY: Special Education Materials, Inc; 1968.

28. Mathiowetz V, Rogers S, Dowe-Keval M, Donahoe L, Rennells C. The Purdue Pegboard: norms for 14 to 19 year olds. *Am J Occup Ther.* 1986;3:174–179.

29. Desrosiers J, Heber R, Bravo G, Dute E. The Purdue Pegboard Test: normative data for people aged 60 and over. *Disabil Rehabil.* 1995;17:217–224.

30. Oxford-Grice K, Vogel K, Le V, Mitchell A, Muniz S, Vollmer M. Adult norms for a commercially available nine hole peg test for finger dexterity. *Am J Occup Ther.* 2003;57:570–573.

31. Mathiowitz V, Weber K, Kushnan N, Volland G. Adult norms for the nine hole peg test of finger dexterity. *Occup Ther J Res.* 2003;5:24–38.

32. Poole J, Burtner P, Torres T, et al. Measuring dexterity in children using the Nine-Hole Peg Test. *J Hand Ther.* 2005;18:348–351.

33. Jebsen R, Taylor N, Trieschmann R, Trotter M, Howard L. An objective and standardized test of hand function. *Arch Phys Med Rehabil.* 1969;70:311–319.

34. *The Minnesota Rate of Manipulation Tests Examiner's Manual.* Circle Pines, MN: American Guidance Service Inc; 1969.

35. *Hand Tool Dexterity Test User Instructions.* Lafayette, IN: Lafayette Instrument; 2002.

36. Crawford Small Parts Dexterity Test. www.creativeorgdesign.com/cspdt.htm. Accessed July 18, 2007.

37. Crawford Small Parts Dexterity Test. http://pearsonassess.com/HAIWEB/Cultures/en-us/Productdetail.htm?Pid=015-8040-805&Mode=summary. Accessed July 18, 2007.

38. *O'Connor Finger Dexterity Test User Instructions.* Lafayette, IN: Lafayette Instrument; 2002.

39. *O'Connor Tweezer Dexterity Test User Instructions.* Lafayette, IN: Lafayette Instrument; 2002.

40. *Roeder Manipulative Aptitude Test User Instructions.* Lafayette, IN: Lafayette Instrument; 2002.

41. Stromberg Dexterity Test. www.creativeorgdesign.com/sdt.htm. Accessed July 18, 2007.

42. Stein C, Yerx EJ. A test of fine finger dexterity. *Am J Occup Ther.* 1990;44:499–504.

43. Grooved Pegboard. www.rehaboutlet.com/dexterity_hand_eye_coordination_tests.htm. Accessed August 5, 2007.

44. Apfel E. Preliminary development of a standardized hand function test. *J Hand Ther.* 1990;3:191–194.
45. Mathiowetz V, Weber K, Volland G, Kashman N. Reliability and validity of hand strength evaluation. *J Hand Surg (Am).* 1984;9A:222–226.
46. Mathiowetz V, Kashman N, Vollard G, Weber K, Dowe M, Rogers S. Grip and pinch strength: normative data for adults. *Arch Phys Med Rehabil.* 1985;66:69–74.
47. Hanten WP, Chen WY, Austin AA. Maximum grip strength in normal subjects from 20 to 64 years of age. *J Hand Ther.* 1999;12:193–200.
48. Coldman F, Lewis J, Lee H. The reliability of one vs three grip trials in symptomatic and asymptomatic subjects. *J Hand Ther.* 2006;19:318–326.
49. MacDermid JC, Evenhuis W, Louzon M. Inter-instrument reliability of pinch strength scores. *J Hand Ther.* 2001;14:36–42.
50. Schreuders T, Roebroeck M, Goumans J, van Nieuwenhuijzen J, Stijen T, Stam H. Measurement error in grip and pinch force measurements in patients with hand injuries. *Phys Ther.* 2003;9:806–815.
51. Kendall P, McCreary EK. *Muscle Testing and Function.* 3rd ed. Baltimore, MD: Williams & Wilkins; 1983.
52. Daniels L, Worthington C. *Muscle Testing Techniques of Manual Examination.* Philadelphia, PA: WB Saunders; 1986.
53. Christopherson B, Hayes P. *Valpar Component Work Samples Uses In Allied Health.* Tucson, AZ: Valpar; 1992.
54. Trossman P, Suleski K, Li PW. Test-retest reliability and day-to-day variability of an isometric grip strength test using the work simulator. *Occup Ther J Res.* 1990; 10:266–271.
55. Shechtman O, Davenport R, Malcolm M, Nabavi D. Reliability of the BTE-Primus Grip Tool. *J Hand Ther.* 2003;16:36–42.
56. Coleman EF, Renfro RR, Cetinok EM, Fess EE, Shaar CJ, Dupace KR. Reliability of the manual dynamic mode of the Baltimore Therapeutic Equipment Work Simulator. *J Hand Ther.* 1996;9:223–237.
57. Brown A, Cramer L, Eckhaus D, Schmidt J, Ware L, MacKenzie E. Validity and reliability of the Dexter Hand Evaluation and Therapy System in hand-injured patients. *J Hand Ther.* 2000;13:37–45.
58. Bellace J, Healy D, Besser M, Byron T, Hohman L. Validity of the Dexter Evaluation System's Jamar Dynamometer attachment for hand grip strength in the normal population. *J Hand Ther.* 2000;13:46–51.
59. Innes E. Hand grip strength testing: a review of the literature. *Aust Occup Ther J.* 1999;46:120–140.
60. King JW, Berryhill BH. Assessing maximum effort in upper extremity functional testing. *Work.* 1991;1:5–76.
61. Shechtman O. Is the coefficient of variation a valid measure for detecting sincerity of effort of grip strength? *Work.* 1999;2:163–169.
62. Schechtman O. Using the coefficient of variation to detect sincerity of effort of grip strength: a literature review. *J Hand Ther.* 2000;14:25–32.
63. Schechtman O. The coefficient of variation as a measure of sincerity of effort of grip strength, part I. *J Hand Ther.* 2001;14:180–187.
64. Shechtman O. The coefficient of variation as a measure of sincerity of effort of grip strength, part II: sensitivity and specificity. *J Hand Ther.* 2001;14:188–194.

CHAPTER 12

65. Stokes HM, Landrieu KW, Domangue B, Kumen S. Identification of low-effort patients through dynamometry. *J Hand Surg (Am).* 1995;20:1047–1056.
66. Shechtman O, Gutierrez Z, Kokendofer E. Analysis of the statistical methods used to detect submaximal effort with the five-rung grip strength test. *J Hand Ther.* 2005;18:10–18.
67. Goldman S, Cahalan TD, An KN. The injured upper extremity and the Jamar Five Handle Position Grip Test. *Am J Phys Med Rehabil.* 1991;70:306–308.
68. Gutierrez Z, Schechtman O. Effectiveness of the five handle position grip strength test in detecting sincerity of effort in men and women. *Am J Phys Med Rehabil.* 2003;11:847–855.
69. Hildreth DH. Breidenbac WC, Liste GD, Hodge AD. Detection of submaximal effort by use of the rapid exchange grip. *J Hand Surg (Am).* 1989;4:742–745.
70. Shechtman O, Taylor C. How do therapists administer the Rapid Exchange Grip Test? *J Hand Ther.* 2002;15:53–61.
71. Taylor C, Shechtman O. The use of Rapid Exchange Grip Test in detecting sincerity of effort, part I: administration of the test. *J Hand Ther.* 2000;13:195–202.
72. Shechtman O, Taylor C. The use of Rapid Exchange Grip Test in detecting sincerity of effort, part II: validity of the test. *J Hand Ther.* 2000;13:203–210.
73. Schapmire D, St James D, Townsend R, Stewart T, Delheimer S, Focht D. Simultaneous bilateral testing: validation of a new protocol to detect submaximal effort during grip and pinch strength testing. *J Hand Ther.* 2002;15:242–249.
74. Shechtman O. Using the "Visual Target Grip Test" to identify the level of effort during grip strength. Presented at the 30th Annual Meeting of the American Society of Hand Therapists; October 6, 2007; Phoenix, AZ.

Postoffer Functional Testing for Injury Prevention: Methodological and Practical Considerations

Eva Schonstein, PhD, MHPEd, AppSc(Phty), Norashikin Mahmud, MSc, BA, and Dianna T. Kenny, PhD, MA, BA (Hons) Dip Ed

Functional capacity evaluations (FCEs) were developed in the late 1970s in response to concern about increasing delays in workers returning to work after injury and consequent increased costs.[1] These delays were attributed in part to the difficulty physicians had in deciding when an injured worker could return to work or determining the level of work that the worker could sustain on his or her return.[1] Allied health professionals responded to the need for standardized tools to assess work capacity by developing the concept of the FCE. This concept resulted in a variety of commercially available FCE protocols[2] whose aim was to assess injured workers' physical capacities and sincerity of effort during the FCE assessment. On the basis of this information, the health care practitioner predicted the timing of return to work and the level of physical work a worker would be able to safely sustain on his or her return to work. Other functions for the FCE also emerged, such as to ascertain the earning capacity of injured workers in case of litigation and in the area of primary prevention as preplacement tools, especially for physically demanding jobs.[3]

In primary prevention, the basic premise of FCE is that a worker's performance during an FCE can predict whether he or she has the ability to safely perform the essential job tasks. As a corollary, it is presumed that if these predictions are accurate and the worker has sufficient physical capabilities to perform his or her prospective job, the risk of injury while performing the job will be decreased.[4,5] Preplacement FCE developed because pre-employment assessment involving medical history (eg, history of back pain) and medical tests such as X-rays, physical examinations, and manual handling training did not provide useful information about risk for future musculoskeletal work injury.[6-13] The use of functional assessments became a significant component in prospective employee selection in many industrialized countries. According to Randolph,[14(p814)] "FCE now stands in some jurisdictions as a mainstay of safe job placement and risk diminution by (theoretically) providing objective data pertaining to an individual's ability to safely perform job tasks."

Legislation such as the Anti-Discrimination Act of 1977[15] and the Disability Discrimination Act of 1992[16] in Australia and the 1990 Americans with Disabilities Act[17] in the United States have made pre-employment testing more specific, ie, assessments before a job offer are contrary to the aforementioned acts. In other words, pre-employment tests must be conducted after a conditional job offer has been made by the employer on the basis of skills and other personal attributes. This legislation protects workers with disability by requiring that reasonable accommodations of the workplace be made by employers.[17] This legal requirement does not exist in all countries. For example, in Malaysia there is no antidiscrimination legislation to protect job applicants with disabilities from being denied employment. However, the Malaysian Occupational Health and Safety Act 1994[18] places strong emphasis on an employer's responsibility to protect employees from physical harm and illness. For that purpose, pre-employment medical tests are compulsory for all government employees.[19] These tests are generally simple, such as chest X-rays and blood tests to prevent communicable diseases in the workplace. Physical or functional tests to screen employees for risk of musculoskeletal injuries are, however, rare.

There is limited and conflicting empirical support for the efficacy of postoffer FCEs in determining workers' physical capabilities with respect to job demands and for its predictive validity with respect to injury prevention.[20-23] The purpose of this chapter is to review the evidence for the effectiveness of FCE as a postoffer functional assessment.

Current Research Evidence

The key elements of a useful FCE are its safety, reliability, validity, and practicality.[20-25] Accordingly, each of these elements is described in this section as it relates to use in postoffer testing. Chapter 21, "The Scientific Status of FCE" discusses these elements as related to FCEs in general.

Safety

Safety during an FCE is critical for prevention of injury during assessment.[25-31] The safety of job applicants may be compromised by their effort level during the assessment because they may feign their capacity and overexert themselves or understate existing musculoskeletal conditions with an intention to be accepted for the job.[26] It has been noted, for example, that low back pain can be exacerbated with isometric tests.[32] Safety can be monitored through physiologic (eg, heart rate and blood pressure), biomechanical (eg, observation of postures and signs of muscle fatigue and weakness), and psychophysical factors such as pain.[27] Readiness of an evaluee for FCE testing is another important aspect of safety during preplacement testing, and the Physical Activity Readiness Questionnaire,[33] as recommended by the American College of Sports Medicine's Guidelines for Exercise Testing and Prescription,[34] can be helpful in this regard.

Reliability

As noted in Chapter 21, the strength of an assessment lies in its reliability (repeatability) and validity (the extent to which a measurement measures what it is expected to measure and covers the domain of interest). Various statistical tests on the reliability of assessment tools can be made. Tests for test-rest reliability assess the degree to which a test produces the same results over time; other tests measure or evaluate the extent to which assessors are reliable in their assessments as individuals (intrarater reliability) and as a group (interrater reliability). The FCE assessment tools that are reliable in the measurement of physical capacity of a prospective employee are not necessarily valid.[35] Without reliability *and* validity, a test may not be useful.[30]

In general, studies of the reliability of FCEs conducted on healthy, noninjured subjects have reported positive or acceptable results in terms of various aspects of reliability of the assessments studied.[36-39] One study reported test "reactivity" of three functional assessments.[40(p43)] *Reactivity* was defined as the extent to which the assessment process affects workers' test performance. For example, workers participating in assessments administered on two occasions may perform better on the second occasion owing to skill development or reduced anxiety associated with the assessment on the second day. High assessment reactivity can reduce the reliability and usefulness of the assessment. In other words, the effect of the assessment on the workers must be evaluated, and efforts to minimize these effects should be made. In FCE testing, establishing intrarater and interrater reliability is important.[21,41,42]

Table 13–1 represents a summary of the reliability studies published using healthy subjects. One study[38] described an assessment specifically designed as a preplacement tool, and the remainder assessed the reliability of FCE used for the return to work of injured workers. See Chapter 21 for a more in-depth discussion of reliability. More studies are needed to determine the reliability of the FCE assessment tools used to determine prospective workers' physical job capacities in relation to job demands.

Validity

There are several types of validity: external validity describes the population group to whom the study results can be applied, and internal validity describes the accuracy of a measurement instrument. External validity is maintained by adhering to the inclusion and exclusion criteria in the study protocol and is a concept that is described rather than measured using statistical methods. Study results have good external validity if a random sample is enrolled and a high response rate is attained. External validity determines the degree to which results can be generalized to other groups.[43]

Internal validity is necessary to ensure that results are interpretable, ie, it ensures that any differences between study or exposure groups can be attributed to the effect under investigation rather than to problems in recording measurements. *Face validity* is the extent to which an instrument appears to measure what it is intended to measure, and *content validity* is the extent to which an instrument covers the domain under investigation. Both of these forms of validity describe the extent to which an instrument fulfills its purpose.

TABLE 13–1   FCE Reliability Studies

Author	Assessment(s) Tested	Results	Types of Reliability Studied	Author Conclusions
Gouttebarge et al[37] (2004)	Ergo-Kit	Intrarater and interrater reliability (8-d interval) was high (ICC, > .80) for the isometric lifting tests, moderate (ICC, < .50) for the manipulation tests. The interrater reliability of the isometric and dynamic lifting tests (4-d interval) was high (ICC, > .80), and it was moderate (ICC range, .50–.80) for both manipulation tests.	Intrarater and Interrater	The isometric and dynamic lifting tests of the Ergo-Kit have a moderate to high level of reliability; the manipulation tests have a low level of reliability.
Legge and Burgess-Limerick[38] (2004)	JobFit System Pre-Employment Functional Assessment Tool	A good to excellent rating was allocated to the overall PEFA score, floor to bench to overhead lift, bilateral carry, and climbing. A moderate to good rating was recorded for squatting, balance, and fitness tests. Test-retest scores were typically lower than intratester and intertester scores.	Test-retest Intrarater and Interrater	ICC scores should be interpreted with consideration of their limitations and in conjunction with the actual test results.

CHAPTER 13

TABLE 13–1 FCE Reliability Studies (continued)

Author	Assessment(s) Tested	Results	Types of Reliability Studied	Author Conclusions
Boadella et al[36] (2003)	Ergos Work Simulator	A learning effect was found in sensibility and coordination subtests. No order effect was observed in terms of the intensity of the subtests. A time effect was found in coordination tasks: keyboarding performance was better in the morning and handling better in the afternoon.	Test-retest	Repeated upper extremity FCE testing in the present pilot study was reliable during a 4-week period in healthy subjects.
Reneman et al[39] (2004)	Isernhagen Work Systems	Acceptable reliability was demonstrated for 7 of 9 tests (78%) of the material handling group and the shuttle walk test. Sixteen out of 17 criterion (94%) showed acceptable reliability. Of these 17 tests, 8 were eligible for further analysis, and of these 8 tests, the reliability of 1 test was acceptable based on ICC analyses (12%).	Test-retest	The test-retest reliability of the material handling group was acceptable. Crude analyses of the ceiling and criterion tests revealed acceptable test-retest reliability of most but not all tests.

Abbreviations: FCE indicates functional capacity evaluation; ICC, intraclass correlation coefficient; and PEFA, preemployment functional assessment.

CHAPTER 13

There are a limited number of studies investigating the content validity of FCE, and none was found specific to postoffer FCE. Most extrapolate work requirements from the US Departments of Labor's O*NET database or its predecessor, the *Dictionary of Occupational Titles* (DOT).[44,45] This extrapolation is problematic because the DOT was developed as a vocational tool and presents generic vocational categories that have not been validated empirically.[31,46,47] Indeed, the physical demands in the DOT were not based on quantitative work task analysis but on consensus among experts in the field.[48] A systematic review[49] concluded that there is strong evidence that there is no relationship between trunk muscle strength and the risk of low back pain and inconclusive evidence about a relationship between physical capacity measures and the risk of neck and/or shoulder pain.

"Functional job analysis is a systematic process of identifying critical demands of specific jobs and should form the basis on which job demands are characterized."[50] It involves identifying the essential functions of the job, necessary equipment and tools, and the performance of work-site measurements (eg, forces, distances, and weights). Results from functional job analysis assist occupational health practitioners in the development of job-specific FCE protocols.[31,51] Job analysis aimed at quantifying the physical demands of a job is best performed by an in-house staff supported by an external consultant for improved structure and objectivity.[50] One study reported improved validity of a pre-employment test in terms of accuracy of job demands for firefighters through use of in-depth, semistructured interviews of six experienced workers.[52] The need for job specificity of worker assessment tools is further demonstrated by a study that described the development of an FCE protocol for hospital nurses.[53] Originally intended as an assessment of injured nurses returning to work, the study described the method used to develop this protocol, ie, systematic on-site observation (task analysis). This study concluded that such an approach to the development of an assessment improves its validity for the specific workplace.

A systematic review that assessed the use of static and dynamic tests to determine specific occupational demands (eg, lifting, pushing, and pulling) concluded that isometric strength testing is not related to the duration, intensity, and frequency of these work demands.[48] Among the dynamic tests studied, some lifting tests only partly considered the relation between the work demands (as defined by the DOT) and the maximally acceptable load lifted by the individual applicant. In regard to push-pull, only the Physical Work Performance Evaluation was found to partially consider the relationship between the applicant's maximally acceptable load and the work demand (based on the DOT). The authors discussed the questionable validity of using the DOT to identify work demands.[48] Another study on workers with chronic low back pain reported on the extent to which FCE activities matched activities observed during workplace assessments and concluded that lifting could not be directly matched with data from workplace assessments owing to differences in duration, frequency, and other parameters of lifts performed in the workplace.[54] The authors concluded that the inclusion of generic (simulated) lifting tasks in a preplacement assessment is not likely to protect the worker or the employer from the risks of musculoskeletal injuries during performance of such tasks.

Criterion-related validity includes concurrent validity and predictive validity. *Concurrent validity* refers to the extent to which FCE assessments can be used interchangeably with other similar instruments. In other words, this refers to the extent to which the results of validity testing of one assessment tool can be generalized to others in different circumstances, such as different employers or jobs. Two studies investigated the levels of concurrent validity of FCE using healthy adults, and both concluded that the concurrent validity was unacceptably low.[55,56] This finding is significant for preplacement assessments because it concurs with the findings of studies cited earlier that suggest that job-specific and not generic assessments are more appropriate.

Predictive validity in the context of postoffer testing refers to the extent to which the assessment and workplace performance are statistically related. The prognostic value of preplacement FCE is essential if the aim of the assessment is to predict the risk of future injury for prospective employees. The prognostic value of preplacement FCE as it relates to future injury has received little attention in the published literature. Most studies investigating the prognostic value of FCE to predict safe return to work of injured workers report a low to moderate relationship.[20,22,30,57-59] One systematic review reported that the predictive validity of only one FCE (the Isernhagen Work Systems) was acceptable.[37] One explanation for this poor correlation between assessment data and the future workplace injury rate could be the association of factors such as age, history of back pain, initial diagnosis, self-report, and psychosocial indicators such as low job satisfaction and worker's negative expectation of return to work with delayed return to work.[35] They may also affect the injury rate. Abdel-Moty et al[25] also suggest that workers' performance is likely to be influenced by work-related attitudes, pain perception, and environmental stressors.

Three studies described the effectiveness of postoffer preplacement functional assessment.[12,60,61] All three reported a strong association between assessment data and postassessment injury rates. One study noted a 30% increase in injury rates for workers who were hired but did not demonstrate physical capacity commensurate with job requirements.[60] This study was a quality prospective study comprising 2482 prospective employees. Another study reported that strength testing was a predictor of future low back pain only when the prospective employee's history of low back pain was also known.[12] Hence, history of back pain, and not physical strength per se, may be the best general predictor of future low back pain in the workplace.[62] However, for jobs involving a high level of physical demands and when preplacement assessment tasks were closely aligned to actual job demands, effectiveness has been demonstrated.[63]

Concern has been raised with respect to practicality of preplacement assessments and their costs in relation to their lack of demonstrated capacity to predict chronic disability (such as chronic low back pain).[31,64] This concern is important because the major costs in work disability are associated with the minority of workers who become chronically disabled rather than with the majority of workers who develop symptoms of musculoskeletal injuries and return to full function (including work) in a timely and durable manner.[62]

Construct validity refers to the degree to which inferences can legitimately be made from a study to the theoretical constructs on which the study was based. Like external validity, construct validity is related to generalizability. But, whereas external validity involves generalizing from one study population to another, construct validity refers to generalizability of a preplacement assessment to the concept of this assessment. For example, when a preplacement assessment states that it aims to prevent musculoskeletal injuries due to manual handling in the workplace, is that what it is really measuring as an outcome? In other words, how well can a study differentiate between low back pain caused by workplace factors only as opposed to other everyday activity factors, such as playing sports, lack of physical activity, and obesity?

There is a conceptual difficulty with establishing the validity of preplacement FCE assessments, namely, they are used as diagnostic tests to identify prospective workers at risk for musculoskeletal injuries. Studies of the accuracy of diagnostic tests involve applying the test to people and determining how well the test's findings correspond with the correct diagnosis. The test used to establish the correct diagnosis is often called the "gold standard" or reference test.[43] The problem with studying the accuracy of FCE assessment in identifying at-risk prospective workers is that there is no gold standard. Therefore, more suitable validity research methods would randomize subjects to a group identified as at risk to an intervention (such as additional strength training) or to a control group[65] and then assess the injury rate in both groups after they have been placed in identical jobs. Another method could be to randomize workers to a group receiving an FCE assessment and an intervention or to a control group receiving no FCE and no intervention, with, again, subsequent tracking of injury rates in both groups.

Medicolegal Considerations

Poor validity of preplacement or postoffer assessments can lead to inappropriate selection or, more important, rejection of prospective employees, which in turn can be considered a form of discrimination. An example of such a potential for discrimination for jobs with high physical demands would be against women applying for such jobs, particularly if the test does not specifically simulate the job requirements. Tests of strength and endurance screen out proportionally more females than males.[66] Pre-employment or postoffer physical tests that simulate the job's lifting requirements avoid potential discrimination because the test has content validity. Selection procedures that are compliant with the Equal Employment Opportunity Commission guidelines may have disparate impact and not violate the law. Chapter 20 provides a more detailed discussion of the legal issues in employment screenings.

Conclusion and Recommendations

The use of FCE in preplacement screening has received inadequate attention in the literature, and further quality research is necessary. Practical and methodological limitations have been associated with preplacement FCEs, despite some evidence of their ability to prevent some musculoskeletal injuries, although predicting chronicity resulting from such injuries has not been demonstrated. Based on current literature, the quality of preplacement FCE assessments could be improved by providing evaluators with accurate definitions and assessments of job demands based on thorough functional job analysis and work simulation conducted by expert evaluators. Assessment protocols based on accurate job demands that closely parallel functional job demands of a workplace would improve their capacity to predict prospective employees' ability to perform the job. Generic assessments have been shown to have poor generalizability and limited usefulness. Antidiscrimination laws requiring employers to offer reasonable workplace accommodations to future employees remain unclear in terms of the definition of what is *reasonable,* and more research is needed to evaluate the effectiveness of worker strength and endurance training, especially for physically demanding jobs. In the absence of evidence for a better method of assessing the degree to which applicants for a given job can meet relevant physical requirements, judicious use of functional testing based on a thorough understanding of job-specific tasks is the best current mechanism.

References

1. D'Orazio BP. *Back Pain Rehabilitation.* Boston, MA: Andover Medical Publisher; 1993.
2. Innes E, Straker L. Workplace assessments and functional capacity evaluations: current beliefs of therapists in Australia. *Work.* 2003;20:225–236.
3. National Council on Compensation Insurance. *Countrywide Workers' Compensation Experience Including Certain Competitive State Funds, First Report Basis.* Boca Raton, FL: NCCI; 1982.
4. Scott LR. Post offer screening. *AAOHN J.* 2002;50:559–563.
5. Snook SH. Approaches to preplacement testing and selection of workers. *Ergonomics.* 1987;30:241–247.
6. Battie MC, Bigos SJ, Fisher LD, Hansson TH, Jones ME, Wortley MD. Isometric lifting strength as a predictor of industrial back pain reports. *Spine.* 1989;14:851–856.
7. Bigos SJ, Battie MC. Preplacement worker testing and selection considerations. *Ergonomics.* 1987;30:249–251.
8. Bigos SJ, Battie MC, Fisher LD, Hansson TH, Spengler DM, Nachemson AL. A prospective evaluation of pre-employment screening methods for acute industrial back pain. *Spine* 1992;17:922–926.
9. Bigos SJ, Hansson T, Castillo RN, Beecher PJ, Wortley MD. The value of preemployment roentgenographs for predicting acute back injury claims and chronic back pain disability. *Clin Orthop.* 1992;283:124–129.
10. Gibson ES, Martin RH, Terry CW. Incidence of low back pain and pre-placement x-ray screening. *J Occup Med.* 1980;22:515–519.
11. Jackson AS. Pre-employment physical evaluation. *Exerc Sport Sci Rev.* 1994;22:53–90.
12. Troup JD, Foreman TK, Baxter CE, Brown D. 1987 Volvo Award in Clinical Sciences: the perception of back pain and the role of psychophysical tests of lifting capacity. *Spine.* 1987;12:645–657.
13. Weil Y, Weil D, Donchin M, Mann G, Hasharoni A. Correlation between pre-employment screening x-ray finding of spondylolysis and sickness absenteeism due to low back pain among policemen of the Israeli police force. *Spine.* 2004;29:2168–2172.
14. Randolph DC. Use of functional employment testing to facilitate safe job placement. *Occup Med.* 2000;15:813–821.
15. Anti-Discrimination Act 1977 (NSW) Web site. www.austlii.edu.au/au/legis/nsw/consol_act/aa1977204/. Accessed November 15, 2007.
16. Disability Discrimination Act 1992. www.law.uiuc.edu/publications/cll&pj/archive/vol_24/issue_4/PatmoreArticle24-4.pdf. Accessed November 15, 2007.
17. US Department of Labor. Americans with Disabilities Act. 1990. www.usdoj.gov/crt/ada/adahom1.htm. Accessed June 15, 2007.
18. Occupational Safety and Health Act 1994. http://dosh.mohr.gov.my/koperat/LAW/Occupational%20Safety%20and%20Health%20Act%201994%20(Act%20514)/a0514.pdf. Accessed October 8, 2007.
19. General Orders Public Services Department. General Order No. 3: Recruitment, Selection, Appointment and Manpower Reporting. www.dpm.gov.pg/GeneralOrders/3/GO03.pdf. Accessed July 28, 2007.

CHAPTER 13

20. Gross DP. Measurement properties of performance-based assessment of functional capacity. *J Occup Rehabil.* 2004;14:165–174.

21. Innes E, Straker L. Reliability of work-related assessment. *Work.* 1999;13:107–124.

22. Innes E, Straker L. Validity of work-related assessments. *Work.* 1999;13:125–152.

23. King PM, Tuckwell N, Barrett TE. A critical review of functional capacity evaluations. *Phys Ther.* 1998;78:852–866.

24. Uniform Guidelines on Employee Selection Procedures. 1978. www.usdoj.gov/crt/emp/uniformguidelines.html. Accessed October 15, 2007.

25. Abdel-Moty E, Campton R, Steele-Rosomoff R, Rosomoff HL, Khalil TM. Process analysis of functional capacity assessment. *Journal of Back and Musculoskeletal Rehabilitation.* 1996;6:223–236.

26. Gibson L, Strong J. A review of functional capacity evaluation practice. *Work.* 1997;9:3–11.

27. Gibson L, Strong J. Safety issues in functional capacity evaluation: findings from a trial of a new approach for evaluating clients with chronic back pain. *J Occup Rehabil.* 2005;15:237–251.

28. Gross DP, Battie MC, Cassidy JD. The prognostic value of functional capacity evaluation in patients with chronic low back pain: part 1: timely return to work. *Spine.* 2004;29:914–919.

29. Hart DL, Isernhagen SJ, Matheson LN. Guidelines for functional capacity evaluation of people with medical conditions. *J Orthop Sports Phys Ther.* 1993;18:682–686.

30. Innes E, Straker L. Attributes of excellence in work-related assessments. *Work.* 2003;20:63–76.

31. Pransky GS, Dempsey PG. Practical aspects of functional capacity evaluations. *J Occup Rehabil.* 2004;14:217–229.

32. Hansson TH, Bigos SJ, Wortley MK, Spengler DM. The load on the lumbar spine during isometric strength testing. *Spine.* 1984;9:720–724.

33. Canadian Society for Exercise Physiology. Physical Activity Readiness Questionnaire PAR-Q. www.google.com/search?source=ig&hl=en&rlz=&q=physical+readiness+questionnaire+&btnG=Google+search. Accessed December 18, 2008.

34. American College of Sports Medicine. *American College of Sports Medicine's Health-Related Physical Fitness Assessment Manual.* Philadelphia, PA: Lippincott Williams & Wilkins; 2005.

35. Schonstein E, Kenny D. The value of functional and work place assessments in achieving a timely return to work for workers with back pain. *Work.* 2001;16:31–38.

36. Boadella JM, Sluiter JK, Frings-Dresen MH. Reliability of upper extremity tests measured by the Ergos work simulator: a pilot study. *J Occup Rehabil.* 2003;13:219–232.

37. Gouttebarge V, Wind H, Kuijer PP, Frings-Dresen MH. Reliability and validity of functional capacity evaluation methods: a systematic review with reference to Blankenship system, Ergos work simulator, Ergo-Kit and Isernhagen work system. *Int Arch Occup Environ Health.* 2004;77:527–537.

38. Legge J, Burgess-Limerick R. Reliability of the JobFit System Pre-Employment Functional Assessment Tool. *Work.* 2004;28:299–312.

39. Reneman MF, Brouwer S, Meinema A, Dijkstra PU, Geertzen JH, Groothoff JW. Test-retest reliability of the Isernhagen Work Systems Functional Capacity Evaluation in healthy adults. *J Occup Rehabil.* 2004;14:295–305.

40. Matheson LN, Rogers LC, Kaskutas V, Dakos M. Reliability and reactivity of three new functional assessment measures. *Work.* 2002;18:41–50.

41. Lechner R, Roth D, Straaton K. Functional capacity evaluation in work disability. *Work.* 1991;1:37–47.

42. Reneman MF, Wittink H. Functional performance evaluation. In: Nordin M, Andersson GBJ, Pope MH, eds. *Musculoskeletal Disorders in the Workplace: Principles and Practice.* 2nd ed. Philadelphia, PA: Elsevier; 2007:397–408.

43. Herbert R, Jamtvedt G, Mead J, Hagen KB. *Practical Evidence-Based Physiotherapy.* Edinburgh, Scotland: Elsevier Butterworth Heinemann; 2005.

44. Information Technology Associates. DOT with O*NET 98 Data & Viewer on CD-ROM. www.theodora.com/new.onet.html. Accessed January 22, 2008.

45. US Department of Labor. *Dictionary of Occupational Titles.* www.theodora.com/new/onet.html. Accessed January 22, 2008.

46. Kersnovske S, Gibson L, Strong J. Item validity of the physical demands from the *Dictionary of Occupational Titles* for functional capacity evaluation of clients with chronic back pain. *Work.* 2005;24:157–169.

47. Lo KS, Lam CW. Validity of the *Dictionary of Occupational Titles* as applied to construction site workers in Hong Kong. *Work.* 2000;14:191–194.

48. Bos J, Kuijer PP, Frings-Dresen MH. Definition and assessment of specific occupational demands concerning lifting, pushing, and pulling based on a systematic literature search. *Occup Environ Med.* 2002;59:800–806.

49. Hamberg-van Reenen HH, Ariens GAM, Blatter BM, van Mechelen W, Bongers PM. A systematic review of the relation between physical capacity and future low back and neck/shoulder pain. *Pain.* 2007;130:93–107.

50. Rayson MP. Fitness for work: the need for conducting a job analysis. *Occup Med (Lond).* 2000;50:434–436.

51. Abdel-Moty E, Fishbain DA, Khalil TM, et al. Functional capacity and residual functional capacity and their utility in measuring work capacity. *Clin J Pain.* 1993;9:168–173.

52. Harley A, James C. Fire-fighters' perspectives of the accuracy of the Physical Aptitude Test (P.A.T.) as a pre-employment assessment. *Work.* 2006;26:29–35.

53. Frings-Dresen MH, Sluiter JK. Development of a job-specific FCE protocol: the work demands of hospital nurses as an example. *J Occup Rehabil.* 2003;13:233–248.

54. Kuijer W, Brouwer S, Reneman MF, et al. Matching FCE activities and work demands: an explorative study. *J Occup Rehabil.* 2006;16:469–483.

55. IJmker S, Gerrits EH, Reneman MF. Upper lifting performance of healthy young adults in functional capacity evaluations: a comparison of two protocols. *J Occup Rehabil.* 2003;13:297–305.

56. Rustenburg G, Kuijer PP, Frings-Dresen MH. The concurrent validity of the ERGOS Work Simulator and the Ergo-Kit with respect to maximum lifting capacity. *J Occup Rehabil.* 2004;14:107–118.

57. Fishbain DA, Cutler RB, Rosomoff H, Khalil T, Abdel-Moty E, Steele-Rosomoff R. Validity of the *Dictionary of Occupational Titles* residual functional capacity battery. *Clin J Pain.* 1999;15:102–110.

CHAPTER 13

58. Gross DP, Battie MC. Does functional capacity evaluation predict recovery in workers' compensation claimants with upper extremity disorders? *Occup Environ Med.* 2006;63:404–410.

59. Matheson LN, Isernhagen SJ, Hart DL. Relationships among lifting ability, grip force, and return to work. *Phys Ther.* 2002;82:249–256.

60. Harbin G, Olson J. Post-offer, pre-placement testing in industry. *Am J Ind Med.* 2005;47:296–307.

61. Reimer DS, Halbrook BD, Dreyfuss PH, Tibiletti C. A novel approach to preemployment worker fitness evaluations in a material-handling industry. *Spine.* 1994;19:2026–2032.

62. Waddell G. *The Back Pain Revolution.* 2nd ed. Edinburgh, Scotland: Churchill Livingstone; 2004.

63. Chaffin DB, Herrin GD, Keyserling WM. Preemployment strength testing: an updated position. *J Occup Med.* 1978;20:403–408.

64. Cohen JE, Goel V, Frank JW, Gibson ES. Predicting risk of back injuries, work absenteeism and chronic disability: the shortcomings of preplacement screening. *J Occup Med.* 1994;36:1093–1099.

65. Taimela S, Laara E, Malmivaara A, et al. Self-reported health problems and sickness absence in different age groups predominantly engaged in physical work. *Occup Environ Med.* 2007;64:739–746.

66. Arvey RD, Landon TE, Nutting SM, Maxwell SE. Development of physical ability tests for police officers: a construct validation approach. *J Appl Psychol.* 1992;77:996–1009.

14

Job-specific Functional Testing for Injury Management

Rick Wickstrom, PT, CPE

When information is needed about a person's general physical abilities for job search or extent of physical disability, generic functional testing protocols are appropriate. However, when information about a person's ability to safely perform a specific job or job tasks is needed, the functional testing protocol must be designed to address the job or job tasks in question. When functional testing is performed to determine a person's ability to safely perform a job or job task, the test protocol is termed a *job-specific FCE (functional capacity evaluation)*. A job-specific FCE is an "evaluation protocol that is designed with emphasis on content validity to measure an evaluee's ability to perform the physical demands of a specific, identified job and to determine whether there are any participation restrictions."[1] Job-specific functional capacity testing may be warranted for the following purposes:

- To evaluate fitness for duty of applicants for employment
- To verify fitness of employees applying for an internal job transfer to a more physically demanding job
- To investigate worker reports of symptoms or difficulty performing assigned job tasks
- To determine readiness to safely return to a specific job following an absence due to injury or illness
- To identify transitional work options that would facilitate return to work
- To evaluate whether an injured worker is likely to benefit from continued participation in a company's transitional work program or outpatient therapy
- To determine the feasibility of requests for temporary or permanent accommodations to address barriers to safe work performance

The decision about whether to proceed with a job-specific FCE is often dictated by consideration of potential benefits to be gained vs expenses (as with any FCE), given that the scope, selection, and administration time for a job-specific FCE can range from a short, 20- to 30-minute work ability fitness screen administered before the start of employment to a more lengthy (and costly) postinjury evaluation that includes functional analysis of job tasks, history and physical examination, and job-specific functional capacity tests to evaluate eligibility and the business impact of accommodation options to prevent needless work disability.

Protocols for assessing a worker's fitness for duty and implementing reasonable accommodations have been greatly influenced by civil rights legislation and court decisions governing employment practices for persons with disabilities. Title V of the Rehabilitation Act of 1973 requires federal departments, agencies, instrumentalities, and federally funded contractors to demonstrate affirmative action during hiring, placement, and advancement of "qualified, handicapped individuals."[2] Title I of the Americans with Disabilities Act of 1990 (ADA) prohibits US employers with more than 15 employees from discriminating against a qualified person with a disability if the person can perform the essential functions of the job, with or without reasonable accommodation.[3] The ADA Amendments Act of 2008 (ADAAA) significantly broadened the scope of protection available under the Americans with Disabilities Act of 1990.[4] The critical inquiry under this amended law is no longer about whether the individual has a disability, instead it's whether covered entities have engaged in an interactive process that supports reasonable accommodation of qualified disabled applicants and employees. Examples of legislation in other countries that prohibits employment disability discrimination include the Disability Discrimination Act of 1992 (Australia)[5] and the Disability Discrimination Act 1995 (United Kingdom).[6] Specific medical screening provisions and Equal Employment Opportunity Commission (EEOC) enforcement guidelines related to Title I of the ADA[3,7] have changed the paradigm from traditional pre-employment medical examinations to a more job-specific FCE process. Chapters 2, 13, 19, and 20 provide further discussion of these tests.

Transitional Work Programs

Many medical providers and employers have discovered the benefit of preventing work disability through proactive, early interventions that support workers in their efforts to stay at work and transition back to regular duties while recovering from an injury or illness. See Figure 14–1. Transitional work programs support the primary relationship between the worker and employer by providing a more effective framework for resolving real or perceived worker performance barriers that interfere with return to safe and productive duty. If medically appropriate, the worker is released to return to work with initial restrictions either in an accommodated or modified duty assignment. The work that employees perform during participation in such programs is based on periodic assessments of physical ability in the context of job-specific tasks, which differs from the traditional medical approach. In the traditional approach, physicians provide progressive return-to-work-restrictions on forms that are primarily based on workers' subjective reports of recovery and readiness to resume their preinjury work and lifestyle demands.

The plan of care under a true transitional model of return to work (based on what the worker actually demonstrates functionally as opposed to solely on physician estimates) is driven by measurement of functional job demands in reference to job-specific FCE. Work becomes a key therapeutic activity, which theoretically

CHAPTER 14

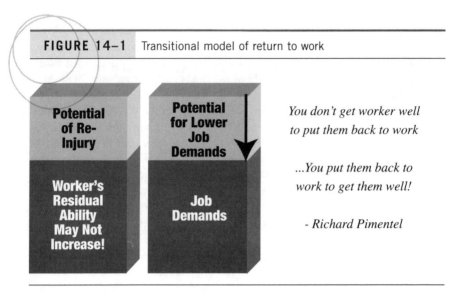

FIGURE 14–1 Transitional model of return to work

results in the need for less treatment and lost time from work. Therapy can also be provided at the job site under the supervision of industrial therapists, the use of actual job tasks in combination with coaching in safe-work–methods and prescribed self-exercises to presumably facilitate a safer and faster return to productive duties. The worker continues to receive his or her salary and also has more time to devote to other important lifestyle activities because most therapeutic tasks can be completed during the regular work shift. Job redesign guidelines by governmental agencies or associations such as the National Institute of Occupational Safety and Health (NIOSH), Regional Employment Medical Adviser (United Kingdom), and American Conference of Governmental Industrial Hygienists, Inc, (ACGIH) may also be applied to identify ergonomic risk and guard against returning an injured worker to a hazardous job.

The job-specific FCE provides a foundation of empirical support for interventions designed to improve productivity and reduce work disability duration and associated costs. Franche et al[8] conducted a systematic review of the literature related to workplace-based return-to-work interventions and concluded that there is strong evidence that the duration of work disability is significantly reduced by work accommodation offers and contact between the health care provider and the workplace. Moreover, moderate evidence shows that it is reduced by interventions that include early contact with the worker by the workplace, ergonomic work-site visits, and the presence of a return-to-work coordinator.

Rationale for Job-specific Functional Capacity Evaluation

Job-specific test results provide the physician with specific functional abilities that will safely guide a worker's return to work. Without this information, the physician might overestimate a worker's physical capabilities, and a premature return to regular duties may result in reinjury. On the other hand, escalating concerns about malpractice liability premiums and patient safety may prompt the physician to set overly conservative restrictions that underestimate a worker's physical capacities, resulting in needless work disability and delayed recovery. Therefore, whenever worker safety, worker restrictions, or disability is an issue, the health care professional should ask screening questions such as the following:

1. If *working*: How does your health status affect your ability to do your regular work activities in the usual way?
2. If *not working*: What specifically is preventing you from working today?

Functional job analysis in combination with job-specific FCE is a "bridge" between health care and the workplace. The analysis and evaluation assist the rehabilitation team and employer in evaluating a worker's recovery in a vocational context. Most typically, a licensed physical or occupational therapist with specialized training is responsible for administering the functional test battery to more objectively establish the worker's ability to perform functional job tasks than would otherwise be possible. Consolidation of the test results with other medical and job analysis findings helps substantiate the worker's medical impairment, disability, and job-performance barriers. This information leads to more effective health care or the delineation of reasonable accommodations that allow an injured worker to meet lifestyle and occupational demands. Figure 14–2 shows an example of a transitional work decision tree[9] that incorporates job-specific FCE as a key component to facilitate earlier return to safe and productive duty.

CHAPTER 14

FIGURE 14–2 Transitional work therapy decision tree

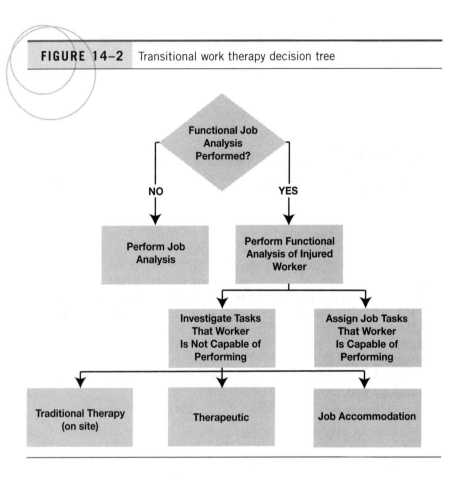

Design Implications for Job-Specific Functional Capacity Evaluation

Many methods have been used to evaluate job-specific functional capacities. In critically evaluating these methods, it is necessary to consider their safety, reliability, practicality, limitations, and relevance to the stated purpose. The job-specific FCE protocol should be flexible in composition and duration to respond to the specific needs and the financial constraints of the referral source. The National Institute for Occupational Safety and Health criteria for evaluating employer screening programs provide a framework for discussion of test methods[10]:

- Is the testing safe to administer? (safety)
- Does the test give reliable, quantitative values? (reliability)

- Is the test related to the specific job requirements? (content validity)
- Is the test practical? (practicality)
- Does the test predict risk of future injury or illness? (utility)

Additional information about functional testing as an injury prevention tool in postjob offer assessments is provided in Chapter 13. Many similar design considerations apply.

Safety

Safety is a concern during administration of job-specific functional testing when there is potential for an overly motivated or deconditioned evaluee to sustain an overexertion injury. Therefore, any activity selected for inclusion in the test protocol must be safe enough to readminister during the subacute and chronic recovery phases. Inclusion of a screening examination of active range of motion before more rigorous tasks can serve as a warm-up and identify any absolute or relative contraindications for activity. Gradual progression and close monitoring of the evaluee is important. For example, rather than starting a test in which the worker performs the regular duty task of lifting a full 50-lb box of copy paper, the evaluator might ask the worker to lift a partially filled box of lesser weight (eg, 10 lb) and progress the test in a gradual and incremental manner. During this process, the evaluator will monitor the worker's lifting style and control and provide coaching in appropriate pacing and body mechanics to improve safety. In addition, the evaluator may evaluate the worker's functional lift and carry strength in various postures and specify which items can be safely handled based on the specific lift and carry conditions required for task performance. When testing people in the acute or subacute stage of recovery, it may be advisable to limit testing to a submaximal level by using a Borg scale of perceived exertion (see Chapter 5) and asking the person to remain within a "somewhat hard" or "hard" threshold of perceived exertion.[11] This approach should help limit the risk of increased symptoms in response to initial functional ability testing and engender a trusting relationship between the injured worker and clinician during the initial phase of rehabilitation services.

During a job-specific FCE, it is usually unnecessary and unwarranted to subject an injured worker to more than the peak lifting or carrying demands required for performance of essential or marginal job functions. Additionally, the evaluator may need to identify hazardous lifting tasks by applying ergonomic assessment tools such as the ACGIH Threshold Limit Values (TLVs®) for Lifting[12] or NIOSH Revised Lifting Equation[13] to determine the task threshold limit value for most workers. Such hazardous tasks should be identified and modified or restructured whenever possible, rather than subjecting an injured worker to unreasonable FCE tasks. Waters et al.[14] studied the correlation between the Lifting Index (LI)* (derived from the NIOSH Revised Lifting Equation) and the prevalence and severity of lifting-related LBP and found "increased risk of having LBP lasting a week or more during any 12-month period" for workers performing continuous lifting where the LI is greater than 2.0.[14(p393)] Therefore, if a job's lifting demands are unclear, then it may be reasonable and prudent to impose a safety limit on lifting tasks during an FCE that avoids subjecting the worker to a lifting index of 2.0 or more. This recommendation is given, *in spite of the results of the study*, which indicated that "for jobs with a lifting index of higher than 3.0, however, the odds ratio was lower (odds ratio = 1.45)." [14(p386)]

Safety concerns for maximum isometric strength tests such as the torso lift or leg lift[15,16] (see Chapter 8) have been largely abandoned in favor of dynamic lift tasks (see Chapter 6) that better simulate work demands and allow for gradual task progression in combination with kinesiological assessment of body mechanics. (Chapter 8 provides further discussion of static testing.) Persons with known or suspected heart disease should have heart rate and blood pressure monitored during test activities. A submaximal step test is an example of a portable and relevant field test that can be administered in a progressive manner at very low risk according to the American College of Sports Medicine[17] (aerobic testing is discussed further in Chapter 10).

Reliability

An objective test must be measurable and reliable. During job-specific testing, the industrial therapist is often designing progressive work samples that do not have established reliability. Within the scope of a work-conditioning program, it is possible to evaluate an evaluee's consistency of performance over multiple days as a measure of reliability. It is also possible to integrate more generic standardized tests within the battery of job-specific tests to determine performance consistency. The inclusion of cross-testing (evaluation of an activity or positional tolerance without the evaluee's knowledge that it is being evaluated) is another method of assessing performance consistency. Repeating trials of activities allows computation of a coefficient of variation, but, as discussed in Chapter 11, there are important limitations to consider with this method. A number of studies have documented the interrater reliability of lifting methods that are based on kinesiophysical assessment.[18–21]

---

*The lifting index, as defined by NIOSH, provides an estimate of the level of physical stress associated with a particular manual lifting task.[14]

Content Validity

Content validity is the hallmark of job-specific functional testing and must be demonstrated for all physical qualification standards, tests, or selection criteria in accordance with the EEOC's Uniform Guidelines for Employment Selection[22] and provisions of the ADA. Under the ADA,[3,7] a job-related standard or selection criterion may evaluate or measure the ability of job applicants or employees to perform one or more essential functions of the job. Chapters 2 and 20 provide further discussion of these requirements.

Functional job analysis is the first and single most important initial step toward establishing content validity. It is only when an individual's disability prevents or impedes performance of marginal job functions that the ADA requires the employer to consider the person's qualifications based solely on his or her ability to perform the essential functions of the job, with or without accommodation. The practical impact of this requirement is that it is perfectly legitimate to test the person's ability to do marginal functions during job-specific functional capacity testing to clarify whether the worker is able to perform such marginal duties if the need arises.

For example, in an accounting office, it is not uncommon for bankers' boxes of files to be moved to storage on an infrequent basis. If an existing employee is qualified to perform this marginal function, the employer would not need to pay additional money for a professional mover. If the employee was hired primarily for clerical expertise and demonstrates the ability to lift only 30 lb, the supervisor would know that is not safe to assign the employee to move 50- to 60-lb bankers' boxes. Likewise, it is not uncommon for employers to use a functional screening process to assist with assignment of employees to appropriate work tasks. If the heaviest assignment required heavy lifting, lift and carry strength could be tested to the highest capacity required for any work assignment, and workers could be assigned to jobs that are safe based on their tested capacities. In institutions such as medical facilities, it is not uncommon to determine whether the worker is additionally qualified to serve on patient transfer teams that earn additional hourly compensation. This is based on demonstration of additional physical prowess and transfer skills that are applicable to working with special populations such as patients undergoing some type of bariatric treatment.

Practicality

Practical considerations for job-specific testing include test length, equipment and space requirements, personnel required for test administration, training, and expense. The ability to adapt a test process to allow evaluation for a range of working conditions is optimal. For example, some employers obtain workers through a temporary employment agency to evaluate worker performance before tendering an employment offer. This practice can prove costly owing to additional wages and training investment and the loss in productivity or quality if the worker does not satisfy performance expectations. Functional testing should also be performed at a location that is convenient for the worker. Portable systems that can be taken to the work site clearly have some advantages in this regard.

Utility

Utility refers to the degree to which a selection procedure is predictive of or correlated with job performance. This criterion is more difficult to meet because it is costly to conduct epidemiologic research of injury and illness data on people who are well-matched to the job vs people who are not. Some longitudinal studies on motivated populations of job applicants[23-25] have demonstrated evidence of predictive validity in functional capacity testing methods, whereas other investigations[26] have not. Disability is a complex phenomenon that is influenced by motivation and other societal factors; therefore, it is not surprising that studies in Canada and the Netherlands have not demonstrated predictive validity for FCEs.[27-29]

Information Needed From a Functional Job Analysis

Accurate knowledge of the full-duty job demands is critical to develop a realistic and job-specific plan of care, including the selection of job-specific functional tests to measure recovery status. This information also helps to evaluate the appropriateness of requested claims allowances following an alleged work-related injury. A properly developed functional job analysis helps the employer clearly communicate functional demands of specific tasks, transitional work options, and program policy to the attending physician and other health care professionals. The job analysis process should address the following key components:

- Purpose of the job
- Environmental conditions and work-schedule issues
- Medical screening needs and physical qualifications
- Interviews of incumbents and supervisors to specify critical job functions, materials, tools, equipment, work aids, and modified duty options

- Observations of incumbents performing critical job functions to determine work methods, work ability demands, and safety concerns
- Production demands and injury trends
- Essential vs marginal functions
- Qualifications (skills, knowledge, and education) and worker screening methods

Performing a Functional Analysis of an Injured Worker

Once the job analysis has been performed, the data are used to evaluate the work abilities of injured workers. Key components of a well-designed, job-specific functional evaluation include the following:

- Comprehensive health, lifestyle, and injury history
- Review of lifestyle and job demands and limitations
- Assessment of diagnostic and other relevant findings in records
- Neuromusculoskeletal examination, including baseline measurements such as active range-of-motion limitations
- Selection of functional tests that relate to critical, specific job functions
- Monitoring of worker performance during real or simulated job tasks
- Summary of worker abilities in comparison with job demands (job match)

Considerations when customizing a job-specific FCE include unique lifting parameters (ie, hand coupling), postural demands, environmental factors, and the use of actual work tools, when possible. The more closely the testing simulates the actual job, the more likely the worker will "buy in" to the program. If the task represents an all-or-nothing work sample such as palletizing 50-lb packages, a dynamic lifting protocol can be administered with gradual addition of weight to the tote pans as a screening measure to improve safety. When cardiovascular endurance is a concern, heart rate can be monitored during task performance to objectively evaluate response to real or simulated work tasks.

CHAPTER 14

Summary of Work Abilities in Comparison With Job Demands (Job Match)

Researchers have shown that many of the activities included in general-purpose FCEs are not directly relevant to the demands of specific jobs.[30] Therefore, a cost-efficient selection of tests must consider the most relevant and critical factors for job placement as a point-in-time assessment of work ability and need for sick leave. The most widely used taxonomy for matching the physical qualifications of workers with job demands is the US Department of Labor taxonomy of 20 physical demand factors.[31] The Department of Labor strength physical demands factor is used to classify workers or jobs as sedentary, light, medium, heavy, or very heavy based on the amount of standing, walking, sitting, lifting, carrying, pushing, and pulling required. Unfortunately, broadly classifying a worker in one of the strength classifications does not provide sufficient information to promote safe and productive job placement. For example, a person with a knee impairment may be able to occasionally handle 50 lb (medium strength rating) at waist level or above but only safely handle 20 lb (light strength rating) near floor level and tolerate standing on a frequent basis. A person with a recurrent shoulder dislocation may be able to handle 50 lb from waist to floor level but only be able handle 10 lb (sedentary strength rating) from shoulder to overhead. For this reason, it is often necessary to evaluate a worker's capacity and job-task demands with respect to a variety of conditions and postures that consider the following:

- Vertical location of the hands at the origin and destination of the handling task
- Horizontal location of the hands at the origin and destination of the handling task
- Frequency and duration of the materials handling task
- Body posture during the task
- Specific dimensions and coupling to the object being handled
- Fitness and underlying impairment of the worker

The frequency rating system used by the US Department of Labor relies on a frequency rating system based on an 8-hour workday for 19 other physical demand factors:

- Constantly (C): Present two thirds or more of the time
- Frequently (F): Present up to two thirds of the time
- Occasionally (O): Present up to one third of the time
- Not present (N): Activity or condition does not exist

One of the obvious limitations with this frequency rating scale is that longer workdays are common in industry; therefore, the scale is not adequate for representing worker capacity and job tolerance requirements for jobs and tasks that last longer than an 8-hour workday. The sitting tolerance demands of an office worker who works an 8-hour shift are clearly different from those required for over-the-road truck drivers who may be required to sit and drive up to 12 hours per day. Another shortcoming in applying this DOT rating scale to physical demand factors such as near vision, far vision, and balancing is that these types of traits are more commonly evaluated by skill level demonstrated than actual tests of tolerance. Criticism can also be applied to many of the forms about worker restrictions that medical providers are asked to complete. For example, review of the Work/Nonwork Capabilities on the MEDCO-14 Physician's Report of WorkAbility form[32] used by the Ohio Bureau of Workers' Compensation (Figure 14–3) reveals the following factors that cannot be directly related to job demands:

- Lift/carry strength is not characterized by the height of the lift, type of lift, or distance carried.
- Push/pull frequency rating fails to consider the amount of force applied.
- Definitions of ability factors are not operationally defined.
- Repetition ranges for frequency categories do not correspond to frequency categories used for risk assessment of materials handling tasks.[12]

The lack of information on this and similar forms makes it difficult for employers to evaluate job match or suitability of modified duty because of difficulty translating the work restrictions prescribed by health care providers. Additionally, most statements of worker restrictions completed by physicians fail to indicate whether they have any insight into a worker's actual full-duty job demands.

FIGURE 14–3 Work Restrictions Section of the Ohio BWC MEDCO-14 Form

Work/Non-Work Capabilities

	None at all	Occasional	Frequent	Continuous
% of Workday (8 hr)	0%	1-33%	34-66%	67-100%
Repetitions per hr		4-6	6-12	>12
Lift/Carry				
Up to 10 lbs	☐	☐	☐	☐
11- 20 lbs	☐	☐	☐	☐
21- 50 lbs	☐	☐	☐	☐
51-100 lbs	☐	☐	☐	☐
Bending	☐	☐	☐	☐
Twist/turn	☐	☐	☐	☐
Reach below knee	☐	☐	☐	☐
Push/pull	☐	☐	☐	☐
Squat/kneel	☐	☐	☐	☐
Stand/walk	☐	☐	☐	☐
Sit	☐	☐	☐	☐
No lifting above shoulders	☐	☐	☐	☐

Hand restrictions ☐ Left ☐ Right | No use of ☐ Left ☐ Right
    ☐ Must wear splint | ☐ Arm
    ☐ No lifting greater than____ lbs | ☐ Hand
    ☐ No repetitive activities | ☐ Finger ____
    ☐ No work with hot or cold substances | ☐ Other

☐ Change positions every ____   ☐ Work activity as splint/bandage permits
☐ Avoid driving ☐ Keep wound clean/dry ☐ Limit working to ____ Hrs./Day

CHAPTER 14

An example of a more direct comparison format for worker abilities with job demands is shown in Figure 14–4 from the FCE Summary Report of Workability developed by WorkAbility Systems, Inc. in West Chester, Ohio. The strength of this approach, and similar approaches used by others, is that every job match factor can be rated or measured for the worker and the job, allowing the job

FIGURE 14–4   WorkAbility eJobMatch Taxonomy

Lift/Carry Abilities	Worker	Job Match
Floor lift strength (0-12")	_____ lbs	_____ lbs.
Knee lift strength (12-30")	_____ lbs	_____ lbs.
Waist lift strength (30-34")	_____ lbs	_____ lbs.
Chest lift strength (34-52")	_____ lbs	_____ lbs.
High lift strength (52-70")	_____ lbs	_____ lbs.
Carry strength (40' or less)	_____ lbs	_____ lbs.
Horizontal push/pull strength	_____ lbs	_____ lbs.
Frequent lift/carry (12-30x/hr)	_____ lbs	_____ lbs.
Constant lift/carry (>30x/hr)	_____ lbs	_____ lbs.

Physical Aptitudes	Worker	Job Match
Dynamic balance	_____	_____
Aerobic stamina	_____	_____
Climbing agility	_____	_____
Wrist-finger speed	_____	_____
Finger dexterity	_____	_____
Manual dexterity	_____	_____
Near vision acuity	_____	_____
Far vision acuity	_____	_____
Hearing sensitivity	_____	_____

Key: **U** = **U**nrated *****V** = **V**ery low (negligible) *****L** = **L**ow
      *****M** = **M**edium *****H** = **H**igh *****E** = **E**xtra high (exceptional)

Work Tolerances	Worker	Job Match
Standing	_____	_____
Sitting	_____	_____
Reaching above shoulders	_____	_____
Twisting or turning head	_____	_____
Stooping	_____	_____
Kneeling or crouching down	_____	_____

Key: **U** = **U**nrated *****N** = **N**ever (0%) *****O** = **O**ccasional (1-33%
      or <12x/hr) *****F** = **F**requent (34-66% or 12-30x/hour)
      *****C** = **C**onstant (67-100% or >30x/hour) *****E** = **E**xtra time
      (=>8 hours per shift)

CHAPTER 14

demands to be visually represented as the objectives for a job-specific plan of care. In addition, many of the Lift/Carry Abilities listed on the WorkAbility eJobMatch taxonomy have descriptors and frequency ranges that correspond closely to the ACGIH Threshold Limit Values (TLVs®) for Lifting.[13]

Summary

Job-specific testing requires an in-depth understanding of functional job demands to develop and select appropriate components based on consideration of safety, reliability, validity, practicality, and utility. The functional job analysis should drive the selection and development of job-specific test components. This analysis must be applied not just to the overall job as a whole but also to each critical job function that contributes to key physical ability requirements or work performance barriers. This information allows health care professionals to advise company representatives regarding the ability of prospective workers to perform a given job and identify what tasks injured workers are capable of performing and what tasks need further investigation during the course of a transitional work program. Performing a functional analysis of job tasks is critical in order to ensure a progressive and safe return to work.

The applications of job-specific functional tests have been discussed in this chapter. They include the following:

■ Injury prevention: Preoffer, postoffer, periodic screening (job placement), and fitness for duty
■ Management of early injury or illness, often as part of a transitional return to work program
■ Management of more complex or chronic injuries or illness, when the issue is whether a patient can perform a specific job

Employers confronted with cases involving lost time or restricted duty should make it a high priority to review functional job demands and identify modified duty options as soon as possible so that treating health care providers can design job-specific care plans. Job demands may be difficult or impossible to simulate in a clinical environment. Therefore, in such cases, occupational health providers may be trained and equipped to provide services, including the FCE, at the work site. Provision of a job-specific FCE at the work site has the added advantage of allowing health care providers to witness the actual job tasks and coach an injured worker in the appropriate pacing and safer work methods. If on-site services cannot be provided, provision for off-site therapy services are more likely to be rendered in a realistic and job-specific care plan in which an adequate and functional job analysis has been completed. A transitional model for return to

CHAPTER 14

work enhanced by the use of job-specific functional testing can expedite safe and productive return to work while reminding all parties involved that job-specific functional restoration is the ultimate goal of therapy in the occupational setting. In those situations when this testing can be performed at the work site, the implicit community-based approach to rehabilitation helps support the primary relationship between worker and employer.

References

1. American Physical Therapy Association. *Occupational Health Physical Therapy Guidelines: Evaluating Functional Capacity.* Amended July 11, 2008 [Note: This document has been approved and is available at www.apta.org].
2. Rehabilitation Act of 1973, Sections 501 (Employment of Handicapped Individuals) and 503 (Employment Under Federal Contracts). (1973). Public Law 93–112 93rd Congress, H. R. 8070. September 26, 1973.
3. The Americans with Disabilities Act of 1990, Section 102 of Title 42 of the United States Code (1990).
4. ADA Amendments Act of 2008.
5. Disability Discrimination Act of 1992. Australia. http://scaleplus.law.gov.au/html/pasteact/0/311/pdf/DDA1992.pdf. Accessed July 13, 2008.
6. The Disability Discrimination Act of 1995. United Kingdom. www.equalityhumanrights.com/Documents/Legislation/DDA1995.pdf. Accessed July 13, 2008.
7. Equal Employment Opportunity Commission. *Enforcement Guidance: Disability-Related Inquiries and Medical Examinations of Employees Under the Americans with Disabilities Act (ADA).* Washington, DC: Equal Employment Opportunity Commission; 2000. EEOC publication 915.002.
8. Franche R, Cullen K, Clarke J, Irvin E, Sinclair S, Frank J, and The Institute for Work & Health (IWH) Workplace-Based RTW Intervention Literature Review Research Team. Workplace-based return-to-work interventions: a systematic review of the quantitative literature. *J Occup Rehab.* 2005;15:607–631.
9. Basich M, Driscoll T, Wickstrom R. Transitional work therapy on-site: work is therapy! *Prof Case Manag* 2007; 12:351–357.
10. National Institute for Occupational Safety and Health. *Work Practices Guide for Manual Lifting.* Cincinnati, OH: US Dept of Health and Human Services, National Institute of Occupational Safety and Health; 1981. NIOSH technical report 81–122.
11. Borg GAV. Psychophysical bases of perceived exertion. *Med Sci Sports Exerc.* 1982;14:377–381.
12. American Conference of Governmental Industrial Hygienists. Threshold Limit Values (TLVs) for Lifting. TLVs and BEIs Book. 2007. Available at: www.washingtonsafepatienthandling.org/images/ACGIH_Lifitng_TLV.pdf. Accessed July 13, 2008.

13. Waters TR, Putz-Anderson V, Garg A. Applications manual for the revised NIOSH lifting equation. DHHS (NIOSH) Pub. No. 94–10. U.S. Department of Health and Human Services. Centers for Disease Control and Prevention, National Institute for Occupational Safety and Health. Cincinnati: OH; 1994.

14. Waters T, Baron SL, Piacitelli LA, et al. Epidemiological evaluation of the revised NIOSH lifting equation: a cross sectional study. *Spine.* 1999; 24(4):386–395.

15. Battie MC, Bigos SJ, Fisher LD, Hansson TH, Jones ME, Wortley MD. Isometric lifting strength as a predictor of industrial back pain reports. *Spine.* 1989;14:851–856.

16. Hansson TH, Bigos SJ, Wortley MK, Spengler DM. The load on the lumbar spine during isometric strength testing. *Spine.* 1984;9:720–724.

17. American College of Sports Medicine. *ACSM's Guidelines for Exercise Testing and Prescription.* 7th ed. American College of Sports Medicine; 2006.

18. Gouttebarge V, Wind H, Kuijer PP, Sluiter JK, Frings-Dresen MH. Reliability and agreement of 5 Ergo-Kit functional capacity evaluation lifting tests in subjects with low back pain. *Arch Phys Med Rehabil.* 2006;87:1365–1370.

19. Gouttebarge V, Wind H, Kuijer PP, Sluiter JK, Frings-Dresen MH. Intra- and inter-rater reliability of the Ergo-Kit functional capacity evaluation method in adults without musculoskeletal complaints. *Arch Phys Med Rehabil.* 2005;86: 2354–2360.

20. Gouttebarge V, Wind H, Kuijer PP, Frings-Dresen MH. Reliability and validity of functional capacity evaluation methods: a systematic review with reference to Blankenship system, Ergos Work Simulator, Ergo-Kit and Isernhagen Work System. *Int Arch Occup Environ Health.* 2004;77:527–537.

21. Reneman MF, Fokkens AS, Dijkstra PU, Geertzen JH, Groothoff JW. Testing lifting capacity: validity of determining effort level by means of observation. *Spine.* 2005;30:E40–E46.

22. Section 60-3, Uniform Guidelines on Employment Selection Procedures (1978); 43 FR 38295 (August 25, 1978).

23. Chaffin DB, Park KS. A longitudinal study of low-back pain as associated with occupational weight lifting factors. *Am Ind Hyg Assoc J.* 1973;35:513–525.

24. Keyserling WM, Herrin GD, Chaffin DB. Isometric strength testing as a means of controlling medical incidents on strenuous jobs. *J Occup Med.* 1980;22: 332–336.

25. Liles DH, Deivanayagam S, Ayoub MM, Majajan M. A job severity index for the evaluation and control of lifting injury. *Hum Factors.* 1984;26:683–693.

26. Bigos SJ, Battie MD, Fisher LD, Hansson TH, Spengler DM, Nachemsen AL. A prospective evaluation of preemployment screening methods for acute industrial back pain. *Spine.* 1992;17:922–926.

27. Gross DP, Battie MC. Does functional capacity evaluation predict recovery in workers compensation claimants with upper extremity disorders? *Occup Environ Med.* 2006;63(6):404–410.

28. Gross DP, Battie MC. The prognostic value of functional capacity evaluation in patients with chronic low back pain, part 2: sustained recovery. *Spine.* 2004;29:920–924.

29. Gross DP, Battie MC, Cassidy JD. The prognostic value of functional capacity evaluation in patients with chronic low back pain, part 1: timely return to work. *Spine.* 2004;29:914–919.

CHAPTER 14

30. Kuijer W, Brouwer S, Reneman MF, et al. Matching FCE activities and work demands: an explorative study. *J Occup Rehabil.* 2006;16:469–483.

31. US Department of Labor Employment and Training Administration. *The Revised Handbook for Analyzing Jobs.* Washington, DC: US Dept of Labor Employment and Training Administration; 1991.

32. Ohio Bureau of Workers' Compensation. MEDCO-14 Physician's Report of WORKABILITY. BWC-3914 (8/29/01). Available at: www.ohiobwc.com/downloads/blankpdf/MEDCO-14.pdf. Accessed July 13, 2008.

15

Functional Capacity Evaluation for Patients With Chronic Pain

Lisa Fore, OTR, Janice Keeley, PT, and Tom Mayer, MD

The earlier chapters of this book have discussed the scientific basis and clinical applications of various components essential to the functional capacity evaluation (FCE). When one comes to the application of the FCE to a person with chronic pain complaints, a paradox arises. The information provided by the FCE in this patient population is important because it can quantify the functional impact of physiologic deficits that may not be easily identified by other forms of testing and help guide decisions regarding treatment and return to work. However, the ability to effectively apply the FCE to this population is severely limited by the confounding effect of pain. It is with this in mind that we need to study the particular characteristics of patients with chronic pain and the associated "deconditioning" and psychosocial recovery barriers. Judicious use of the FCE can assist in guiding the management of people who may benefit from rehabilitative efforts and also may help identify people with pain complaints who would be best served by expediting return to work and claim resolution.

Patients With Chronic Pain

Following occupational injuries to the musculoskeletal system, chronic pain occurs in 5% to 15% of patients. *Chronic pain* is pain extending beyond the normal "healing period" from the trauma sustained and is often associated with persistent work disability despite the receipt of seemingly appropriate medical interventions. The problems of patients with chronic pain represent a disproportionate amount of the cost to the workers' compensation system. In time, these patients also account for disproportionate costs for long-term financial benefits from insurers, government agencies, and retirement schemes.

Chronic pain is inherently a subjective phenomenon and has been found to have a multifactorial development process. As a result, medical approaches have evolved to treat this costly and complex phenomenon, but not always with results beneficial to society or, over the long run, to the patient. Palliation of chronic pain, regardless of whether this leads to improved function, may become the primary focus of sympathetic medical providers and result in overuse of opioid medications or development of a codependent therapeutic alliance between patient and physician. The latter may lead health providers to abet escalating physical disuse and a psychological retreat from usual realities of earning a living and other customary social responsibilities. Protective physical disuse may then lead to a *deconditioning syndrome*, which can be substantially modulated by pain perception and patient fears. Deconditioning is discussed in more detail later in this chapter.

Certain musculoskeletal disorders have a predilection for becoming chronic disabling conditions. Spinal disorders, particularly those affecting the low back, usually begin as sprains and strains and are more prevalent among people with chronic pain and disabling work-related injuries than disorders involving other musculoskeletal joints or regions. Upper extremity neurocompressive complaints, particularly those termed *repetitive motion* or *cumulative trauma disorders* (CTDs), also have a higher rate of developing chronicity, with CTD claims known to be 1.8 times more expensive than non-CTD claims.[1-7] By contrast, lower extremity injuries, particularly if they involve fractures, tend to resolve more completely within a usual tissue healing period.

Chronic pain is more likely to result when the diagnosis and mechanism of injury are more subjective and vague. Failed efforts to identify the source of the pain ("pain generator") then often result in the identification of "psychogenic" or "functional" pain. These are terms attributed to pain for which no physical source can be found and, therefore, for which psychological or "nonorganic" causes are suspected. Patients in whom chronic pain develops have often been found to have a number of psychological difficulties (eg, depression, anxiety, and substance use) and social losses (eg, inability to work, family role changes, and financial stressors), which are now known to modulate the pain experience. Turk and Rudy[8] helped popularize the biopsychosocial model of pain, asserting that pain is engendered not only by physical insult but also by cognitive, affective, psychosocial, and behavioral influences.

Much controversy exists regarding the development of chronic pain and disability syndromes after work-related musculoskeletal injuries. A variety of psychosocial host factors, secondary gain, and socioeconomic predictors have been variably reported in the literature.

Psychosocial Factors in Chronic Pain

When work-related musculoskeletal injury is associated with compensation for disability, physical problems are rarely the only factors that should be considered in organizing a treatment approach. Many psychosocial and socioeconomic problems may confront patients recovering from a painful disorder, particularly if inability to lead a productive lifestyle is associated with the industrial injury. The patient's inability to see a "light at the end of the tunnel" may produce a reactive depression, often associated with anxiety and agitation. The musculoskeletal injury itself may be associated with emotional distress as expressed by rebellion against authority or job dissatisfaction. Poor coping styles associated with reaction to stress or underlying personality disorders may be manifested as anger, hostility, and noncompliance directed at the therapeutic team. Brain dysfunction related to age, alcohol, drugs, or an underestimated minor head injury or limited intelligence may cause cognitive dysfunctions that make patients difficult to manage and educate. A full discussion of these topics is beyond the scope of this chapter.

A number of self-report validated questionnaires about pain and function have shown associations with various important objective outcomes of chronic pain treatment in the PRIDE (Productive Rehabilitation Institute of Dallas for Ergonomics, Dallas, TX) occupational setting.[9–11] A number of these validated questionnaires may be useful to clinicians treating patients with chronic pain because they can be used as adjuncts to the FCE to get a sense of how the patients see themselves and their limitations. The self-report scales also provide a counterpoint to test performance, over and above the response to pain. Many experienced therapists recognize the impact of patient-specific psychosocial factors on disability or depression without the use of validated questionnaires, but even skilled clinicians can benefit from comparing their experience and intuition with patients' own perceptions. Having validated questionnaires available that deal with the relationships among pain, function, and disability in the musculoskeletal system is useful. The questionnaires, like patient behaviors, can be guides to the degree of psychosocial disturbance associated with chronic pain and disability and are described further in Chapter 5. The questionnaires most useful in the population with chronic pain are as follows:

- The Pain Disability Questionnaire[11–13]: Measures functional deficits throughout the musculoskeletal system
- Oswestry Disability Index[14–16]: Measures lumbar spine–related functional deficits
- Disabilities of the Arm, Shoulder, and Hand (DASH) and *Quick*DASH[17–22]: Measure upper extremity functional deficits
- Short-Form (SF) 36 and SF-12[23–25]: Measure health-related quality of life
- Beck Depression Inventory[26]: Measures self-assessed depressive symptoms

Factors That Impact FCE Performance in Patients With Chronic Pain

A number of factors can affect how a person with chronic pain performs during an FCE. These factors include "weak link," deconditioning, fear-avoidant beliefs, and reliance on palliation (especially opioids). It is helpful to understand these factors before attempting to apply principles of the FCE to a patient with chronic pain.

Impact of a Weak Link

Following the apparent resolution of injury, some patients are left with a specific *weak link* in the biomechanical chain related to a specific site of injury. Normal functional capacity may often be preserved, as one stronger link *substitutes* for a weaker one. A typical example is a person with mild, residual low back pain who squats and lifts with his or her legs and, when evaluated briefly, performs a test at the desired level. It is not difficult to intuit, however, that if the FCE actually observed the worker performing this task throughout an 8-hour day (rather than during a brief test period), endurance problems or "biomechanical breakdown" might occur because the low back is weaker than the other links of the biomechanical chain that transmit forces from the hands to the foot-floor contact. These effects can be observed during the FCE if the patient is tested using protocols that avoid the substitution of the stronger links (hips and knees). One such method is to use the National Institutes of Occupational Safety and Health (NIOSH) Isometric Torso Lift, comparing performance with the NIOSH Leg Lift. In a patient with chronic pain or a person with multiple-joint involvement, the weak link problems may be magnified because multisite involvement may preclude substitution of a healthy biomechanical link for a weaker one. When the evaluator recognizes that performance during the FCE is suboptimal and is specifically affected by one or more weak links, the idea of performing longer tests arises. Assessing a patient's performance for a longer period, especially in patients whose functional capacity is almost sufficient to allow full-duty or transitional work return, may better address the presence of localized strength or endurance deficits, which compromise overall performance, even though the patient can do well in a short test. In some cases, an 8-hour or 2-day test may be used. In others, more sophisticated computerized testing equipment (see Chapter 7) might characterize and quantify the weak link, leading to a corrective therapeutic approach that would address performance deficits attributable to a weak link identified in the FCE.

Impact of Deconditioning

The term *deconditioning* refers to the loss of mobility, strength, endurance, and/ or coordination associated with prolonged disuse of an injured limb or spinal region. With an acute injury, pain is almost always associated with limitations of motion and strength, but these limitations resolve spontaneously if prompt healing occurs. With longer periods of disuse and the development of chronic pain, protective joint splinting leads to recalcitrant joint stiffness. Loss of normal joint function leads to decreased muscle fiber recruitment, creating strength and endurance deficits in the peri-articular muscles and, ultimately, to muscle atrophy and fatty replacement. Deconditioning is a relative term in the sense that every healthy person demonstrates a balance between the physical demands of daily life and functional capacity for handling activities of daily living (ADLs).

CHAPTER 15

When there is an imbalance, the person's status is termed *deconditioned*. The term is also used when a person has shown a decrease in levels of physical capacity and ability to meet daily demands due to sequelae of injury or inactivity for a period, even if a new balance point has been reached. Obviously, people of the same sex, age, and size may have vastly different balance points, as is commonly seen when comparing the condition of high-performance athletes with that of sedentary (or relatively inactive) people.

It has been proposed that chronic pain typically induces inactivity, disuse, and deconditioning. Kottke[27] stated, "The functional capacity of any organ is dependent within physiologic limits upon the intensity and frequency of its activity. Although rest may be protective for a damaged organ it results in progressive loss of functional capacity for normal organs." The decrease in function will be proportional to the duration, degree, and type of limitation of activity. Hasenbring et al[28] proposed physical disuse as a risk factor for chronicity in patients with lumbar disk disorders. *Disuse* or *disuse syndrome* and deconditioning are terms associated with this loss of functional capacity. Mayer and Gatchel[29] introduced the term *deconditioning syndrome* to represent the cumulative disuse changes, physical and psychological, produced in chronically disabled patients with spinal and other chronic musculoskeletal disorders. They considered deconditioning a response mediated physically by the injury, injury-imposed inactivity, neurologically mediated protective reflexes, iatrogenic medication dependence, nutritional disturbance, and psychologically by tension and stress, vocational adjustment problems, and/or limited social coping resources.[9]

Ultimately, physical deconditioning is characterized by muscle inhibition and atrophy, decreased cardiovascular conditioning, decreased neuromuscular coordination, decreased ability to perform complicated repetitive tasks, and musclotendinous contractures, leading to even further restrictions in activity level and worsened physical status. A recent review of the deconditioning process was written by Sawchuk and Mayer.[30] Some controversy remains about the concept of physical deconditioning,[31,32] which may not be present in all patients with chronic pain and, if it is present, may not be the primary cause of their limitations. However, considering the wide acceptance of the concept as applied to multiple organ systems, especially the cardiovascular system, denial of the medical evidence for this basic physiologic process is not tenable.

In the absence of any psychosocial barriers to recovery, patients in a deconditioned status often recover spontaneously or with limited advice from health care providers to participate in a home exercise program. When a person with no obvious physical disabilities takes part in an FCE, performance on the FCE is dependent on the degree of deconditioning, modulated by factors such as age, sex, body weight, and psychosocial status. As stated, while deconditioning is not uniformly seen in all patients with chronic pain, it is reasonable to expect that the FCE will reveal some evidence of this process in many patients with chronic pain. In fact, a benefit of the FCE in this population is its ability to identify physical evidence of true muscle weakness, abnormal recruitment patterns, and decreased aerobic fitness that otherwise may not be readily discerned. On the other hand, if deconditioning is primarily due to complaints of chronic pain and the ensuing physical inhibition produced by fear avoidance, or secondary gain leading to illness behaviors and embellishment, performance on the FCE may be markedly diminished even when an objective physiologic explanation is not apparent.

Impact of Fear-Avoidance Beliefs and Other Psychosocial Factors

In a patient with chronic pain, physical activity is generally equated with pain, and pain avoidance, in and of itself, has become a goal of the patients. To a greater or lesser extent, all patients with chronic pain fear the pain, with the appearance of that fear leading to guarding against, or avoidance of, the perceived painful activity. Thus, pain limitation is often equated with *fear avoidance*, which has led to a type of psychotherapy termed *fear avoidance belief training*. Another commonly used term for the guarding is *inhibition* because the pain is thought to inhibit the patient's ability, or motivation, to perform *positional activity* deemed potentially harmful. Inherent to all these terms for pain-limited *abilities* is the patient belief that "hurt means harm."

Minimal performance during an FCE may be a combination of multiple factors, many of which have a psychosocial origin. Lack of instruction about the importance of exerting maximal effort and uncertainty or trepidation about how the results may be used (including threatening current socioeconomic stability) may also be factors. The latter are real patient concerns but are not the traits that would characterize a sociopath attempting to profit by "fooling the system." Rather, these factors represent the psychosocial baggage of patients mired in defeat and degradation in the majority of cases.

Impact of Pain Palliation

A focus on pain therapies that rely on *palliation* rather than *functional recovery* is another factor frequently encountered in the workers' compensation system that can affect the results of the FCE. Once patients accept that they have a chronic pain syndrome, regardless of intelligence, socioeconomic status, or educational level, they are highly prone to suggestion and education received from trusted health care providers. If pain palliation becomes the patient's primary goal, the information received may include advice against participating in hurtful activities, cessation of these activities as soon as pain occurs, reliance or dependence on passive care provided by a clinician (eg, acupuncture, electrical stimulation, and massage), or over-reliance on medications. Foremost among the palliative medications are the opioids. While they are the most potent analgesics, their mechanism of action is in the brain on the so-called pain centers, rather than at the injury or inflammatory site (as with anti-inflammatory agents). *Opioid-induced hyperalgesia,* in which patients experience a heightened sensitivity to pain when taking regular doses of opioids, is an unfortunate potential side effect of all opioids. It has been argued that the hyperalgesia itself is part of the reason for inhibition because a decreasing level of opioid at the brain's pain center leads to perception of increased pain and to greater pain sensitivity with activity. In a sense, these medications may disrupt our cognitive ability to process pain stimuli that are really being messaged from the injury site in the periphery. Thus fear-avoidance behaviors coupled with a history of having received primarily palliative treatments coupled, when applicable, with the use of opioids can profoundly influence the degree to which an evaluee is willing to perform the physical testing that is generally the focus of FCEs.

The FCE in Chronic Pain

General Concepts

In a patient with chronic pain, any or all of the factors discussed up to this point may intervene to produce what is generally called "pain limitation." This finding leads to controversy about the usefulness of the FCE in patients with chronic pain. Some clinicians, dismayed by the negligible performance levels seen in many patients in initial testing, judge the entire enterprise as worthless. Although many think of FCEs as tools to facilitate disposition of a case at the termination of a patient's treatment, and they can, indeed, be used for this purpose, FCEs can also be used to plan treatment or to progress treatment that has already begun. Using baseline FCE performance as the basis for the initial exercise prescription increases patient's confidence in the therapist's initial exercise dosing and allows the therapist to develop a regimen that is tailored to the needs of the patient. By facilitating the identification of the *degree* of deficit in ADLs, as well as the association of this deficit with nonanatomic factors rather than focusing solely on demonstrating that deficits are present, the FCE permits individualization of all aspects of the interdisciplinary program and enhances the likelihood of successful outcomes. The essential purposes of the FCE for patients with chronic pain are not markedly different from the goals in other patients. They are to:

- Match functional ability to desired vocational or recreational physical demand requirements;
- In the event of a mismatch, identify ADLs (performance deficits) requiring rehabilitation; and
- Judge the degree to which rehabilitation of specific ADLs is required to achieve the targeted performance levels.

When treatment is not an option, the FCE will be performed specifically to facilitate the following:

- Case settlement or closure by identifying a "minimum the patient can do" despite pain inhibition; or
- Setting work restrictions by identifying the "minimum the patient is able to demonstrate."

When a therapist begins an FCE, he or she may be completely unaware of how the patient will perform. It is only when specific *pain behaviors* occur that the therapist is alerted that test performance may be surprisingly low due to pain limitation. Clues may be derived from early test anxiety, high pretest pain ratings, obsessive reporting of symptoms, or patient concerns about what he/she will *not* be able to do. Pain behaviors may be detected within the early phases of the FCE through groaning or pain displays, perceived exertion by the patient that fails to match heart rate during activity, severe complaints with minimal activity levels, or simple refusal to perform requested activities. Use of the psychometric questionnaires described previously, coupled with observation of the patient during the FCE, can help shed light on whether psychosocial factors may be operant and the degree to which they inhibit performance. When extensive pain behavior leads to extremely low performance levels, it becomes clear to the therapist early in the FCE that diligent completion of every aspect of the FCE is unnecessary to draw an appropriate conclusion. The hope that this test will lead to meaningful information on current physical capabilities will not be realized, and the test itself then becomes an opportunity to observe the degree to which pain inhibits the patient's performance. Such information may be useful if future treatment is to be provided, in which case the FCE becomes the baseline from which subsequent physical performance tests or FCEs are judged for progress. In other cases, as in the situation of patients previously having demonstrated noncompliance after opportunities for rehabilitation, the FCE may simply become the final demonstration of a particular patient's intransigence.

Even if the clinician believes he or she is observing the latter, attention should be given to the psychosocial and other factors to see whether the noncompliance might have a correctable cause. Given the reason for the assessment and the initial patient performance, it is safe to say that testing can be completed

CHAPTER 15

with a shorter range of assessments whenever severe pain appears. Specifically, this means that the FCE may be shortened with the explanation that guarding and inhibition are so severe that meaningful testing cannot be performed on relevant ADLs. For example, once a patient has demonstrated a zero score on any computerized testing equipment or performs minimally on tests of dynamic material handling, continuing to test at different speeds (for isokinetic testing) or positions (for dynamic material handling) is unnecessary. Extensive FCEs may not be necessary or valid for assessing the physical performance of patients with chronic pain because estimates regarding their level of ability will ultimately need to be based on the clinical judgment of the evaluator.

Consistency of effort has been discussed in previous chapters, and well-trained therapists become excellent observers of pain behaviors and physical inhibition. Technology may be helpful in providing more mathematical or objective measures (eg, coefficient of variation on isokinetic isolated strength and lifting tests, or variance of repeated active goniometric extremity joint or inclinometric true regional spinal motion measurements). An argument can be made that the difficulty of accurately identifying the degree of physical decrement or quantitatively assessing the degree of psychosocial recovery ambivalence warrants a greater reliance on technology for clinicians dealing frequently with patients with chronic pain. However, high-tech devices are not absolutely necessary for the majority of tests and, indeed, may be primarily of benefit in situations when the evaluator and/or referral source can use objective documentation of self-limited behaviors to better determine management options or when the patient is participating in a rehabilitation program.

Principles and Components of Functional Capacity Evaluation

Certain principles help patients to do their best during an FCE, particularly patients with chronic pain. These principles are generalizable to all FCEs, but are of particular importance when evaluating people with disabilities with work-related injuries. Here are some pointers:

- *Standardized initial information:* It is important that evaluators present consistent and standardized information to the patient regarding the content and process of the FCE. This story should not be delivered in a script that is read to the patient, but should generally be presented by the therapist who obtains the history and performs the musculoskeletal examination. Patients should initially be provided information about the test itself, the report that will be generated, and the expected duration of the test. If isokinetics are used, patients should be told about "accommodating resistance" and the way that isokinetic devices work. Patients should also be provided specific safety information and encouraged to "do the best you feel is safe for you at this time."

- *FCE atmospherics:* Because many patients are typically nervous, and are afraid they will be injured in some way, reassurance and a calm demeanor among the testing staff are important. Patients should be given opportunities to ask questions and to receive direct responses, insofar as possible.
- *Pain ratings:* Pain ratings are noted by the evaluators before and after each task. Although this information is useful in correlating to test performance, it also provides reassurance to patients that their pain concerns and guarding are being noted by the testers. The evaluator should not spend significant time "focusing" on pain. Rather, simple questions should be asked related to pain level and what change was noted, if any, on completion of each subtest.
- *Voluntary task discontinuation:* Patients will voluntarily stop performance of certain tasks they consider painful or dangerous. The tester should ascertain the reasons for stopping and how long it took the patient to reach that point.
- *Observed effort:* The evaluator should use all acquired clinical skill to observe for consistency of effort, correlation between similar tasks, and patterns of motivation or inhibition during each task performed. Even without the use of computerized testing, observation of performance and complementary tests to measure consistency of effort can help to distinguish pain inhibition from a complete lack of effort and motivation to perform (eg, negligible increase in heart rate and zero weights lifted on materials handling tasks). The evaluator should also be sure to note when the patient demonstrates limitation of activities that predominantly require the use of body parts that are normal on clinical examination and would not have been affected by injury.
- *Inconsistent behaviors:* The examiner should note tolerance of sitting during paperwork completion and walking, if possible, while the evaluee is in the lobby of the facility and on entrance and departure from the clinic and examining room. Changes in demeanor, such as an increase in apparent physical distress, when the evaluee enters the testing site or when other family or significant others are present or enter the room may also provide useful information.
- *Responsiveness:* The tester should assess not only what the evaluee does at the initiation of each task, but also the ability, or willingness, of the evaluee to be educated in pain management techniques by applying information provided during an initial task to tasks that are performed later in the sequence. Apparent unwillingness to do so in the context of continued complaints of pain should be noted.

The components of an FCE for patients with chronic pain are similar to the components used in other FCEs.

CHAPTER 15

- *The clinical examination*, discussed in Chapter 4, is important. Joint motion is generally best measured by assessing active motion. In some cases, passive motion may be gently evaluated to help the examiner validate findings attained through active motion to differentiate joint restriction, weakness, and pain. Joint motion can be assessed with a goniometer in the extremities and an inclinometer in the spine. Muscle bulk can be assessed by tape measurements. Right-left comparisons between affected and unaffected sides can be made. Besides assessing range of motion (ROM), strength, and cardiovascular fitness, the clinical examination should also assess balance, coordination, and endurance. Neuromuscular residuals of paresis, tremor, spasm or cognitive dysfunction may limit recovery and create uncorrectable deficits in performing certain ADLs. Identification of these types of neuromuscular deficits can contribute to understanding patients with chronic pain.

- *Measurements of aerobic fitness* relate to lower extremity strength, as well as to cardiovascular fitness, because the standard measurement techniques involve exercise protocols on bicycles, treadmills, or measured walking courses that require good lower limb function. Major deficits in lower extremity strength or cardiovascular fitness may seriously limit aerobic fitness or even hamper performance of the test.[33] Chapter 10 reviews methods of aerobic assessment more broadly. Assessment of aerobic fitness should be a component of FCEs performed on patients with chronic pain.

- *Heart rate monitoring* is a very important clue to how hard individuals are willing to push themselves during the evaluation, especially when attempting to determine whether there is a physiologic basis for low or inconsistent observed effort. Heart rate, ie, when higher than anticipated based on age norms, can also be a guide to the level of aerobic fitness currently maintained, providing "evidence" of deconditioning.

- *Isokinetic strength testing* may be added to compare potential weak-link performance with the functional capacity of the whole body. Chapter 7 provides a discussion on the use of computerized testing in FCEs.

- *Materials handling and non–materials handling components* are used in the PRIDE FCE in addition to the clinical examination and use of self-report questionnaires. The PRIDE FCE looks at standard materials handling tasks, such as the Progressive Isoinertial Lifting Evaluation (PILE),[34–35] and non–materials handling assessment, such as sitting, standing, balance, stair climbing, and fitness testing. The NIOSH isometric lift tests and isokinetic lifting may also be added to the range of tests provided. Testing is usually performed in a single day during a range of 3 to 5 hours, depending on the musculoskeletal areas involved and/or pain experienced by the patient.

Pain Behaviors

Pain behaviors that are disproportionate to objective findings are almost uniformly observed when an FCE is used for people with chronic pain. Patterns typically seen in people with chronic pain include the following:

- Global pain, ie, all over pain complaints or complaints that are not fully consistent with the diagnosis or length of disability, which may include the following:
  - Pain complaints extending from the low back in a nonphysiologic way to the neck or arms
  - Spinal pain that radiates to toes or fingertips bilaterally with nondermatomal sensory deficits or nonmyotomal weakness
  - High reports of generalized pain (often seen with opioid-induced hyperalgesia)
- An obligation to tell "their story," despite multiple health care providers already being aware of it, which includes the following:
  - Inability to follow directions because of a compulsive need to retell their story to each listener
  - Failure to be reassured by the therapist or to feel rapport with the therapist
- Inconsistent performance when the patient is aware of being observed vs unaware, including the following:
  - Inconsistency in active ROM between specific goniometry measurements and observed functional activities
  - Ability to sit answering questionnaires for an extended period, but unable to sit when that ADL is being tested
- Testing at different percentiles of "normal" performance based on age, sex, or height and weight, which includes the following:
  - Performing weak but qualitatively reasonable manual muscle testing, but testing at an isokinetic strength of zero when strength is quantitatively measured
  - Demonstrating a weak link by showing lower strength testing levels at a specific joint or spinal region (eg, 10% of normal) compared with lifting capacity from floor-to-waist or waist-to-shoulder (eg, 40% of normal)
- Accommodation to disability, which generally takes place within 3 or 4 years of the injury and is manifested by a relative indifference to the disability, loss of interest in societal reintegration, and a generally low, but not negligible, level of physical performance
- Reluctance or refusal to perform tasks due to the belief that they will harm themselves
- Self-limitation during lifting and functional activities that does not correlate with the injury area or other screening findings during the musculoskeletal evaluation, such as the following:

CHAPTER 15

- - Upper limb injury with limitation in lower limb tasks, such as in walking, standing, or squatting despite no history of lower limb injury
  - No evidence of injury found in a musculoskeletal examination, yet extreme inhibition in the performance of functional tasks with the examined musculoskeletal area
  - Refusal to perform an activity because a health provider imposed a restriction or because of a reported likelihood of experiencing severe pain if a very limited performance level is exceeded
- Demonstrated high intensity and frequency of pain complaints throughout testing without observed changes in exertion or biomechanical loading patterns, often accompanied by excessive pain displays, which can include the following:
  - Crying, groaning, or grimacing
  - Rubbing the extremity after use
  - Slowly lowering a weight to show how difficult the task was, even though greater exertion is required to do this than would be necessary to lower the weight normally
- Complaints of excessive exertion with little change in heart rate or respiratory rate
- Patient statements that "nothing decreases the pain" from high levels but that some activities can "increase the pain" even if it is rated as 10 of 10 at rest. Patients who make these statements are frequently users of significant amounts of opioids.
- Consistently poor performance throughout the FCE, including areas that should be unaffected by the injury, often accompanied by inconsistency between similar test items

Interpretation of the Functional Capacity Evaluation

The FCE in patients with chronic pain can provide useful information even when pain behaviors are present. However, it is important to not focus on individual tasks or test components and instead look at the "big picture." Pain levels before, during, and after testing reveal much about pain perception. Aerobic fitness and the patient's actual performance on individual tasks of materials handling or non–materials handling are less important than consideration of the consistency of performance in comparing results from one test to another and in the context of information obtained from observation of pain behaviors, the clinical examination, heart rate monitoring, and the evaluator's assessment of whether all tests are inhibited or only tests involving the injured areas.

Although extreme pain limitation is only uncommonly caused by intentional efforts to mislead examiners or noncompliance, when the initial FCE suggests the possibility that submaximal performance is volitional, the one-on-one therapy provided early in interdisciplinary rehabilitation can foster identification of patients motivated to fail. In other words, cost-effectiveness is enhanced by early identification of patients unwilling to seize the opportunity for functional recovery. Alternatively, the identification of volitional submaximal performance can be used in conjunction with the independent medical evaluation and other information that may be available to guide termination of care for patients deemed unsuitable for referral to interdisciplinary rehabilitation. In certain circumstances, people performing poorly in an FCE will already have been observed to perform at higher levels in physical training that is part of rehabilitation programs before the FCE. When such inconsistencies arise, poor effort and motivation demonstrated in the FCE may lead to a recommendation for termination of medical care and claim closure to avoid additional ineffectual intervention.

When terms such as pain or illness behaviors, exaggeration, and embellishment are used to characterize a patient, the issue of *malingering* often arises. This is a term applied to people who feign illness or demonstrate *intentional* efforts to defraud the examiner (and others). One of the difficult tasks in interpreting FCEs of people with chronic pain is determining whether limitations are truly reflective of chronic pain or represent malingering. This determination is difficult because the "red flags" already discussed are similar. However, patients with chronic pain typically have limited activity owing to high pain perception, fear of injury, or fear of increased pain with activity. Generally, they seem overwhelmed by their present status. Malingerers are typically less likely to show the usual psychological manifestations of chronic pain that were discussed previously. Although this difference may cause the evaluator to suspect that the person's behaviors may represent malingering, applying this label to a patient is problematic. Although skilled examiners can identify exaggeration, embellishment, inconsistency, and psychosocial overlay and, may also be aware of *secondary gain factors* that relate to compensation, medical care, and avoidance of usual social responsibilities (eg, work and family responsibilities), for observers to assert that they can identify these behaviors as *intentional* is fraught with risk. *Speculating* on what a patient may be thinking and *knowing* that this is indeed so are clearly two different matters. The *malingering* label is also emotionally potent and, when applied in a typical adversarial system (like workers' compensation), may create disputes that obscure the relevant issues that the FCE is attempting to address. That having been said, poor performance and effort in an FCE in the presence of medical treatment (or surveillance) in which a patient has been covertly observed to do better on the performance of ADLs than when aware of being watched may result in a recommendation that further therapeutic efforts are likely to be ineffectual, with claim closure the most appropriate strategy. The therapist does not need to raise the issue of *intent* or use the term malingering to provide such a recommendation.

CHAPTER 15

Application of the Functional Capacity Evaluation

FCEs are often used at a point when a person with chronic pain is presumed to have reached maximum medical improvement (MMI), that is, the point when further medical care is not expected to materially result in further functional improvement. The FCE can also be used before this time as a component of a rehabilitation program or, when in doubt, as part of the MMI determination process. Although the initial FCE of a patient with chronic pain referred for rehabilitation may sometimes demonstrate a match between vocational demands and the demonstrated performance by the close of treatment, such a match is definitely anticipated. Patients who have been noncompliant or failed to make progress with exercise, medication, or goal setting will likely have dropped out or been terminated from the program as noncompleters, while others may have completed a rehabilitation program and discharged early because of rapid progress to a point of confidence about return to work. In certain cases, disposition of both groups may not involve another FCE. In other cases, documentation of the ability to return to the desired job demands or the patient's failure to have demonstrated effort on testing despite opportunities for rehabilitation may suggest the need for a short, repeated FCE. In these cases, the FCE should include only the components of the FCE that demonstrate the particular issue at hand (eg, consistency of effort, specific materials handling tasks, or positional tolerances that were not achieved previously).

The correlation between FCE performance and recommendations and the patient's ultimate vocational reintegration is difficult to assess. Ideally, the final FCE for a person who completes an interdisciplinary program will always demonstrate disinhibition, elimination of fear-avoidance, and a positive display of excellent pain management techniques. In practice, a few surprises always occur in terms of poor performance. These cases are usually the exceptions to the rule and become important case examples for program quality improvement. For example, some patients continue to believe that poor performance on the FCE will somehow enhance their permanent partial disability financial settlement. Even though the treatment team may be confident that these patients with such beliefs are headed back to work and that case closure will occur at a reasonable interval after the final FCE, the patients may have received contrary information from family members or other trusted advisors and perform poorly on this basis, thus leading one to question the cost-effectiveness of having instituted the rehabilitative program at all. In other cases, patients may have made below-average progress but performed sufficiently well to permit them to limp along in the program, just above the threshold for noncompletion. This group of patients frequently has already engendered uncertainty in the treatment staff about whether their commitment to vocational reintegration is valid. They frequently perform poorly on the final FCE and also frequently fail to implement their vocational plans after treatment. Again, the risk factors cannot be fully discussed in this chapter, but have previously been discussed extensively in the published literature.[36-38]

Regardless of the behaviors and remaining uncertainties in situations such as these, these patients can now be considered as having reached MMI. The same is the case when FCEs are performed as part of an independent medical evaluation process as there may be no interdisciplinary rehabilitation program available or the quality and outcomes of such programs may be in question. The requesting organization may consequently be prepared to deal with work assistance for the patient at his or her current level of performance, but not to provide interdisciplinary rehabilitation (a situation that occurs frequently when FCEs are performed in the context of long-term disability policies). In these cases, the requesting organization simply wants to know the minimum capabilities of the patient, along with some assessment of consistency of effort to give guidance on the accuracy of the reported test results. This situation also occurs when there is a financial dispute about ability to work in a workers' compensation jurisdiction where payments are based on the patient's ability to demonstrate *work incapacity*. In a sense, this is also the criterion by which patients are accepted for federal Social Security Disability Income (SSDI). These situations are not infrequent, and determining minimum capacities and effort may be the focus of assessments when identification of persons who are totally incapable of work is the primary goal of the FCE.

Example A 52-year-old man has been disabled for 5 years after a low back injury resulting in an initial diskectomy and a subsequent L4-S1 fusion 3 years ago. The patient's workers' compensation benefits have been discontinued, but he is receiving SSDI and takes significant daily doses of sustained release oxycodone supplemented by immediate-release oxycodone for "breakthrough pain." He is referred for FCE, but performs with extreme pain limitation, demonstrating "0" scores on isokinetic back and lift testing and lifting a maximum of 8 lb floor to waist and waist to shoulder on the PILE test. His only skills are in carpentry and roofing. He is referred for treatment, but demonstrates extreme skepticism. He draws a line about any "tampering" with his medications. Because of high pain sensitivity, possibly related to opioid-induced hyperalgesia, he fails to make progress and leaves complaining of exhaustion after 4-hour sessions. He drops out after eight part-day visits.

Analysis Although this patient had initially stated interest in returning to work to supplement his SSDI payments and in reducing his reliance on narcotics, he was unwilling to comply with attempts to reduce his medication, which ultimately

CHAPTER 15

led to treatment failure. The staff was alerted to the problem by the extreme level of pain limitation in conjunction with an absence of objective findings. Despite attentive treatment, the patient's actions during therapy were not aligned with his stated goals of reduced narcotic use or work reintegration. Although the patient was provided a treatment opportunity, he demonstrated noncompliance. The insurance carrier pursued medication weaning through other means.

Example A 47-year-old woman injured her right shoulder 1 year ago and underwent a rotator cuff repair and subacromial decompression 7 months ago. She completed a postoperative reconditioning therapy process and came in for an FCE as a prelude to returning to work. During the evaluation she cradled her right arm and reported extreme pain and tenderness throughout the cervical scapular and right upper extremity areas. There was no objective sign of swelling, redness, or color/temperature change. She resisted active ROM to no more than 30° of flexion or abduction during goniometric measurements (when she was aware of being observed), but was able to don and remove her jacket with minor modification (slowing the pace of dressing, but moving the shoulder to 90° of abduction at times). Grip strength was better with her right (nondominant) hand than the unaffected left hand. However, when observed during isokinetic strength testing for the right arm or doing two-arm lifting tests, she was unable to develop any force on the right side alone or when both arms are used.

Analysis This patient's testing was pain-limited but also inconsistent and fully inhibited. She demonstrated inconsistency between ADLs performed when she was aware of being observed vs when she was distracted. She did not simply demonstrate a decrease in strength performance with her affected arm, but could develop no force whatsoever. Yet, grip strength was surprisingly well preserved, with performance actually better than her unaffected (dominant) left hand grip. This was an invalid performance in the FCE, and the patient demonstrated persisting psychosocial barriers to recovery and return to work. Without an adequate history of treatment and the training levels she has participated in, no conclusions can be drawn about whether the current FCE demonstrated the maximum effort of which the patient is currently capable. However, if supplied with information that the patient's postoperative rehabilitation, which ended 1 month ago, had demonstrated 135° of flexion and abduction and active ROM with frequent lifting to 40 lb waist to shoulder, voluntary limitation of effort would be suspected. In this situation, it is recommended that the therapist "call it like it is" based on limited information, identifying mildly deficient motion associated with an adequate demonstration of ability to perform at the observed physical demand level.

Summary

This chapter has been a brief review of the FCE as applied to patients with chronic pain. Potentially, the FCE can be very useful, as long as one understands the nature of chronic pain, particularly in an occupational injury disability system. The chapter discussed the nature of chronic pain and the biopsychosocial model, which is now the accepted means of clinically analyzing the status of patients with chronic pain. There was also a review of psychosocial barriers to recovery for patients with chronic pain, including a brief description of some validated self-report questionnaires that may aid therapists providing an FCE. The deconditioning syndrome and the tendency of the injured area to become a weak link (with loss of localized ROM, strength, and endurance) as chronicity progresses was discussed, as was the application of these principles to FCE testing. Finally, this chapter discussed the benefits and limitations of FCEs in prerehabilitation and postrehabilitation situations. In particular, the FCE's utility at the initiation of chronic pain treatment as an alternative that may provide information leading to return to work, recreation, or improved home function was described, as was its use outside of the rehabilitation setting, where the evaluation may be part of an independent medical evaluation in which the output may not include opportunities for rehabilitation (as in workers' compensation financial disputes or long-term disability cases). In these cases, because rehabilitation may not be available even if deemed medically desirable, establishing minimum performance levels permits dispute resolution or some type of work accommodation on return to the job. In the uncommon case of clear evidence of fraudulent intent (inconsistent surveillance videos or documentation of high levels of performance in a prior rehabilitation program), claim closure may be the most appropriate recommendation. Under these circumstances, when a patient essentially produces zero force output on multiple tests, a shortened FCE is justifiable. The goal of the therapist in this situation is to demonstrate that the extremely poor performance appears volitional rather than tied to a legitimate extreme weak link deficit in mobility or strength.

In the case of the finding that a patient is work-ready, the FCE may obviate the need for treatment. In some cases, extremely low functional capacity will be demonstrated, associated with *pain limitation,* in which case, therapists can recognize obvious psychosocial barriers, including physical inhibition and fear-avoidance. In other cases, performance of the weak link is selectively much lower (as a percentage of "normal" for the tested person) than the manual handling tasks capabilities (eg, lifting, carrying, pushing, and pulling) or the ability to perform whole-person functional tasks (eg, bending, reaching, twisting, and climbing). In situations when the FCE can be used as the initial step in designing a patient-specific treatment regimen, treatment should result in resolution of most physical inhibition and fear avoidance, with production of a valid FCE showing good consistency of effort. In these cases, a legitimate measurement of

CHAPTER 15

the patient's functional capacity for work or recreation should be identifiable by using the FCE after rehabilitation, although nonphysical factors will always have a role in ultimate return-to-work outcomes.

It is important that the FCE for patients with chronic pain be tailored to the individual situation being assessed and performed by a health provider who is experienced in the evaluation of patients with chronic pain. Although the initial FCE of patients with chronic pain will ideally be the first step in a rehabilitative effort, there are also cases in which results (of physical assessment and psychometric testing) may be so inconsistent as to cause the evaluator to question their credibility. In situations such as this, all parties are best served if the FCE provides a detailed description and analysis of relevant findings and applies test results and the results of the physical examination to arrive at an estimate of what minimum safe capacities should be.

References

1. Mayer T, Gatchel R, Polatin P, Evans T. Outcomes comparison of treatment for chronic disabling work-related upper extremity disorders and spinal disorders. *J Occup Environ Med.* 1999;41:761–770.
2. Vender M, Kasdan M, Truppa K. Upper extremity disorders: a literature review to determine work-relatedness. *J Hand Surg.* 1995;20A:534–541.
3. Association of Schools of Public Health/National Institutes for Occupational Safety and Health. Proposed national strategies for the prevention of leading work-related diseases and injuries, part 1. Washington, DC: Association of Schools of Public Health; 1986:19.
4. Bureau of Labor Statistics. Workplace Injuries and Illnesses in 1994. Washington, DC. US Department of Labor; 1995. US Dept of Labor publication 95–508. www.osh/osnr0001.txt. Accessed February 2, 2008.
5. Bureau of Labor Statistics. Workplace Injuries and Illnesses in 1996. Washington, DC. US Department of Labor; 1997. US Dept of Labor publication 97–453. www.osh/osnr0005.txt. Accessed February 2, 2008.
6. Brogmus G, Sorock G, Webster B. Recent trends in work-related cumulative trauma disorders of the upper extremities in the United States: an evaluation of possible reasons. *J Occup Environ Med.* 1996;38:401–411.
7. Webster B, Snook S. The cost of compensable upper extremity cumulative trauma disorders. *J Occup Med.* 1994;36:713–727.
8. Turk D, Rudy T. Toward a comprehensive assessment of chronic pain patients. *Behav Res Ther.* 1987;25:237–249.
9. McGeary D, Mayer T, Gatchel R. High pain ratings predict treatment failure in chronic occupational musculoskeletal disorders. *J Bone Joint Surg Am.* 2006;88:317–325.

10. Anagnostis C, Mayer T, Gatchel R, Proctor T. The million visual analog scale: its utility for predicting tertiary rehabilitation outcomes. *Spine.* 2003;28:1051–1060.

11. Gatchel R, Mayer T, Theodore R. The Pain Disability Questionnaire: relationship to one-year functional and psychosocial rehabilitation outcomes. *J Occup Rehabil.* 2006;16:75–94.

12. Gatchel R, Mayer T, Theodore B. Proceedings of the NASS 20th Annual meeting, The clinical utility of the Pain Disability Questionnaire in predicting functional restoration socioeconomic outcomes in chronic spinal patients: a 1-year prospective outcome study. *Spine J.* 2005;5(4)(suppl):S6–S7.

13. Anagnostis C, Gatchel R, Mayer T. The Pain Disability Questionnaire: a new psychometrically sound measure for chronic musculoskeletal disorders. *Spine.* 2004;29:2290–2302.

14. Fairbank J, Couper J, Davies J, O'Brien J. The Oswestry low back pain disability questionnaire. *Physiotherapy.* 1980;66:271–273.

15. Roland M, Fairbank J. The Roland-Morris Disability Questionnaire and the Oswestry Disability Questionnaire. *Spine.* 2000;25:3115–3124.

16. Hakkinen A, Kautiainen H, Jarvenpaa S, Arkela M, Ylinen J. Changes in the total Oswestry Index and its 10 items in females and males pre- and post-surgery for lumbar disc herniation: a 1-year follow-up. *Eur Spine J.* 2007;16:347–352.

17. Hudak P, Amadio P, Bombardier C. Development of an upper extremity outcome measure: The DASH (disabilities of the arm, shoulder, and hand) [published correction appears in *Am J Ind Med.* 1996;30:372]. The Upper Extremity Collaborative Group. *Am J Ind Med.* 1996;29:602–608.

18. Beaton D, Davis A, Hudak P, McConnell S. The DASH (disabilities of the arm, shoulder and hand) outcome measures: what do we know about it now? *Br J Hand Ther.* 2001;6:109–118.

19. Beaton D, Katz J, Fossel A, Wright J, Tarasuk V, Bombardier C. Measuring the whole or the parts? validity, reliability and responsiveness of the disabilities of the arm, shoulder and hand outcome measure in different regions of the upper extremity. *J Hand Ther.* 2001;14:128–146.

20. McDermid J, Richards R, Donner A, Bellamy N, Roth J. Responsiveness of the Short Form-36, disability of the arm, shoulder and hand questionnaire, patient related wrist evaluation, and physical impairment measurements in evaluating recovery after a distal radius fracture. *J Hand Surg [Am].* 2000;25:330–340.

21. Beaton D, Wright J, Katz J; Upper Extremity Collaborative Group. Development of the *Quick*DASH: comparison of 3-item reduction approaches. *J Bone Joint Surg Am.* 2005;87:1038–1046.

22. Matheson L, Melhorn J, Mayer T, Theodore B, Gatchel R. Reliability of a visual analog version of the *Quick*DASH. *J Bone Joint Surg Am.* 2006;88:1782–1787.

23. Ware JE, Kosinski M, Keller SD. *SF-36 Physical and Mental Health Summary Sales: A User's Guide.* Boston, MA: The Health Institute, New England Medical Center; 1994.

24. Luo X, George M, Kakouras I, Edwards C, Pietrobon R, Richardson W. Reliability, validity, and responsiveness of the Short Form-12-item survey (SF-12) in patients with back pain. *Spine.* 2003;28:1739–1745.

25. Grotle M, Brox J, Vollestad N. Functional status and disability questionnaires: what do they assess? a systematic review of back-specific outcomes questionnaires. *Spine.* 2004;30:130–140.

CHAPTER 15

26. Beck AT, Ward CH, Mendelson MM, Mock J, Erbaugh J. An inventory for measuring depression. *Arch Gen Psychiatry.* 1961;4:561–571.

27. Kottke FJ. The effects of limitation of activity upon the human body. *JAMA.* 1966;196:117–122.

28. Hasenbring M, Marienfeld G, Kuhlendahl D, et al. Risk factors of chronicity in lumbar disc patients: a prospective investigation of biologic, psychological, and social predictors of therapy outcome. *Spine.* 1994;19:2759–2765.

29. Mayer TG, Gatchel RJ. Quatitative Lumbar Assessment to Address the Deconditioning Syndrome. In: *Functional Restoration for Spinal Disorders: The Sports Medicine Approach.* Philadelphia, PA: Lea and Febiger; 1988:8–9.

30. Sawchuk T, Mayer E. Deconditioning. In: Slipman C, Derby R, Simeone F, Mayer T, eds. *Interventional Spine.* London, England: Elsevier Global Publications; 2007: 113.

31. Wittink H, Hoskins Michel T, Wagner A, Sukiennik A, Rogers W. Deconditioning in patients with chronic low back pain: fact or fiction? *Spine.* 2000;17:2221–2228.

32. Verbunt JA, Seelen HA, Vlaeyen JW, van der Heijden GJ, Knottnerus JA. Fear of injury and physical deconditioning in patients with chronic low back pain. *Arch Phys Med Rehabil.* 2003;84:1227–1232.

33. Protas E, Mayer T, Dersh J, Keeley J, Gatchel R, McGeary D. Relevance of aerobic capacity measurements in the treatment of chronic work-related spinal disorders. *Spine.* 2004;29:2158–2166.

34. Mayer T, Barnes D, Kishino N, et al. Progressive isoinertial lifting evaluation, part I: a standardized protocol and normative database [published correction appears in *Spine. 1990; 15:5*]. *Spine.* 1988;13:993–997.

35. Mayer T, Barnes D, Nichols G, et al. Progressive isoinertial lifting evaluation, part II: a comparison with isokinetic lifting in a disabled chronic low back pain industrial population [published correction appears in *Spine. 1990; 15:5*]. *Spine.* 1988;13:998–1002.

36. Proctor T, Mayer T, Theodore B, Gatchel R. Failure to complete a functional restoration program for chronic musculoskeletal disorders: a prospective 1-year outcome study. *Arch Phys Med Rehabil.* 2005;86:1509–1515.

37. Proctor T, Mayer T, Gatchel R, McGeary D. Unremitting health-care-utilization outcomes of tertiary rehabilitation of chronic musculoskeletal disorders. *J Bone Joint Surg Am.* 2004;86-A:62–69.

38. Garcy P, Mayer T, Gatchel R. Recurrent or new injury outcomes after return to work in chronic disabling spinal disorders: tertiary prevention efficacy of functional restoration treatment. *Spine.* 1996;21:952–959.

16

Data Analysis and the Functional Capacity Evaluation Report

Jill Galper, PT, MEd, and Jerry N. Fogel, MS, PT, CHQCM

Data analysis is a dynamic process that is performed by the functional capacity evaluation (FCE) evaluator during and after the FCE. Data are obtained from multiple sources that include the diagnosis, medical history, available medical records, results of psychometric questionnaires, reported symptoms, musculoskeletal evaluation findings, observation of the evaluee throughout the FCE, and the evaluee's performance during functional testing. A number of FCE models are commercially available (see Appendix), as are FCE protocols developed by individual clinicians. Test procedures and the methods used to analyze and score test performances vary widely amongst FCEs.

The variety of FCE protocols and reports can be a challenge for the end user of this information, who frequently is not aware of the protocol's procedures or scoring methods (this information is usually considered proprietary) and does not understand the technical data contained within the FCE report. If a report does not clearly delineate an evaluee's abilities, or there are apparent inconsistencies within the report, it can be difficult or impossible for the requestor to use the information.

As discussed in previous chapters, most FCE protocols include the same general categories of test components (eg, dynamic material handling and movement and positional tolerance tests), but there are no universally agreed-on standardized methods for collecting, analyzing, and reporting the data. In Australia, Innes and Straker[1] grouped FCEs into three types (job-specific, general, and work assessment performed at the workplace) and found differences in standardization among them. In addition, the FCE evaluator's skill, judgment, and bias have been found to impact data analysis.[1-3] The existing guidelines for FCEs (eg, from the American Physical Therapy Association[4]) list *what* should be included in an FCE but do not specify *how* the test should be performed, analyzed, or reported.

One would expect consistency in testing methods, data analysis, and report format within a specific model, but there may be some variation that depends on the version of the model used. For example, if an evaluator attended FCE training but did not attend subsequent training or obtain protocol updates, the FCE protocol may be outdated and not include modifications or changes in the method. However, the outdated protocol may continue to be used because there are no requirements that the evaluator obtain the relevant training or updates. Factors inherent to evaluees may also influence FCE results. This possibility was illustrated by a study performed by Reneman et al[5] who found differences among results of FCEs performed in three countries using the same model (IWS/WorkWell FCE). This finding suggests that evaluators were not observing performance and/or analyzing data in the same manner or that there were differences inherent to the evaluees that affected the results.

Further investigation is needed to identify the reasons for the different findings between countries.

In this chapter, we discuss the general principles an FCE evaluator should use in determining an evaluee's functional ability. As stated, each FCE protocol has its own method of data analysis. The owners of most commercially available FCE models will not share their specific method or evidence base because the information is considered proprietary. Comparing how different FCE models analyze performance data is, therefore, difficult. That said, there are general principles that FCE evaluators should use when analyzing and reporting functional test data. General principles of data analysis are discussed first, followed by discussion of the FCE report.

The Significance of Clinical Correlation

An FCE is requested to provide answers to the requestor's questions about a person's physical abilities in the context of a medical condition. (Chapter 2 discussed this in detail.) In the absence of a clinical or medical condition, such as when performing agility testing for prehire determinations, functional testing does not need to be performed by a health care provider. *The FCE evaluator must always consider the evaluee's abilities (and limitations) relative to a medical condition(s). Therefore, it logically follows that the FCE is a type of clinical evaluation, because the evaluator determines functional ability in the context of an injury or illness.*

Unfortunately, based on a number of reports that we have reviewed, it is evident that clinical correlation with function does not always occur. In fact, some evaluators seem to have the following beliefs:

- An FCE is a totally "objective" test process that, if performed correctly, will allow determinations to be made by "plugging" results into the relevant formulas.
- Functional testing protocols and scoring procedures allow an evaluee's physical abilities to be determined independent of clinical judgment. Clinical judgment is viewed negatively because it is considered subjective, as opposed to functional test performance, which is considered to be objective (ie, the evaluee does or does not do the activity or does so at an easily quantifiable level).
- The FCE evaluator's role is more technical than clinical. The evaluator's primary functions are to observe the performance, record the results, and move on to the next test procedure.

CHAPTER 16

These beliefs suggest that the evaluator is superfluous to the functional testing process, when, in fact, the opposite is true. Functional evaluation was not intended to supersede clinical evaluation and judgment; rather, functional evaluation *requires* it.

Given this clinically based functional assessment perspective, the FCE evaluator's responsibility is to identify whether there are activities the evaluee *cannot do* or *should not do* because of the underlying health condition. The FCE evaluator should determine whether there are activities that might worsen the health condition, substantively delay or interfere with recovery from the health condition, or place the evaluee or others at risk by performing an activity. In other words, for an activity to be limited or restricted, it is critical for the evaluator to demonstrate that the underlying clinical condition is correlated, ie, has an effect on, functional performance or that performance of a given function has an effect on the underlying clinical condition. Consequently, when the evaluator is asked to establish whether there are functional implications to the evaluee's clinical condition, the evaluator needs to identify what that evaluee cannot do or should not do vs what he or she *will not do*. These determinations can only be made by professionals who are knowledgeable in anatomy, pathology, physiology, kinesiology, and other relevant topics; have skill in clinical and functional evaluation methods; and are able to triangulate multiple data sets in the context of the evaluee's injury or illness. (Chapter 17 discusses selecting an FCE evaluator.)

Use of Cross-testing and Retesting in Evaluator Determinations

Cross-testing and retesting assist the evaluator in identifying patterns and trends during the FCE. *Retesting* refers to repeating the *same* test within an FCE to determine whether there is a change in performance. *Cross-testing* refers to the use of a *different* test or method to assess the *same* element of performance. Retesting allows the evaluator to determine the following:
- Whether the evaluee's performance was consistent
- Whether there is a pattern of inconsistent performance that has clinical rationale
- Whether there are commonalities of functional limitations related to an underlying dysfunction or health condition
- The impact of the performance on the evaluee (tolerance)

Cross-testing will allow the same determinations as retesting, with the additional advantage that the evaluee does not know (at least theoretically) that he or she is performing the "same test," thereby controlling for the variables of perception and motivation. For example, an evaluee's sitting tolerance may first be tested indirectly while the evaluee completes a variety of paperwork. The evaluee is usually unaware that sitting tolerance is being evaluated. Later in the protocol, sitting is reassessed with the evaluee's knowledge that this tolerance is being evaluated. Cross-testing may even be retested when the evaluee performs other test activities, such as finger dexterity or hand strength tests. There are two important cautions associated with cross-testing. First, the activities used must be comparable in terms of the clinical performance variable(s). If additional variables are unknowingly introduced into the analysis, erroneous conclusions may be drawn. Second, evaluator bias can impact results, so it is important that the evaluator is aware of any existing biases. For example, if the examiner believes that the evaluee is trying to "fool" him or her, the evaluee's future communication, observations, interpretations, and conclusions may all be significantly biased by that belief and affect the accuracy of the test. This effect of bias is discussed in Chapter 3 in more detail.

Finally, it should be noted that cross-testing and retesting are different constructs and are not interchangeable. Each serves a different function in the overall scheme of the test battery. For example, retesting is more helpful in assessing the effect of motor learning or anxiety on performance of an evaluee, whereas cross-testing better identifies performance inconsistencies. Cross-testing and retesting are used in FCEs because both are typically necessary to obtain a complete clinical and functional picture.

Framework for Analyzing Evaluee Effort

How can an evaluator decide if the performance he or she observes is the evaluee's maximum? If performance is not consistent during testing, what do the trends and patterns suggest? To answer these questions, evaluators can use the following four criteria: (1) performance consistency, (2) commonalities of functional limitations, (3) patterns of inconsistency, and (4) clinical substantiation. These criteria should be integrated and not used in isolation, allowing the evaluator to perform an objective, in-depth analysis on multiple data that will strengthen his or her ultimate conclusions about evaluee performance. To accomplish this synthesis, a conceptual framework for analyzing these criteria is presented herein.

Consistency of Effort

Every FCE evaluator determines an evaluee's performance consistency, although the specific methods for doing so may vary between protocols. The most common methods for determining consistency are analysis of repeated test trials and observation of evaluees' movement patterns during the test. In regard to repeating test trials, the concept is that if an individual produces and later reproduces the same performance *values* on a given test or functional task, the performance is acceptable. Some evaluators draw two conclusions from this finding: First, consistent performance means the person "was really trying" and that the performance was the evaluee's maximum effort. The second conclusion frequently drawn is that any limitation identified during the functional test battery is directly related to a somatic dysfunction or deficit. Although these assumptions may sometimes be correct, sometimes they are not. Performance can be consistent at low effort levels, so additional factors have to be considered by the evaluator. In addition, a number of factors can impact performance consistency, such as motor learning, fatigue, anxiety, communication and perception, and provocation. There is also a significant distinction between conscious manipulation of the test results and behavioral dysfunction (eg, fear-avoidant beliefs). It is therefore inappropriate to "lump" them into the same category. Later in this chapter, these issues are critically analyzed, and a comprehensive framework for interpreting performance data is proposed.

The next step in analyzing performance is to identify performance patterns by evaluating consistency in conjunction with other test results, ie, the criteria of pattern analysis and clinical substantiation. Determining whether there are similar findings (*commonality of findings*) during different activities may allow additional trends to be identified. For example, it may be noted that similar limitations were observed for all tasks that required lumbar flexion beyond 20° or during any activity requiring hip extensor strength. Identification of these patterns has significant relevance in establishing a more well-defined relationship between the specific somatic dysfunction (physical impairment) and the resultant functional limitation. When commonalties of functional limitations (patterns and trends) are identified, they will have a significant impact on the nature of treatment intervention and problem resolution. If there are consistent limitations in performance values but the clinical evaluation does not reveal specific somatic dysfunction, one possible interpretation is that the limitations are the result of the evaluee's overall physical status (eg, weakness) and not the result of any specific lesion or musculoskeletal dysfunction. This possibility is relevant if causation is an issue or apportionment required.

Inconsistent performance may also be pattern-specific. There are three typical patterns: (1) linear improvement, (2) linear decline, and (3) erratic. Linear improvement occurs when a performance value improves with continued testing. If the improvement is noted during the testing process (eg, during a period of 3 hours or day 2 of a 2-day FCE), the inconsistency may be the result of a learning curve, decreased anxiety or fear, or other similar variables. If improved performance is measured for a period (eg, > 1 week), the change may be the result of training (if the evaluee is receiving an intervention) or improvement or resolution of the impairment. A decrement in performance can be gradual or abrupt. Gradual decay may be attributed to fatigue. An abrupt decrease in performance may be associated with acute provocation or irritation of the involved tissues or even reinjury. Erratic ups and downs in the performance values or inconsistent performances between cross-testing tasks are typically associated with conscious manipulation of the test results.

The final and, possibly, most significant criterion is *clinical substantiation*. Simply stated, when a performance limitation is observed (typically a cessation of an activity), clinical substantiation occurs when the evaluator can identify clinical findings or signs accounting for the performance deficit.

There are three scenarios for task limitation:
1. The evaluee self-terminates the task, without substantiation by the evaluator.
2. The evaluee self-terminates (or self-terminates concurrently with the evaluator's recommendation) the activity, with substantiation.
3. The evaluator substantiates a performance deficit and terminates the task (typically to avoid provocation or reinjury).

For example, an evaluee is performing unloaded overhead work for a given duration. When the evaluee terminates the task, the evaluator must determine whether there is a "reason" for the "limitation." In this case, the evaluator observed a unilateral, asynchronous, involuntary tone change in the lower cervical paraspinal and/or the scapulothoracic musculature before the evaluee terminated the test activity. The evaluator can correlate the apparent musculoskeletal dysfunction as the cause of or response to the activity termination. Either way, this clinical pattern would strongly suggest that a somatic component (impairment) was contributing to the resultant functional limitation. In addition, the evaluator would probably also observe a change in the evaluee's performance before task termination, such as a change in the rate of activity or a change in the evaluee's body mechanics. For this reason, evaluators should be knowledgeable and trained in evaluation of musculoskeletal dysfunction. Many of the changes and signs observed during functional testing can be subtle and complex, requiring a trained observer to identify and interpret them. In addition, it is also important that the evaluator be able to rule out insignificant and/or unrelated changes and signs so as not to "overread" the test and report false findings.

discussion of substantiation as a criterion, here is a case
there are no observed clinical signs or proportionate change in
......n. In this example, the evaluee, who was performing a test activity
at a given level of function (eg, load, rate, and exertion of movement), abruptly
terminated the activity with a report that the activity was too painful. It would be
reasonable to expect the evaluator to observe some change in the evaluee's body
and performance vs no indication of any signs of difficulty. If acute provocation
resulted from the activity, one would expect a commensurate change in external
physiology, especially if the provocation was severe enough to terminate the
activity. Therefore palpation, inspection, and a thorough knowledge of the clinical aspects of biomechanics and neuromuscular physiology are prerequisites for
an FCE evaluator.

Issues in Determining Evaluee Ability

The aforementioned principles should be applied to any determination made
during functional testing. In this section, we discuss some common issues that
evaluators face when analyzing test data. In most FCEs, there is determination
of the following:

- Manual material handling abilities
- Positional tolerance for a variety of activities, eg, sitting,
  standing, and overhead work
- Movement abilities, eg, walking, kneeling, reaching, and
  fingering
- Aerobic fitness level
- Evaluee performance effort and consistency

In a job-specific test, evaluee performance is compared with the specific job
requirement. This discussion is focused on the considerations made during a
general FCE. Chapter 14 discusses job-specific testing.

Manual Material Handling Ability

Manual material handling refers to the lifting, carrying, pushing, and pulling
tests performed during the FCE. For each activity, the evaluee's ability to perform occasionally, frequently, and constantly is reported. In some FCE protocols frequent and constant abilities are extrapolated from occasional abilities,
other protocols, these abilities are determined within the specific test

protocol. (See Chapter 6 for further discussion of evaluation of lifting ability.) In a job-specific FCE, the evaluee is asked to simulate the job-specific task(s) to the level required by the job.

Users of material handling test data should be aware that lifting results have not been shown to be interchangeable among different lifting protocols. Three studies comparing the lifting tests of two FCE protocols found that the results were not comparable.[6-8] Ijmker et al[6] found significant differences between the upper body lifting results of two FCE models, and Soer et al[7] concluded that the lumbar PILE and WorkWell System's floor-to-waist lifting test could not be used interchangeably. Rustenburg et al[8] investigated the maximum lifting capacity of healthy firefighters using the ERGOS Work Simulator and the Ergo-Kit lifting protocols and concluded that the concurrent validity for lifting between FCE methods was poor. The Ergo-Kit lifting protocol results were higher than the ERGOS Work Simulator test results for lower and upper lifting tests. Therefore, if an evaluee undergoes two FCEs during treatment that use different methods of assessing lifting ability, any change in the reported performance cannot necessarily be attributed to a change in the evaluee's health condition. Therefore, consistent testing protocols are recommended when an evaluee's abilities are being assessed.

Considerations in Identifying a Physical Demand Level

Based on an evaluee's demonstrated strength to perform material handling tasks, most FCE evaluators identify an overall physical demand level for the evaluee based on the US Department of Labor's *Dictionary of Occupational Titles* (DOT; eg, sedentary, light, and medium).[9]

TABLE 16–1   Physical Demand Characteristics of Work

Physical Demand Level	Occasional (0%–33% of Workday), lb	Frequent (34%–66% of Workday), lb	Constant (67%–100% of Workday), lb	Typical Energy Required (MET)
Sedentary	1–10	Negligible	Negligible	1.5–2.1
Light	11–20	1–10	Negligible	2.2–3.5
Medium	21–50	11–20	1–10	3.6–6.3
Heavy	51–100	21–50	11–20	6.4–7.5
Very Heavy	> 100	> 50	> 20	> 7.5

Abbreviation: MET indicates metabolic equivalents.

CHAPTER 16

Each demand level represents a range of ability. For example, within the medium level, occasional ability is defined as 21 to 50 lb. The evaluee is assigned a strength category based on his or her demonstrated ability. Many evaluators use their discretion in assigning a demand level, particularly when evaluee performance is slightly over the cutoff level (eg, occasional lift at 25 lb). There is no standardized criterion based on published research to guide the evaluator, who uses his or her clinical judgment in determining the appropriate level. The decision to downgrade an evaluee to a lower demand level (or vice versa) is usually based on the clinical examination results and the evaluee's symptom reports or manifestations during testing, effort during testing, and aerobic fitness level. The rationale for the evaluator's decision should be clearly stated in the report.

Another challenge for the evaluator in identifying a physical demand level is deciding which lift to use to reflect overall strength when there are significant differences between lifting ability at different heights. Some evaluators use the floor-to-waist (or knuckle) lift to make this determination, but, at present, there is no research or standardized method to guide evaluators. The muscles used, their relative strength, and the biomechanical stresses on the tissues and structures involved are all significantly different and change with the vertical height of the lift. A simple example is the difference between the relatively powerful lower quarter musculature and lumbar flexion used in a floor-to-waist lift vs the relatively weaker upper quarter muscles and lumbar extension used when lifting overhead. Assignment of one physical demand level may not adequately represent an evaluee's ability. Some evaluators will identify two demand levels based on lifting height (eg, floor to waist height and waist height and above), but, again, no standard exists for the determination or the reporting of the information. The evaluator's clinical reasoning for these determinations should be explained in the FCE report.

Impact of Aerobic Capacity

The FCE evaluator should take the evaluee's aerobic capacity into account when determining lifting ability and identifying a physical demand level. Each demand level has an associated energy requirement in metabolic equivalents (MET), as shown in Table 16–1. These MET requirements can be used as a guide in determining an evaluee's abilities. An evaluee who is deconditioned from a cardiovascular standpoint may not have the ability to sustain lifting at higher frequencies. Aerobic testing is recommended to determine an evaluee's aerobic capacity, but, currently, this testing is not standard practice among all FCE evaluators. Many evaluators rely on an evaluee's heart rate response during the FCE to reflect aerobic response, but, again, there is no demonstrated reliable or valid method for determining aerobic capacity from these data.

Impact of Movement Ability

When an evaluee is limited in performing a particular activity, eg, walking constantly, the evaluator should also discuss this limitation in terms of the evaluee's ability to perform other tasks that involve that activity (eg, carrying and dynamic pushing and pulling activities). Some FCE reports extrapolate an evaluee's carrying, pushing, and pulling abilities to a constant level, even though the evaluator has limited walking to a frequent basis.

To summarize, an evaluee's ability to perform manual material handling activities should be based on more than how much the person lifted during the lifting evaluation. All of the factors discussed (aerobic ability, joint motion, movement abilities, and effort level) must be considered.

Positional Tolerance and Movement Abilities

In most FCE protocols, an evaluee's ability to perform a particular activity (eg, reach, stoop, squat, walk, sit, or stand) is assessed for a relatively brief period. The method used for testing depends on the specific testing protocol used. The evaluator extrapolates the demonstrated performance to a specific frequency. The method of extrapolation depends on the specific FCE protocol. For example, the sitting ability of an evaluee who can sit comfortably for 45 minutes may be identified as "constant," based on the FCE model's criterion. Evaluee report of symptoms, quality of motion, and heart rate response are also taken into consideration in determining movement ability. (Chapter 9 provides further discussion.)

Assessment of positional tolerance is usually determined by observing the evaluee while in the target posture. Retesting and cross-testing are used to obtain more information, as previously discussed. Observation of the evaluee in the target posture and the evaluee's symptom reports are used to help guide determination of ability. The FCE models have different criteria for determining activity frequency and positional tolerances, so that what is considered "frequent" ability in one model may be "constant" or "occasional" in another. For example, an evaluee who sits comfortably for 45 minutes may be classified as having constant ability by one model, frequent in another, and occasional in a third model. There are some commercial FCEs that do not assign constant ability for some movement and positional tolerance tests in a general FCE. The rationale for this is that constant ability, other than sitting, is rarely required by most occupations and is difficult to determine given the time constraints in FCE. Some FCE providers routinely test positional tolerance to a predetermined level. One of us (J.G.) spoke with an FCE evaluator who said that she only tests positional tolerance within occasional ability owing to the time constraints in testing. In her testing model, the frequency cut points were 5 minutes for occasional ability, 40 minutes for frequent ability, and 1 hour for constant ability. Given these criteria, testing an evaluee to constant ability would take hours or even days, if cross-testing and retesting are included in the protocol. Someone requesting an FCE from this evaluator must specifically request that abilities and tolerances be tested to a higher level to obtain this information.

Another challenge in assigning activity frequency using the DOT framework (occasional, frequent, and constant) is the nonspecific nature of the criteria. For example (Table 16–1), if an evaluee was categorized as being able to perform certain activities occasionally defined as up to 33% of the workday, does that mean he can perform the activity for 2.5 hours nonstop at the beginning of the work day; 2.5 hours nonstop at the end of the work day; three 1-hour bouts at the beginning, middle, and end of the day; or bouts of 15 minutes on and 15 minutes off throughout the entire day? Clearly, each pattern would create a completely different set of biomechanical and cardiovascular demands on the person, yet all would be categorized the same in the nonspecific DOT framework. Therefore, it is suggested that when use of these categories is required, the evaluator include additional details to further define the evaluee's ability (eg, can sit for 30 minutes at a time and then needs a 10-minute break by walking or standing).

There is much diversity in the methods used to assess and analyze an evaluee's movement abilities and positional tolerances. Performance standards for movement testing and positional tolerance are needed, and this area requires further research and development.

Aerobic Capacity

Aerobic assessment methods were covered in detail in Chapter 10. In that chapter, Wittink and Takken stated that an evaluee's aerobic capacity should be evaluated in a general FCE. At present, many FCE models do not require the evaluator to specifically assess aerobic capacity. Many FCE evaluators monitor heart rate response during the test and make judgments about aerobic capacity based on the observed heart rate response during and following activity. As discussed in Chapter 10, the method of aerobic assessment is an important consideration, with some methods (ie, treadmill vs step test vs bicycle) better tolerated by particular evaluees than other methods. For example, a treadmill walking protocol has been found to be better tolerated by people with chronic low back pain than bicycle or step tests.[10] The use of aerobic testing in FCEs should be further developed to improve consistency between FCE evaluators and protocols when discussing an evaluee's physical abilities.

Software Computation and Evaluator Judgment

Many commercial FCE models have software that assists the evaluator by tabulating the data and performing computations (eg, coefficient of variations, percentage of maximum heart rate, MET levels, and percentage of consistent test results). Commercial FCE models generally have guidelines for data interpretation for determining the acceptable level of effort and activity frequency. For example, the evaluee's consistency of performance is often determined by calculating the percentage of tests within acceptable parameters. If the percentage meets the FCE model's cutoff score, consistency is considered acceptable or unacceptable. The specific percentage is dependent on the FCE model. Caution is needed when effort determination relies on the percentage of tests found "acceptable" based on coefficients of variance because evaluees can consistently perform at low effort levels.[11]

Although software programs may "calculate" an evaluee's sincerity of effort and ability to perform various movements and sustain positions, the FCE evaluator can (and should) modify the software's determination based on consideration of other data and clinical findings that the software might not take into account (see previous discussion about retesting, cross-testing, and clinical substantiation). For example, if an evaluee has poor aerobic fitness demonstrated by submaximal treadmill testing results or by elevated heart rate response to activity, slow heart rate recovery after activity, and a significantly increased resting heart rate at the end of the FCE, the evaluator should consider these findings during data analysis and recommend activity frequencies and lifting levels that are consistent with the evaluee's aerobic capacity, if the software does not take this into account. The FCE report should include the evaluator's rationale. The FCE evaluator has the ultimate responsibility for the FCE findings, and software computation should not be substituted for clinical judgment.

The Impact of Patterns of Performance on Functional Capacity Evaluation Interpretation

When the various criteria discussed thus far are applied across a broad spectrum of performance tests, objectivity and relevance of the FCE are enhanced. There are several reasons for this benefit. First, and probably most significant, is the resultant decrease in dependency on the subjective responses of the person being tested. Also significant is the decrease in examiner subjectivity, because there are well-defined criteria and an accompanying rationale for interpretation. Finally, there are principles in place to allow for the assimilation of large quantities of data into a well-organized, criteria-based analysis system for interpretation and recommendations.

Earlier in this chapter, we discussed the importance of evaluator observation and clinical correlation during all test components. This observation and clinical correlation are particularly important because there is controversy about the methods commonly used to make effort determinations. When consistency of performance (values and patterns) is combined with clinical substantiation, four general categories of performance outcomes can be identified:
  1. Consistent-Substantiated
  2. Inconsistent-Unsubstantiated
  3. Consistent-Unsubstantiated
  4. Inconsistent-Substantiated

Of course, the determinations for evaluees may fall somewhere between these categories or there may be different combinations associated with each individual functional task. The principles and patterns used to place evaluees into these categories still apply. A discussion of each category and the clinical implications will demonstrate the significance of this type of framework in analyzing overall functional assessment results.

Consistent-Substantiated

This category describes an evaluee who, during an FCE, consistently performed most or all of the functional tasks on retesting and cross-testing. In addition, the evaluator identified a clinical phenomenon that explained an identified limitation or supported its existence. This pattern strongly suggests that the performance levels demonstrated were as a result of the evaluee's current somatic status. In other words, any limitations noted were connected to a specific musculoskeletal dysfunction or deficit. Furthermore, the tasks that were problematic could be analyzed for patterns, such as common denominators, providing further clarification and insight as to the nature and extent of the dysfunction. In general, these results can be used to define the evaluee's safe parameters of function with some degree of confidence that this definition will not impact negatively on the evaluee's clinical condition, recovery, or safety. In other words, staying below or within the physical and functional demands should be safe and appropriate. This determination will give an evaluee confidence to remain optimally functional during his or her rehabilitation or after treatment has ended.

Inconsistent-Unsubstantiated

This category describes an evaluee whose performance was essentially inconsistent and clinically unsubstantiated. In other words, the values were erratic, and the evaluator found little or no reason for difficulty with or termination of the test activities. In addition, there was no apparent pattern to the demonstrated limitations. This scenario is characteristic of a person who is consciously manipulating the test results. If the test is well constructed, it is very unlikely that the evaluee would be able to "second guess" the process, certainly not with any consistency or logical pattern. In addition, it is believed that when human movement and performance are generated by conscious control, as opposed to integrated automatic behavior, it is less efficient and reproducible. There are two cautions, however, about the interpretation of this type of performance: First, it cannot be stated categorically that the evaluee has no true impairment or resultant disability, only that the evaluee's performance did not reveal any such findings. The second caution relates to the assumption of motivation of such a performance. Other factors besides conscious intent could produce this pattern, but most FCE evaluators cannot make this determination.

Historically, some evaluators have been hesitant to interpret these findings as such. They have chosen to report that the FCE findings represent the evaluee's minimal abilities, whereas other evaluators report the FCE as "invalid." The term *invalid* is confusing because the FCE itself is not invalid; it is the evaluee's performance that did not meet the FCE's criteria for acceptable performance effort and consistency. When an evaluee demonstrated gross inconsistencies and poor effort, some evaluators will write that the evaluee's physical abilities must be left to conjecture. Some question whether an evaluator can estimate an evaluee's abilities at a higher level than what was demonstrated when gross inconsistencies have been documented and there is no basis for limitation based on the clinical examination. Many evaluators shy away from such estimations of ability, deferring to a physician or the administrative or legal process. Although some would argue that the construct of the FCE should be seen as an extension of the clinical evaluative process and that the "normal until confirmed ill" standard be used, evaluators often do not have access to medical records or other clinical information besides what was obtained through their physical examination. It is consequently difficult for many to feel confident in stating that the absence of pathology on physical examination combined with inconsistent-unsubstantiated FCE performance implies that there are no limitations whatsoever. In situations such as this, it is often necessary for a physician to review the FCE results in conjunction with other clinical information to arrive at a final determination. The evaluator can, however, be of assistance in identifying what the expected level of functional performance might typically be for similar evaluees based on the evaluee's clinical diagnosis, examination findings, and body habitus.

Consistent-Unsubstantiated

This classification is one of the most common patterns observed. This category describes results that are characterized by fairly consistent performance levels, with low effort demonstrated during many test items and the evaluee's performance limited by reports of symptoms. The evaluator generally cannot identify any clinical reasons for the various expressed limitations. This category may describe people with fear-avoidance beliefs or "functional overlay." Consistent performance may occur because the evaluee truly believes that he or she has a problem, so the behavior, expressed as functional performance, will be an "automatic," if not integrated, expression of that belief. The consistency may be less than if caused by a somatic variable, but certainly more than if generated by conscious control. However, the limitations will be relatively unsubstantiated because there is no identifiable somatic origin. This is not to suggest that there is no somatic component, just that the limiting factor seems to be behavioral. In fact, many evaluees described by this category have some, even if minor, somatic dysfunction. As with the previous category, the FCE evaluator is not equipped to explain *why* an evaluee exhibits the observed behavior, only what behavior was demonstrated during testing. Insight into the behavioral factors affecting performance could have a beneficial effect on potential treatment options and overall management (see Chapters 3, 5, 15, and 18). At the very least, in most cases, the FCE results will represent the evaluee's minimal abilities. Minimal abilities may be regarded as being within an evaluee's tolerance level and well within the evaluee's physical capacity, because physical effort based on observed physiologic and biomechanical parameters was not observed. The evaluator can, therefore, have confidence that the evaluee can perform this level of activity on a safe and dependable basis. It is, however, important to discuss in the FCE report that these limitations are not substantiated by somatic clinical dysfunction, and, therefore any treatment, vocational, administrative, and legal determinations should be considered accordingly.

Inconsistent-Substantiated

This category may occur least often. This group describes people whose performance limitations are substantiated by clinical signs, yet their performance levels are inconsistent. If examined more closely, the inconsistency pattern is almost always a linear decline (as discussed earlier), suggesting fatigue, provocation, or reinjury. This category may describe people with unstable or unresolved lesions that may require further intervention.

A careful examination of the FCE findings and patterns, as has been outlined in this section, in conjunction with other clinical assessments, should clarify the problem and allow for the appropriate intervention. Again, just as with the consistent and substantiated pattern, staying below or within the functional parameters identified as problematic should provide a safe set of functional guidelines for the evaluee. Figure 16–1 summarizes the four performance categories and their significance.

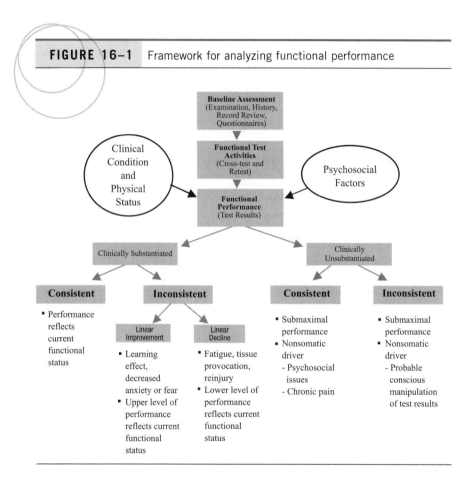

FIGURE 16–1   Framework for analyzing functional performance

The aforementioned categories illustrate the variations in evaluee performance and clinical findings. In some cases, evaluees may demonstrate effort on some test components but perform inconsistently or submaximally on others, so their effort level and consistency are varied within the FCE. For example, an evaluee may perform consistently and demonstrate physical effort on movement and grip tests but perform at a low level during lifting tests. In this case, the evaluator may find that some of the tests represent the evaluee's physical abilities, whereas others represent minimal abilities. If the evaluator analyzes performance as discussed in earlier sections of this chapter, commonalities of limitations may be identified that provide clinical rationale for the observed performance. Clinical correlation and careful observation during the test will help make this differentiation. At present, clinical substantiation and analysis of multiple test procedures within the FCE will best identify the evaluee's level of participation.

The Functional Capacity Evaluation Report

The FCE report is the product produced by the FCE evaluator. Functional capacity evaluation reports vary widely among providers in their content, style, and organization. The report should answer the referral questions, document the FCE findings, state how conclusions were reached (ie, include the evaluator's clinical reasoning), and provide references to support the testing and data analysis methods used. The report should be clearly written and easily understood by nonmedical persons; the use of abbreviations and jargon should be avoided. The report should be more than a listing of test scores; it should provide a picture of the evaluee's performance. If the FCE is a job-specific test, the report should discuss the evaluee's ability to perform the job tasks and indicate the source of the information about the job task requirements (job analysis vs evaluee's or employer's report). The report pages should be numbered. The report should be completed in a timely manner, generally within 7 days.

Results should be discussed in clear terms. For example, if an FCE report states that the FCE is invalid, as many reports state, how should this be interpreted? Is it the test that was invalid or the evaluee's performance? We suggest that terminology such as valid or invalid be avoided in the context of describing performance effort because the meaning can be misconstrued. The framework discussed earlier, in which performance consistency is analyzed in the context of clinical substantiation, may be more useful.

Table 16–2 lists the information that should be included in most FCE reports, although not necessarily in the order given.[2,12–15]

TABLE 16–2	Components of a Functional Capacity Evaluation Report

1. Reason for the referral (questions the requestor posed)

2. Outline of evaluee's demographic and background data
   a. Personal data: age, sex, height, weight
   b. Diagnosis
   c. Occupation
   d. Hand dominance
   e. Splints, braces, or assistive devices worn during the test

3. List and summary of medical records reviewed

4. Summary of information from the evaluee interview

5. Summary of results of activities of daily living or psychometric questionnaires; discussion of the significance of the results or any commonalities in reported limitations

6. Musculoskeletal examination findings (including computerized "iso" tests, if done)

7. Results of the functional tests performed
   a. List of results: performance values (how much, how fast, repetitions)
   b. Physiologic response during the test (heart rate and blood pressure)
   c. Report test end points

8. Discussion of evaluee effort and performance consistency
   a. Retest/cross-test findings (eg, consistency, evidence of fatigue, learning effect)
   b. Clinical substantiation of results
   c. Patterns of consistency
   d. Physiologic evidence of effort (eg, heart and respiratory rate, perspiration)
   e. Movement-based changes demonstrating effort (muscle recruitment, movement speed)
   f. Evaluee's overall effort level

9. Summary of functional abilities (most often in tabular format)

10. Summary of functional limitations and restrictions, including identification of commonalities noted

11. Comparison of evaluee performance with job tasks, if appropriate

12. Recommendations, if appropriate
    a. Accommodation(s) that will lessen limitations
    b. Transitional work recommendations
    c. Treatment

CHAPTER 16

TABLE 16–2 Components of a Functional Capacity Evaluation Report (continued)

---

13. Conclusion: summary of findings, including overall physical demand level, if appropriate (this may often appear in front of report with supportive data following)

14. Completed estimated physical abilities form, if requested

---

As noted, there is a wide variation between report quality and content. Many FCE evaluators do not have direct communication with the referral source and do not receive feedback on their reports. However, communication between the FCE evaluator and referral source may occur after the report is released, especially when the referral source needs clarification. A good working relationship between the FCE evaluator and referral source is important to ensure that the information needs of each are fulfilled.

Summary

Analyzing and interpreting the data obtained in an FCE requires the FCE evaluator to draw conclusions from multiple data points in the context of an evaluee's diagnosis, medical history and condition, and performance. How the evaluator draws his or her conclusions is affected by the type of FCE, the specific model used, and the evaluator's qualifications, skill, and bias. In this chapter, we have provided a clinical framework for data analysis that evaluates whether any patterns of performance and consistency of performance observed have clinical substantiation. This process requires a knowledgeable and skilled evaluator. Some FCE evaluators may not have the background knowledge and clinical expertise to perform a musculoskeletal evaluation, and there may be no clinical context in which results are analyzed.

There are some FCE evaluators who have this clinical background knowledge but believe that this type of data interpretation goes beyond what the FCE is intended to do, and they simply report evaluee performance. These evaluators may defer estimating an evaluee's physical abilities to other medical providers, most commonly physicians. The basis for this deferral is not clear—who better to estimate an evaluee's function than the highly trained and skilled FCE evaluator who has spent hours testing the evaluee? We are not discounting the value of physician analysis and review of the FCE report. The physician who reviews the FCE report does so in the context of the evaluee's medical examination and history and may have reason to modify the FCE evaluator's estimates. However, it is our belief that it is the FCE evaluator who must consider the clinical context to define and give meaning to the functional data. Furthermore, we believe that the FCE report must contain the evaluator's clinical reasoning and interpretation of data for the report to be meaningful and useful.

References

1. Innes E, Straker L. Workplace assessments and functional capacity evaluations: current practices of therapists in Australia. *Work.* 2002;18:51–66.
2. Strong S, Baptiste S, Cole D, et al. Functional assessment of injured workers: a profile of assessor practices. *Can J Occup Ther.* 2004;71:13–23.
3. James C, Mackenzie L, Higginbotham N. Health professionals' attitudes and practices in relation to functional capacity evaluations. *Work.* 2007;29:81–87.
4. American Physical Therapy Association, *Occupational Health Guidelines: Evaluating Functional Capacity.* Alexandria, VA: American Physical Therapy Association; 2001.
5. Reneman MF, Kool J, Oesch P, Geertzen JH, Battie MC, Gross DP. Material handling performance of patients with chronic low back pain during functional capacity evaluation: a comparison between three countries. *Disabil Rehabil.* 2006;28:1143–1149.
6. Ijmker S, Gerrits EH, Reneman MF. Upper lifting performance of healthy young adults in functional capacity evaluations: a comparison of two protocols. *J Occup Rehabil.* 2003;13:297–305.
7. Soer R, Poels BJ, Geertzen JH, Reneman MF. A comparison of two lifting assessment approaches in patients with chronic low back pain. *J Occup Rehabil.* 2006;16:639–646.
8. Rustenburg G, Kuijer PP, Frings-Dresen MH. The concurrent validity of the ERGOS Work Simulator and the Ergo-Kit with respect to maximum lifting capacity. *J Occup Rehabil.* 2004;14:107–118.
9. US Department of Labor, Employment and Training Administration. *Dictionary of Occupational Titles, Revised.* Vol 1 and 2. 4th ed. Washington, DC: US Department of Labor Employment and Training Administration; 1991.
10. Wittink H, Michel TH, Kulich R, et al. Aerobic fitness testing in patients with chronic low back pain: which test is best? *Spine.* 2000;25:1704–1710.
11. Robinson ME, Mac Millan M, O'Connor P, Fuller A, Cassisi JE. Reproducibility of maximal versus submaximal efforts in an isometric lumbar extension task. *J Spinal Disord.* 1991;4:444–448.

12. King PM, Tuckwell N, Barrett TE. A critical review of functional capacity evaluations. *Phys Ther.* 1998;78:852–866.

13. Innes E, Straker L. Strategies used when conducting work-related assessments. *Work.* 2002;19:149–165.

14. Clifton DW, Burnett RA. Functional capability evaluation. In: *Physical Rehabilitation's Role in Disability Management: Unique Perspective for Success.* St Louis, MO: Elsevier Saunders; 2005. Chapter 9:132–146.

15. Lechner D. The well-designed functional capacity evaluation: application in forensic vocational analysis. *J Forensic Vocational Anal.* 2004;7:83–96.

CHAPTER

17

Choosing a Functional Capacity Evaluation Evaluator

Jill Galper, PT, MEd, and Elizabeth Genovese, MD, MBA

The quality of an FCE is in large part dependent on the qualifications, skill, experience, and training of the FCE evaluator. As discussed in the previous chapters of this book, functional capacity evaluation (FCE) protocols differ in terms of their approach, instructions and equipment used, specific test items included, test order or administration, specific equipment and environment, and how results are scored, interpreted, and reported. In addition to these differences in FCE methods, there is diversity in the professional background, training, attributes, and personal biases of FCE evaluators. Because the FCE evaluator is central to the quality of an FCE, it is important to identify the attributes of a "good" evaluator. This chapter discusses the attributes of good FCE evaluators and provides practical recommendations for identifying them.

Evaluator Qualifications

Evaluators come from a variety of professional backgrounds, each with its specific educational requirements, emphasis, and training. In addition to physical and occupational therapists, other professionals who perform FCEs include exercise physiologists and people with educational background in exercise science, athletic trainers, chiropractors, vocational evaluators, nurses, physical therapist assistants, certified occupational therapy assistants, kinesiologists, psychologists, and physicians.[1] State practice acts regulate the practice of some of these providers (ie, physical and occupational therapists and assistants, athletic trainers, nurses, and physicians), and FCE evaluators from these disciplines must practice within the rules and regulations specified by the state in which they practice. In addition, insurance carriers, who pay for FCEs, may restrict who is reimbursed for performing them.[2]

Some professional associations also have guidelines about the qualifications of people providing evaluation services. For example, the American Physical Therapy Association's *Occupational Health Physical Therapy Guidelines: Evaluating Functional Capacity* (section 3.7) identifies a licensed physical therapist with the requisite education, training, and competencies as the appropriate provider of an FCE (as opposed to a physical therapist assistant).[3] Commercially available FCE models also can require specific qualifications in the people they accept for training. These models differ in evaluator qualifications and in the length (and content) of their training programs. The FCE model descriptions in the Appendix provide additional details.

A survey of FCE evaluators in southern Ontario (Canada) conducted by Strong et al[4] found that the data collection methods the evaluators used were diverse.

Although all evaluators reported using a consistent approach in their FCEs, some evaluators varied the specific tests included in a given FCE based on the FCE referral question(s) and the evaluee's symptoms and/or complaints. Other evaluators used a more rigid protocol. Some of the provider organizations relied solely on what was included in a specific commercially available FCE model (requiring less clinical understanding; directed by tools and/or technology), whereas other providers used a commercially available model in addition to other methods of data collection (flexible delivery of protocol; assessor plans an individualized assessment). The use of a more rigid vs flexible approach seemed to depend on the FCE evaluator's educational background. Kinesiologists did not stray from their FCE model's protocol, whereas physical therapists and occupational therapists did. Although one could intuit that a more flexible approach, directed by the referral sources' needs and by the nature of the evaluee's injury or illness, would result in a more meaningful report for the referral source, this assumption has not been formally investigated.

Single Evaluator vs Team Approach

An FCE can be performed by one evaluator or by two or more evaluators. There are differences between functional testing providers in the composition of the team and in how the team functions. One commonly used approach to team evaluation has one clinician perform the musculoskeletal evaluation while the other evaluator(s) oversees the performance-based testing. In their survey of FCE evaluators in southern Ontario, Strong et al[4] found that the majority of physical therapists performed the musculoskeletal screening examination after which occupational therapists and kinesiologists carried out the performance-based tests. The method and extent of communication between team members when analyzing FCE results would seem to depend on the provider's specific operating procedures; no standard exists as to how this communication is done. We are not aware of any published studies investigating whether FCE results and quality differ when tests are performed by one vs a team of evaluators. However, detailed communication between members of an FCE team is critical when analyzing performance data because this analysis requires integration of multiple sources of data (discussed in Chapter 16). In addition, team members must base their observations on the same operational definitions and scoring criteria to ensure intrarater consistency. Although it is therefore not impossible for an FCE to be performed using a team approach, facilities that do so should be prepared to explicitly describe the protocols used to integrate data, especially when accurate identification of submaximal effort is required (see Chapter 11).

Important Attributes of Functional Capacity Evaluation Evaluators

Innes and Straker[5] identified a core of strategies used by Australian therapists in performing all types of FCEs. Their results suggest that the therapist "should be an experienced professional with appropriate qualifications and training who engages in self-reflection and obtains impartial feedback through peer debriefing."[5(p161)]

Based on their survey of therapists in southern Ontario, Strong et al[6] wrote that FCEs are "tools that are only as good as the way they are used, and because of the complexity of human performance needing to be considered within a particular context, FAs [functional assessments] rely heavily on the assessor's training and experience. This points for the need for reflective clinicians who are aware of personal bias, limitations of the FA instrument and who have training in clinical reasoning."[p72] "The assessor has an important role in orienting the worker to the FA, creating a constructive atmosphere, developing rapport and addressing the safety and emotional security needs of the worker. The assessor has a responsibility to conduct a fair, objective assessment according to ethical, evidence-based practice."[6(pp68–69)]

In addition to good communication with the evaluee, the evaluator must be able to communicate well with the referral source and other professionals involved in the treatment and evaluation of the evaluee and write a readable and understandable report. The evaluator should be accessible if there are questions about the report.

The following outline summarizes the attributes of a good FCE evaluator:

1. Evaluator has knowledge of and expertise in clinical evaluation, functional testing, and the application of this testing to injury prevention, injury management, and medical-legal settings. Specifically, the evaluator has knowledge of:
   a. The impact of injury and illness on function
   b. Clinical assessment methods (educational background in the musculoskeletal system, movement, and pathologies)
   c. Processes used to measure function
   d. The demands of occupation within the workplace environments
   e. Occupational analysis and workplace demands
2. Evaluator has expertise in functional testing methods

3. Evaluator is a reflective clinician
   a. Is aware of his or her personal bias
   b. Knows the limitations of the FCE instrument
   c. Has training in clinical reasoning
4. Evaluator is able to develop and maintain a good working relationship with the referral source and the evaluee
   a. Is an effective verbal and written communicator
   b. Is responsive to questions

Evaluator Training

King et al[1] identified evaluator training as a means for ensuring quality and consistency in the performance, scoring, and reporting of FCEs. Training in how to perform FCEs is generally not included as part of an evaluator's academic curriculum in the chosen profession. Most programs do not include training in FCEs or include only a couple of lectures on the topic of industrial rehabilitation, which includes FCEs. Training in FCE is generally provided by the vendors of commercial FCE systems purchased by the evaluator. As shown in the Appendix, the length of evaluator training and requirements for ongoing evaluator training vary between commercial models. The FCE evaluator training programs are not standardized and there are no requirements for quality, although there are general guidelines about the quality of continuing education programs by professional organizations, like the American Physical Therapy Association and the American Occupational Therapy Association. Some commercial models require evaluator certification. The certification process and its requirements differ among vendors.

Some facilities provide in-house training of FCE evaluators by a staff member who completed training in a commercial FCE protocol or who has experience performing the facility's FCE protocol. The level of expertise of the trainer and his or her skill as an educator is not controlled and may vary widely.

No research exists about the optimal length, content, and type of training needed for FCE evaluators to develop and maintain expertise in FCE administration, data analysis, or reporting. This area needs further development. Matheson,[7] in discussing the future direction of functional evaluation, has described the development of a formal certification procedure as a goal. Consideration of this possibility appears warranted.

Issues Specific to the Functional Capacity Evaluation Provider and/or Model

The FCE is always ordered in a clinical context, and, as such, must provide information that is useful to the referral source. Hence, regardless of evaluator identity, qualifications, training, or attributes, the FCE provider must be able to produce a defensible report addressing the specific questions of the referral source within an acceptable period. Although differences in state regulations for physical and occupational therapy evaluators mandate when a prescription or referral is needed for the FCE, this requirement also depends on a facility's specific policies and procedures (liability concerns). Lead time for obtaining a prescription, if required, needs to be built into the time required to receive FCE results.

As discussed throughout this book, there are a number of methods used to assess an evaluee's functional ability, each with varying degrees of support by quality research. Models also differ in their ability to fully complete an estimated physical capacities form. Some models and providers test only to a specific frequency level in their FCE. For example, some models and/or providers will not provide any estimations of ability within a "constant" level, while others will not perform any testing to identify frequency estimates above an occasional level for some activities unless this testing is specifically requested (and sometimes it is not provided even when requested). There are also scenarios in which the FCE provider and/or model is simply not capable of addressing specific referral needs (eg, inability to evaluate activities specific to complex upper extremity function or evaluee effort).

The referral source should be aware of these protocol restrictions in advance. Providers who use models that do not allow projections above the occasional or frequent level for some activities and are unwilling or unable to provide this information based on clinical expertise will identify limitations on the physical capacities estimate form, regardless of what one would expect the activity levels or abilities to be given the evaluee's diagnosis, symptoms (including stated or observed activities of daily living), and/or objective findings. Before scheduling the FCE, the requestor should discuss with the evaluator whether it is possible to address specific questions regarding activity tolerance and the highest frequency level in which the evaluee should be tested. This approach should help identify providers unwilling or unable to obtain the necessary information. (Chapter 2 discusses issues in requesting an FCE.)

Overall Considerations

The following checklist, which incorporates and extrapolates from the preceding considerations, is useful to review when choosing an FCE provider:

1. General evaluator and facility information
   a. Obtain credentialing information: professional liability insurance, resume or curriculum vitae, relevant professional license
   b. Is a physician prescription or referral required?
   c. How much lead time is needed to schedule an FCE?
   d. How long after the FCE until the report is completed?
   e. What is the cost of the FCE?
2. Model-specific information
   a. What model does the FCE provider use?
   b. Is it one that is commercially available or one developed by the FCE evaluator?
   c. What research exists in support of the model?
   d. What physical abilities are (and are not) assessed?
   e. How does the FCE model and evaluator handle frequency projections?
   f. How long is the test process (time with evaluee and time to generate the report)? Can the evaluator perform a 2-day FCE if needed? If so, will the report integrate the findings of both test days?
   g. Is there follow-up with the evaluee after the test? (Follow-up is helpful in a half-day or 1-day FCE to determine the evaluee's response to testing.) If the evaluee reports increased symptoms, how is this information used by the evaluator?
   h. Does the evaluator consider evaluee effort and performance consistency? If so, how are determinations made and reported?
   i. If desired by the referral source, can the evaluator use the model to *fully* complete an estimated physical capabilities form?
3. FCE evaluator and facility information—quality assessment and control
   a. How does the facility ensure quality?
   b. Is the FCE performed by one person or by a team? If the latter, what procedures exist to be certain that information from the clinical evaluation and other observational data are accurately integrated into the final report (particularly important when determining evaluee effort)?
   c. Does the provider perform any quality assurance on the report before it is released? Is it reviewed for content in addition to grammar and spelling?
   d. Who performs the quality assurance?
   e. How does the provider respond to the referral source's questions after report is sent? If there are questions with the report once it's released, how does the provider handle this? What is the average response time?
   f. Will the provider send a sample FCE report?

CHAPTER 17

Summary

The quality of an FCE is highly dependent on the evaluator. In this chapter, we addressed considerations for choosing an FCE provider, including the professional attributes of a good FCE evaluator and other considerations for choosing an FCE facility to meet the requestor's needs. As discussed in Chapter 2, it is important that the requestor of the FCE specify the issues the FCE should address. The Appendix provides information about a number of commercially available FCE models that, when compared, may be helpful in choosing an FCE provider capable of meeting a referral source's specific needs.

References

1. King PM, Tuckwell N, Barrett TE. A critical review of functional capacity evaluations. *Phys Ther.* 1998;78:852–866.
2. Lechner DE. The well-designed functional capacity evaluation: application in forensic vocational analysis. *J Forensic Vocational Anal.* 2004;7:83–96.
3. American Physical Therapy Association. *Occupational Health Physical Therapy Guidelines: Evaluating Functional Capacity.* Alexandria, VA: American Physical Therapy Association; 2001.
4. Strong S, Baptiste S, Cole D, et al. Functional assessment of injured workers: a profile of assessor practices. *Can J Occup Ther.* 2004;71:13–23.
5. Innes E, Straker L. Strategies used when conducting work-related assessments. *Work.* 2002;19:149–165.
6. Strong SA, Baptiste S, Clarke J, et al. *Assessment of a person's ability to function at work.* WSIB research grant 98 0028. Funded by Research Advisory Council, Workplace Safety & Insurance Board. June 2002.
7. Matheson L. The functional capacity evaluation. In: Demeter S, Anderson G, eds. *Disability Evaluation.* 2nd ed. Chicago, IL: Mosby; 2003.

18

CHAPTER

Clinician and Insurer Application of Functional Test Results

Elizabeth Genovese, MD, MBA

This chapter discusses how to apply the results of functional tests to various clinical scenarios, with a focus on situations in which this application is not straightforward. Although appropriately requested, performed, and interpreted FCEs can provide useful information to supplement what is available from other sources, (such as the history, physical examination findings, and diagnostic test results) there are many circumstances when the interpretation or relevance is problematic. These may reflect problems with the test components selected by the examiner, problems with how the test was performed, problems with how the test was interpreted by the examiner, submaximal effort by the evaluee, or problems with how the test was requested, including the possibility that the test should not have been requested at all.

As stated in the introduction to this book, the results of studies assessing the ability of functional capacity evaluations (FCEs) to predict return to work (RTW) or reinjury have been mixed. Certain functional tests were demonstrated to be predictive of low back pain in a prospective cohort study of 430 workers, although different tests predicted outcome depending on whether there was a history of back pain.[1] Performance on the floor-to-waist lift or the total number of failed tasks was weakly associated with RTW in a historical cohort study of workers with low back pain.[2] However, successfully passing more than 8 of 11 (but not all 11) tests in an FCE was actually associated with an increased rate of long-term injury compared with passing fewer than 8 tests; people who passed all 11 tests were not reinjured.[3,4] Similar findings were noted in a subsequent study of workers with upper extremity disorders, with, once again, better FCE performance a weak predictor of RTW but, after controlling for confounders, unrelated to sustained recovery.[5] A study that attempted to match 11 FCE activities with work demands successfully matched 7 of these activities with demands but found no relation among FCE performance, work demands, and sick leave during follow-up.[6]

While yet another study found that greater lifting ability in a floor-to-waist lift was associated with an increased likelihood of RTW and ability to do two other dynamic lifts in addition to the floor-to-waist lift further associated with the level of RTW (full as opposed to modified duty), sex and time away from work were still the strongest predictors of RTW.[7] Similar results were obtained in another study that identified age, lifting ability, pain duration, depression level, and reported disability as individually related to RTW but found only the level of depression and patient age to predict posttreatment work status when variables were evaluated relative to one another.[8] A study of patients receiving rehabilitative services found improved functional capacity measures in a treatment group associated with twice the RTW as seen in a comparison group receiving no treatment; however, positive changes in psychological measures were also seen in the former group.[9] Given studies indicating that psychological factors can affect the results of functional testing,[10,11] the relationship between the two is likely to be one of the reasons why studies evaluating the relationship between functional test results and RTW have been unimpressive. This is not surprising given the substantial body of literature indicating that RTW is predominantly reflective of time off work and psychological and socioenvironmental factors,[12-22] including the attitude of health care providers.[23]

Although the relatively poor performance of functional testing in predicting RTW could be used as justification for eliminating the use of functional testing as a component of RTW planning, studies evaluating the ability of physicians to predict fitness for duty or RTW have also been inconclusive. One study found a lack of consensus on the medical fitness of an applicant, suggesting that the validity of such judgments might be questionable even when detailed fitness criteria were available.[24] A later study found that use of a standardized evaluation similar to a comprehensive history and physical examination with special attention to the neuromuscular examination, pain behaviors, and activities of daily living, when compared with a functional assessment consisting of maximal and sustained lifts, repetitive activities, and a grip dynamometry test, provided a reasonably accurate estimate of work-related functional ability.[25] Of particular interest is a study that in a comprehensive medical evaluation, found no variables to account for significant proportions of variance in RTW. The subjective interpretations and appraisals of injured workers more powerful predictors of the course of postinjury recovery than the exclusive use of medical assessments.[26] The impact of factors other than physical capacity on RTW and the development of musculoskeletal pain may also explain failure of a recent systematic review of the literature to demonstrate anything more than an inconclusive relationship between trunk muscle strength or mobility of the lumbar spine and the risk of low back pain, or physical capacity measures and the risk of neck and/or shoulder pain.[27] The literature about the relationship between the results of postoffer functional capacity assessments and the development of musculoskeletal disorders was discussed in Chapter 13. *Guides to Evaluation of Disease and Injury Causation* provides additional information.[28]

Literature about the use of functional capacity assessment to evaluate movement and positional tolerance, aerobic capacity, sincerity of effort, upper extremity function, and patients with chronic pain was addressed in Chapters 9, 10, 11, 12, and 15, and the scientific status of FCEs as a whole is discussed in Chapter 21. As was the case for RTW, the literature was often inconclusive. On the other hand, even if one accepts that a number of factors other than measurement of physical capacity can assist in predicting RTW and risk of injury, the ability of functional testing to provide qualitative and quantitative information about the ability of workers to perform various tasks provides objective information that otherwise would not be easily available and intuitively would seem to be of some value. It hence seems best to simply accept that FCE is an imperfect tool and to ascertain how to best consistently optimize its application to various clinical scenarios. Chapters 2, 3, 4, and 16 should be reviewed before reading this chapter.

Application of Functional Capacity Evaluation to Specific Scenarios

Physicians, chiropractors, claims adjustors, nurses, case managers, and employers are often asked to review the results of functional testing. As stated in Chapter 2, these tests can be thought of as falling into three overall categories:

- Injury prevention
- Work-related injury or illness management
- Chronic injury or illness management (usually at maximal medical improvement)

Injury Prevention

Employers or health care providers (with whom an employer has contracted) are generally the recipients of the results of tests ordered for the purpose of injury prevention. Application of results from preoffer, postoffer, periodic screening, and fitness-for-duty evaluations designed to address questions such as "Can this person do these job-related activities?" or "Does this person demonstrate the physical ability to perform the essential functions of the job?" is relatively straightforward. If an applicant cannot perform the essential functions of a job and requests accommodation, it is first necessary to establish whether the person has a disability as defined in the Americans with Disabilities Act or is a member of a class that may have been unfairly excluded from consideration for employment by the job requirements. Depending on the outcome, it may be necessary to arrange for a formal job analysis followed by additional focused functional testing.

Periodic screening evaluations are generally done on employees who must maintain a specific level of fitness to perform their jobs. Although it may be difficult to make the argument that employees who are regularly doing all of their job duties no longer meet necessary criteria to continue doing so, it is reasonable to screen employees who must sporadically be capable of performing strenuous activity. The functional evaluations should only "fail" employees who cannot perform well-defined tasks that are clearly relevant to their jobs. Whether these employees are given the opportunity to rehabilitate, transfer, or are discharged would optimally be based on the nature of the physical deficit, the employee's wishes, employer policy, union rules, and the availability of alternative work.

Work-related Injury or Illness Management

Functional testing performed to facilitate early RTW is relatively easy to apply if employees provide full effort. When an employee does not give full effort, submaximal test results ("consistent-unsubstantiated"; see Chapter 16) can represent an opportunity for the treating physician (or other health care provider) to initiate a discussion with the employee to identify any relevant physical, psychological, or socioenvironmental factors. Often the employee has made less progress than expected based on the nature of the injury and the clinical findings. The early RTW evaluation or mini-FCE may then represent an opportunity for the treating physician and/or rehabilitation professional to continue care after a certain point contingent on the worker demonstrating clear functional evidence of progress. This progress can be identified in the course of treatment or by repeated functional testing. The RTW FCE can be applied in a similar manner, ie, as a way of providing an evaluee with ongoing feedback about his or her progress or the lack thereof. Regardless of the length or timing of the FCE, if testing finds no objective evidence of clinical disease or is consistently inconsistent (or, to use the terminology in Chapter 16, inconsistent-unsubstantiated) and the worker's progress has been minimal or nonexistent and not in keeping with the usual natural history of the injury or disease, the treating physician may use the results as the basis for terminating care. The justification for doing so is that the FCE represented an opportunity for the worker with seemingly normal physical examination results (at least as related to the initial injury) to demonstrate that there was an objective explanation for his or her delayed recovery. Inconsistent and nonphysiologic test results that were unsubstantiated by physical findings would suggest that no objective cause existed because if one did exist, it presumably would have been identified by testing.

Chronic Injury or Illness Management

FCEs performed to identify residual functional abilities as part of the job-placement process for motivated employees who are still at their initial place of employment are generally requested with a particular position in mind. The results are then easily applied to determinations about work abilities because submaximal effort is not an issue in this context. Dispositional FCEs that appropriately address the questions asked by the referral source and identify evaluees as having functional abilities consistent with objective clinical findings (consistent-substantiated) that explain the rationale for their conclusions are, likewise, relatively easy to apply. Applying the information provided by dispositional FCEs when there is not a clear match between objective findings and the physical capacities estimate (PCE) completed by the functional capacities evaluator is, on the other hand, sometimes problematic. There are several potential reasons:

1. The evaluator used a model that did not include extrapolations for various positional tolerances and was unwilling to provide a clinical estimate in excess of what was "allowed" by the model used. One example would be a situation in which an evaluee was seen for a diagnosis related to the knee and foot with no upper body diagnoses of symptoms, yet the evaluator only cleared the evaluee for occasional reaching because the model used did not allow the evaluator to state otherwise.

2. The pattern of performance was consistently submaximal and unsubstantiated (see Chapter 16), and the evaluator did not release the evaluee to do activities other than the activities that were demonstrated. In this situation, it would have been more helpful if the evaluator's conclusion included statements such as, "These results reflect what the evaluee did during the test, but based on my clinical examination and the observed physiologic and biomechanical responses during testing, I *would have expected....*"

3. The pattern of performance was submaximal, unsubstantiated, and inconsistent, and the evaluator did not complete a PCE beyond what was demonstrated, despite an apparent absence of objective findings. This is a situation in which there clearly appears to have been justification for the evaluator to state that the information obtained was so inconsistent as to suggest that submaximal effort was at least in part volitional, with no consequent basis for imposing limitations. This statement ideally would have been followed by the evaluator's estimate of what the evaluee should be capable of doing based on information from the history and physical examination, as opposed to simply defaulting to the minimum. If there were objective physical findings (but findings were not adequate to allow classification of the limitations demonstrated during the FCE as "substantiated"), restrictions that were consistent with these findings should have been provided without, again, automatically taking the "safe" route and defaulting to the minimum (see Chapter 16).

4. The pattern of performance was inconsistent but substantiated, and the evaluator indicated that the evaluee, whose functional abilities decreased during the FCE, was capable of only the minimum demonstrated level of function. (Evaluees whose function increases are generally thought to be exhibiting a learning effect, improved confidence, etc, and their FCE results are not problematic.) As noted in Chapter 16, situations such as these are rare and demand that the evaluator assess whether decreased performance corresponds with a pattern reflecting a linear decline (suggestive of fatigue, provocation, or reinjury) or is seemingly erratic. In the latter situation, careful clinical assessment may ultimately suggest (or reveal) the presence of a "weak link" in the biomechanical chain related to a specific site of injury (see Chapter 15) that became apparent only when the area was biomechanically and/or repetitively stressed or the evaluee was tested using protocols that minimized or precluded the substitution of stronger links for the weak one. In all cases in which the pattern of performance is inconsistent yet substantiated, the FCE report should include the evaluator's clinical assessment of the evaluee. When recommendations for treatment have been requested, the evaluator should include potential rehabilitative interventions. In the absence of this information, the physician or insurer, who was not with the evaluee

during testing, is hard-pressed to retrospectively ascertain the exact physical causes of the inconsistencies or how to manage them.

5. The evaluator failed to recognize inconsistencies or misinterpreted results, which led to a PCE below what would be expected given the diagnosis and objective findings.

Although these scenarios are different, they all are characterized by FCEs in which the evaluator failed to draw on his or her clinical training to move past the constraints of the model used or to interpret an evaluee's abilities in the context of the physical examination and other relevant clinical factors (such as whether effort was consistent or reports of symptoms substantiated). The net result was failure to provide the referral source with meaningful information above and beyond what could have probably been obtained by simply asking the evaluee what he or she thought he (she) could do. The FCE reports containing conclusions that are essentially meaningless are, unfortunately, common. If one is unable to engage in a constructive conversation about the report with the evaluator, the alternative is to attempt to work with the report in the context of other information that may be available, including information in the medical record, results of independent medical evaluations (IMEs) or even consultations, and information that can be obtained from other sources, such as surveillance.

Working With a Suboptimal Report

Because suboptimal FCE reports often reflect failure of evaluators to integrate information from functional testing with objective information derived from the physical examination; adequately incorporate tests for sincerity of effort, cross-testing, and retesting; and/or neglect (or refuse) to draw on their clinical expertise in translating the results of the FCE to a PCE, the people who need to "work with" these reports are obliged to try to interject the missing elements retroactively. This can be difficult, but is not impossible, especially when a physician is involved. It is mandatory that the FCE evaluator provide all of the raw data used as the basis for his or her conclusions and not just the final report. It is also important for physicians and insurers to be cognizant of the same factors that should have been considered by the evaluator when completing his or her report, ie, that function should be considered limited or restricted only when there is a direct measure demonstrating correlation between the functional performance and an underlying clinical condition and that it is entirely reasonable, and, indeed, consistent with the premise of "functional restoration" as the cornerstone of injury management, to indicate that an evaluee can perform a function if there is no evidence indicating that this performance would have an adverse effect on the underlying clinical condition. Physicians and insurers are strongly advised to be thoroughly familiar with the concepts and recommendations in Chapter 16 before attempting to apply FCE reports for which there are concerns about the accuracy of the PCEs that were provided. The following suggestions may be of value:

1. When evaluators use a model that does not include extrapolations for various positional tolerances and are unwilling to provide a clinical estimate in excess of what was allowed by the model used because they do not want to rely on their clinical judgment, the recipient should ask that this information be clearly stated in written form—preferably via a notation on the PCE. It is then reasonable to ask a physician who has already (or will) see the evaluee (which is preferable) or a physician who is willing to review the medical record (which will include prior evaluations) to use this information in conjunction with the FCE report to provide a supplemental report and PCE. These should summarize all clinical information relevant to determinations regarding function, discuss the reasons for the failure of the evaluator to provide a release to activities in excess of those provided initially, and update the PCE accordingly.

2. Submaximal consistent but unsubstantiated patterns of performance are generally seen in patients with chronic pain complaints. Although it is possible that an occult medical condition could be present (and this must be ruled out), it is important for people reviewing FCE reports characterized by submaximal effort to remember that the physical capacities demonstrated by evaluees classified as exerting submaximal effort are, by definition, nonphysiologic. The FCE has demonstrated only what the evaluee is willing to do, not what he or she can do. Hence, as was the case in item 1, it is optimal for a physician (or other clinician) to review the FCE report in the context of all available clinical data and issue a supplemental report that integrates this information into a revised PCE. The physician should, as stated earlier, classify function as limited or restricted only if there is a direct measure demonstrating correlation between performance during testing and an underlying clinical condition. It is also entirely reasonable and consistent with the premise of functional restoration to release an evaluee to perform a given function in the absence of evidence indicating that this performance would have an adverse effect on the underlying clinical condition.

3. Most evaluators who have adequately evaluated consistency of effort and described it in their final report clearly identify when the pattern of effort has been inconsistent and unsubstantiated (although they may use other terminology). Evaluators with strong clinical skills are also sometimes willing to provide a PCE that is not based solely on demonstrated abilities but also reflects their clinical judgment. If the evaluator is not willing to do this, an external reviewer can summarize the information in the FCE report, stressing the inconsistencies, and discuss these in the

context of the clinical evaluation performed during the FCE and other available clinical information. Consistent evidence of inconsistencies in demonstrated performance and between performance during functional testing and other clinical information should lead an external reviewer to base a revised PCE solely on objective findings and the "usual" natural history of the medical problem that initiated the request for the FCE. Stating that the evaluee has completely recovered from his or her problem is not unreasonable but must be substantiated (or at least explained).

4. The other problematic pattern of performance, "inconsistent-substantiated," is optimally interpreted by the FCE evaluator who may also, if requested by the referral source, make treatment recommendations. In the absence of a thorough clinical examination and appropriate analysis of the data by the evaluator, it is difficult for a recipient of the FCE to do so retrospectively. Review of medical records, especially IMEs that are roughly contemporaneous, may be useful. The decision about what level of activity to recommend would depend on whether performance had improved or declined during the FCE in the context of information in the medical record about the evaluee's diagnosis, physical examination findings, and prior response to treatment. Determinations regarding the ability of the evaluee to sustain a given level of performance should be conservative and reflect relevant information in the FCE.

5. The situation previously described, ie, when the evaluator seems to have failed to recognize inconsistencies or misinterpreted results, is particularly difficult to manage because the conclusions are, by definition, erroneous and should, if possible, be corrected. The recipient of the FCE report should consider the possibility that this may have occurred when the PCE is grossly less than would be expected given the evaluee's diagnosis and other information in the medical records and the evaluator has failed to state that effort seemed to be submaximal or inconsistent. Review of the raw data from the FCE report will generally allow the external reviewer to ascertain whether the evaluator incorporated testing for consistency of effort (with specific tests or through the use of retesting and cross-testing) into the FCE. If there was testing incorporated, each test should be individually reviewed and evaluated in the context of other tests and the evaluee's clinical manifestations. Clear errors in judgment by the evaluator may be amenable to discussion. Otherwise, the only options are to prepare a separate supplemental report describing flaws in the FCE data analysis or consider using additional sources of information such as an IME (if one was performed), surveillance, or even a repeated FCE with another evaluator. Use of surveillance and other special circumstances is described subsequently.

Special Circumstances

Sometimes, FCEs are used to evaluate people who claim to be limited by chronic fatigue or similar diffuse systemic complaints that are not accompanied by relevant objective pathology. (The evaluation of patients with chronic pain was discussed in Chapter 15.) No model has been developed for widespread use in these cases. As noted in Chapter 2, it is logical to expect that people with debilitating chronic fatigue will exhibit decreased endurance and poor aerobic conditioning. Although the need to obtain this type of information will have optimally been considered before performance of the FCE (leading, often, to the decision to do a 2-day or even longer study), use of an FCE model that does not adequately evaluate the degree to which fatigue limits the evaluee can be supplemented by performing surveillance before and after testing and, preferably, on the next day (or next few days). This surveillance may allow an external reviewer to get a better sense of whether the evaluee is or is not capable of sustained minimum effort. Surveillance may also be useful in other circumstances when the consistency of limitations is in question. Review of the surveillance data by the person who performed the FCE and by physicians who examined the evaluee and/or reviewed the medical record is valuable. In some circumstances, it may be useful for a kinesiologist and/or ergonomist to compare the activities documented via surveillance with the abilities demonstrated in the FCE and/or IME.

The other special circumstance is one that can be encountered as part of the evaluation of patients with chronic pain, chronic fatigue, or other debilitating complaints that seem to exist in the absence of confirmatory physical findings. Although the FCE evaluator is not capable of recommending this, evidence of inappropriate emotional responses to requests to perform activities or prior psychological problems in the context of a report documenting submaximal effort may warrant that a physician or insurer refer the evaluee for a psychological evaluation or at least for testing, such as with the Minnesota Multiphasic Personality Inventory. Although these evaluations and tests will not be useful in most situations, they may be of value when it is necessary to form an accurate assessment of all factors that may be contributing to an evaluee's non-physiologic limitations, especially in light of the contribution of factors other than physical capacities to RTW.

Summary

When a functional assessment is appropriately requested and performed and the situation is relatively straightforward, results can be easily used to address relevant issues. Failure to communicate exactly what one wants to assess to the evaluator or request specific FCE components of interest (see Introduction and Chapter 2) may lead to a suboptimal FCE, as may error on the part of evaluators and/or their inability (or unwillingness) to reach conclusions about evaluee abilities that reflect the synthesis of information from the FCE with that obtained through their clinical evaluation or other objective sources of data.

Because it seems that a number of factors other than physical capacities per se affect RTW and the risk of injury, functional testing may be most easily applied when the evaluee is motivated and the testing ordered to answer simple questions such as "How much can this person lift?" Conversely, functional test results are likely to be most difficult to apply when effort is submaximal (suggesting the presence of underlying psychological and socioenvironmental factors) and the goal was to address whether the evaluee could do some form of work. Reports that describe evaluee limitations that are in excess of what would be expected can still be used constructively. This usually requires involvement of a physician or similarly skilled clinician because the FCE report needs to be reviewed in the context of other information in the record and interpreted accordingly. The ultimate result may be a report that captures the complexities of a given "case" far better than would the clinical evaluation and medical record alone. The use of supplemental evaluations such as surveillance, psychological testing, and assessment of results by an ergonomist or kinesiologist may also be of value.

References

1. Takala EP, Viikari-Juntura E. Do functional tests predict low back pain? *Spine.* 2000;25:2126–2132.
2. Gross DP, Battie MC, Cassidy JD. The prognostic value of functional capacity evaluation in patients with chronic low back pain, part 1: timely return to work. *Spine.* 2004;29:914–919.
3. Gross DP, Battie MC. The prognostic value of functional capacity evaluation in patients with chronic low back pain: part 2: sustained recovery. *Spine.* 2004;29:920–924.
4. Gross DP, Battie MC. Functional capacity evaluation performance does not predict sustained return to work in claimants with chronic back pain. *Journal of Occupational Rehabilitation.* 2005;15:285–294.
5. Gross DP, Battie MC. Does functional capacity evaluation predict recovery in workers' compensation claimants with upper extremity disorders? *Occupational and Environmental Medicine.* 2006;63:404–410.
6. Kuijer W, Brouwer S, Reneman M, et al. Matching FCE activities and work demands: an explorative study. *Journal of Occupational Rehabilitation.* 2006;Sep;16(3):469–483.
7. Matheson LN, Isernhagen SJ, Hart DL. Relationships among lifting ability, grip force, and return to work. *Physical Therapy.* 2002;82:249–256.

8. Vowles KE, Gross RT, Sorrell JT. Predicting work status following interdisciplinary treatment for chronic pain. *European Journal of Pain.* 2004;8:351–358.

9. Mayer TG, Gatchel RJ, Kishino N, Keeley J, Capra P, Mayer H, Barnett J, Mooney V. Objective assessment of spine function following industrial injury: a prospective study with comparison group and one-year follow-up. *Spine.* 1985;10:482–493.

10. Cutler RB, Fishbain DA, Steele-Rosomoff R, Rosomoff HL. Relationships between functional capacity measures and baseline psychological measures in chronic pain patients. *Journal of Occupational Rehabilitation.* 2003;13:249–258.

11. Geisser ME, Robinson ME, Miller QL, Bade SM. Psychosocial factors and functional capacity evaluation among persons with chronic pain. *Journal of Occupational Rehabilitation.* 2003;13:259–276.

12. Wasiak R, Verma S, Pransky G, Webster B. Risk factors for recurrent episodes of care and work disability: case of low back pain. *Journal of Occupational and Environmental Medicine.* 2004;46:68–76.

13. Hunter SJ, Shaha S, Flint D, Tracy DM. Predicting return to work: a long-term follow-up study of railroad workers after low back injuries. *Spine.* 1998;23:2319–2328.

14. Oleinick A, Gluck JV, Guire K. Factors affecting first return to work following a compensable occupational back injury. *American Journal of Industrial Medicine.* 1996;30:540–555.

15. McGeary DD, Mayer TG, Gatchel RJ. High pain ratings predict treatment failure in chronic occupational musculoskeletal disorders. *Journal of Bone Joint Surgical (American).* 2006;88:317–325.

16. Haldorsen EM, Indahl A, Ursin H. Patients with low back pain not returning to work: a 12-month follow-up study. *Spine.* 1998;23:1202–1208.

17. Shaw WS, Pransky G, Patterson W, Winters T. Early disability risk factors for low back pain assessed at outpatient occupational health clinics. *Spine.* 2005;30:572–580.

18. Fritz JM, George SZ. Identifying psychosocial variables in patients with acute work-related low back pain: the importance of fear-avoidance beliefs. *Physical Therapy.* 2002;82:973–983.

19. Watson PJ, Booker CK, Moores L, Main CJ. Returning the chronically unemployed with low back pain to employment. *European Journal of Pain.* 2004;8:359–369.

20. Katz JN, Keller RB, Fossel AH, Punnett L, Bessette L, Simmons BP, Mooney N. Predictors of return to work following carpal tunnel release. *American Journal of Industrial Medicine.* 1997;31:85–91.

21. Fishbain DA, Cutler RB, Rosomoff HL, Khalil T, Steele-Rosomoff R. Impact of chronic pain patients' job perception variables on actual return to work. *Clinical Journal of Pain.* 1997;13:197–206.

22. DeBerard MS, Masters KS, Colledge AL, Holmes EB. Presurgical biopsychosocial variables predict medical and compensation costs of lumbar fusion in Utah workers' compensation patients. *Spine Journal.* 2003;3:420–429.

23. Houben RM, Ostelo RW, Vlaeyen J, Wolters W, et al. Health care providers' orientations towards common low back pain predict perceived harmfulness of physical activities and recommendations regarding return to normal activity. *European Journal of Pain.* 2005;9:173–183.

24. Hamberg-van Reenen HH, Ariens GA, Blatter BM, van Mechelen W, Bongers PM. A systematic review of the relation between physical capacity and future low back and neck/shoulder pain. *Pain.* 2007;130:93–107.

25. de Kort WL, Uiterweer HW, van Dijik FL. Agreement on medical fitness for a job. *Scandinavian Journal of Work and Environmental Health.* 1992;18:246–251.

26. Walker WC, Cifu DX, Gardner M, Keyser-Marcus L. Functional assessment in patients with chronic pain: can physicians predict performance? *American Journal of Physical Medicine and Rehabiliation.* 2001;80:162–168.

27. Hunt DG, Zuberbier OA, Kozlowski AJ, Berkowitz J, Schultz IZ, Milner RA, Crook JM, Turk DC. Are components of a comprehensive medical assessment predictive of work disability after an episode of occupational low back trouble? *Spine.* 2002;27:2715–2719.

28. Melhorn JM, Ackerman WE. *Guides to the Evaluation of Disease and Injury Causation.* Chicago, IL: American Medical Association; 2007.

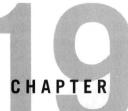

CHAPTER

Application of the Functional Capacity Evaluation by Vocational Experts

Jasen M. Walker, EdD, CRC, CCM

Vocational experts (VEs) are rehabilitation professionals who testify in court matters about a person's capacities to perform competitive employment following the onset of injury or illness. Vocational experts inform the court as to how an injury or disease causes changes in a person's occupational potentials and earning capacity. A rehabilitation professional serving as a VE is generally trained as a counselor or psychologist, skilled in vocational assessment and/or job analysis and placement, and customarily certified by one or more relevant professional associations,[1] such as the American Board of Vocational Experts. Vocational experts are the only rehabilitation professionals who are specifically trained to evaluate an injured person's postinjury occupational disability and employability.

Forensic vocational or disability evaluation does not involve a helping relationship between the VE and the injured party. It consists of the VE executing an independent review of pertinent medical information (including an understanding of the injured person's functionality), a clinical interview, preferably vocational testing (ie, aptitudes and interests), and a resultant assessment of the injured person's transferable skills and residual employability.

In formulating an analysis of residual employability, the VE relies on medical documentation about the injured person's impairment(s) and residual functional capacity (RFC), or what the impaired person is able to do physically and/or mentally despite the medically defined impairment. In vocational disability evaluation, the RFC report bridges the gap between the existence of medical impairment and the assessment of occupational disability and residual employability. The RFC for people who have physical or exertional impairment has customarily been established by health care providers and is an evolving method.

For many years, members of the legal system and employers relied on a physician to make statements as to whether an injured person could work. Concerned parties would ask physicians whether an injured employee, for example, could work without considering issues of what the person might be qualified to do or what the demands of the job might be. All too frequently, exclusive of laboratory methods, the physician responded to items on a checklist and provided only a "guesstimate," or best clinical judgment, of the patient's physical abilities to perform work-related tasks. Unfortunately, this fairly subjective process of delineating RFC continues in some cases. Rehabilitation professionals, however, have long known that vocational "disability is a relational outcome, reflecting the individual's capacity to perform a specific task or activity, contingent on the environmental conditions in which they are to be performed," as stated in an Institute of Medicine Report in 1997.[2]

In its *Guides to the Evaluation of Permanent Impairment,* the American Medical Association speaks to the difference between impairment and disability. According to the *Guides, impairment* is defined as "a loss, loss of use, or derangement of any body part, organ system, or organ function."[3(p2)] On the other hand, *disability* is "an alteration of an individual's capacity to meet personal, social, or occupational demands because of an impairment,"[3(p3)] which is best evaluated by nonmedical means. Still, vestiges of expecting or charging medical personnel with determining vocational disability remain in the health care, legal, and disability systems. Time and experience indicate that confusion of medical impairment with vocational disability has been waning.

As disability determinations, particularly within the Social Security Admin-istration, have become more refined, a growing awareness has emerged that physicians are not formally trained to define a person's occupational capabilities and, therefore, are unable to accurately declare a person as totally disabled for working or, conversely, capable of gainful employment. Many practitioners believe that a patient's RFC is better assessed with a formal functional capacity evaluation (FCE). The VE, who determines the vocational impact of medically determined physical impairment, relies on the functional capacity data that details the impaired person's safe physical capabilities in terms of lifting, carrying, reaching, handling, bending, and other exertional worklike behaviors. The FCE is regarded by many as the state-of-the-art method of determining a person's exer-tional capabilities within the work classifications of sedentary, light, medium, etc. Regardless of whether this statement about FCEs is correct, the FCE is one of the only tools available for use to provide VEs with measured functional capacities that can be applied toward determining a person's employability.

Vocational experts providing opinions in court matters are divorced from the provision of vocational rehabilitation services to the person being examined. As a result, forensic VEs generally do not have the opportunity to observe the injured person's work behavior for an extended period and, therefore, are unable to document what a person can physically do in a work setting by trial and error or through work-adjustment processes. Therefore, VEs must rely on data from other sources about the person's physical capacities. As Dakos[4] states, "The role of the VE in considering the findings of a functional capacity evaluation is that of interpreter/translator." With information about a person's residual functional capacities, the VE can predict, with professional certainty, the examinee's specific employment options and occupational potentials, with or without job accommodation. Ethical standards and case law mandate that the VE provide these opinions about a person's employability on the basis of reliable methods.

Vocational experts, as well as other forensic experts, are required to present "scientific evidence" that helps a judge or jury determine if occupational disabil-ity and economic damages follow personal injury. This requirement is codified in the Federal Rules of Evidence.[5] The Rules help to define what evidence is admissible. Rule 702 states:

If scientific, technical, or other specialized knowledge will assist the trier of fact to understand the evidence or to determine a fact in issue, a witness qualified as an expert by knowledge, skill, experience, training, or education, may testify thereto in the form of an opinion or otherwise, if (1) the testimony is based upon sufficient facts or data, (2) the testimony is the product of reliable principles and methods, and (3) the witness has applied the principles and methods reliably to the facts of the case.

All forensic experts are further challenged by court rulings, such as *Daubert, Joiner,* and *Kumho,*[6] demanding greater relevance and reliability in their assessment methods. Increasingly, all forensic experts are being compelled to establish with the court that their evaluation methods are valid and reliable and, most significant, are based on "scientific" and "reproducible" methods.

This dilemma, as described in the context of FCE, was clearly outlined in a recent editorial in the American Board of Vocational Experts newsletter. In the editorial, the ethics committee chairperson wrote, "…our opinions must be based upon reliable and defensible data and it is our responsibility to investigate whether those assessment tools fit that description. Given that condition and the body of research questioning the validity, reliability, and efficacy of functional capacity evaluations (FCE), is there sufficient evidence to support their use in their current state as a foundation upon which to base one's opinions regarding sustained functional capacity and, therefore, employability and labor market access?"[7] Similar concerns regarding the validity and reliability of FCEs have been expressed by VEs in other venues, and refinement of FCEs may be dependent on developing a meaningful dialogue between the professionals measuring RFC and the professionals charged with the responsibility of defining residual employability.

As the interpreter or translator, the VE relies on others, including the professionals who carry out well-designed FCEs, for accurate data. The importance of FCEs is increasing as vocational and medical experts realize the inadequacy of medical personnel reporting functional limitations based on office examinations, injured workers' self-reports, and other subjective means. The continuing refinement of how an impaired person's physical capacities for competitive employment are defined includes the advancement of the FCE.

As stated, however, the development of valid and reliable tools for measuring an impaired person's physical capacity remains a concern for VEs. The December 2004 issue of the *Journal of Forensic Vocational Analysis* focused exclusively on the use of FCEs in vocational forensics. According to contributors to that issue of the journal, troublesome issues in state-of-the-art FCEs include the following:

- validity and reliability,[8]
- generalizing performance from a 4-hour assessment to an entire workday,[9,10]
- sincerity of effort,[4,9] and
- whether FCEs meet legal standards of relevance and reliability.[11]

No effort is being made here to revisit the concepts of test validity and reliability; they are more than adequately covered elsewhere. However, qualified VEs are cognizant of the basic concepts of validity and reliability and are ethically bound to consider test standardization, reliability, and validity in formulating their forensic findings and opinions.

Every VE knows that the merit of a standardized measure is determined by its reliability and its validity. The assessment of reliability invariably boils down to a simple summary statistic, the reliability coefficient. If test results are highly consistent, the scores of persons taking the test on two occasions will be strongly correlated. Although never reaching the theoretical upper limit of +1.00, the reliability coefficient provides a quantitative description not only of test-retest reliability, but also of interexaminer reliability, alternate-forms reliability, and internal reliability. Reliability speaks to consistency, and if FCEs are to be of value to VEs, injured people, the court system, and employers, they must be consistent not only from test to retest, but also when administered by two or more different examiners and between parts of an assessment. As King[8] states, "To the clinician, reliability means that changes in a client's performance can be attributed to real change in function rather than to measurement error."

The FCE must also be capable of accurately providing a foundation from which to infer appropriate, meaningful, and useful behavior regarding physical functioning in the workplace. That is, FCEs must be valid. In research, validity and reliability are essential aspects of an experiment that has merit. Validity is the ability of the test or experiment to accurately measure what it purports to measure, and ecological validity is a subset of test validity. Ultimately, no matter how reliable, findings from a measure must also be ecologically valid.

To have ecological validity, the methods, materials, and settings of an experiment must approximate the real-life situation under study. The data from an FCE are often interpreted in an accompanying narrative report that includes language such as, "Results obtained indicate this client performed with determined, consistent effort and demonstrated appropriate pain behaviors." It is difficult to understand the meaning of these words exactly in terms of what the FCE measures or what it purports to measure (ie, the person's physical capacities) and, whether if re-tested at another time or by another examiner, this language would appear again in the narrative report. However, the primary concern must be whether the measured behaviors have application to the workplace.

The FCE tends to present inconsistent information regarding physical capacity definitions and classifications of strenuousness defined by the US Department of Labor.[12] The classifications are sedentary, light, medium, heavy, and very heavy. Some FCE reports combine these definitions (as in sedentary-light) and, by doing so, confuse the issue of whether the examinee is capable of one exertional level or both levels. This combination of definitions could represent a substantial difference in both RFC and employability.

Moreover, FCE reports sometimes cloud assessment findings by misrepresenting accepted vocational terms, such as sedentary, light, and medium work, language that is clearly defined by the US Department of Labor[12] and recognized by occupational experts as state-of-the-art terms. Vocational experts rely heavily on this terminology to make accurate and reliable assessments of a person's residual employability. Language in an FCE report such as, "Based on results obtained, the client is able to perform sedentary-light physical demand component work with occasional lifting below waist height to 25 lb, and the client lifted 35 lb to shoulder and 20 lb overhead," potentially confuses the VE's assessment. By definition, lifting 25 and 35 lb places the person beyond the light work domain and into the medium category of work as defined by the US Department of Labor.[12] In offering quantitative data about lifting and then mislabeling that data with the incorrect physical work classification, the FCE report can lead to a potentially inaccurate vocational evaluation and an incorrect forensic conclusion. A standardization of language must be basic to the FCE and congruent with accepted definitions of physical strenuousness. Efforts to consistently use the federal definitions of work in FCEs would prove helpful to the process of conducting accurate vocational assessments.

Among the different FCEs used in determining how a person's exertional impairments translate into RFC, one of the more significant variables is whether the FCE relates to a full day and/or a full week of work. The VE considers this distinction as the difference between part-time and full-time employment. Vocational experts generally remain at a loss as to how FCEs can predict part- or full-time employment. For example, language such as, "In a valid representation of physical capabilities based on consistencies and inconsistencies when interfacing grip dynamometer graphing, resistance dynamometer graphing, pulse variations, weights achieved, and selectivity of pain reports and pain behaviors," the person manifested a "sitting tolerance" of 23 minutes "demonstrated during keyboard activity and history review." In this actual case, the functional capacity assessment specialist "recommended" a workday "tolerance" of only 2 hours. Within weeks of these FCE findings, when examined for vocational evaluation, the same person was able to remain seated for more than 2 hours without interruption while completing standardized paper-and-pencil tests. Considerably more discrepancies between FCE "recommendations" and actual vocational assessment behaviors were observed.

In still another FCE using a different protocol than used in the preceding example, the document reporting the FCE data contains a "functional capacity summary" that describes the examinee's sitting job demands as frequent (34%–66% of the time). However, additional comments read, "It is recommended that he take short standing/stretch breaks during periods of prolonged sitting (eg, >1 hour)." No reason was given for this added comment, but the vocational ramifications are potentially significant. The examinee was a tractor-trailer truck driver, and even though he could perform medium work with frequent sitting, it was "recommended" that he not sit for longer than 1 hour without taking a "short" standing/stretching break, undoubtedly inconsistent with his job demands and not at all explained in the FCE report.

Sincerity of effort remains one of the most controversial and unresolved issues associated with the efficacy of FCEs, according to Lechner[9] and others.[4,13] According to Lechner,[9] "The standardization, reliability, and validity of some of the methods used to determine sincerity of effort are questionable." As an example, Lechner[9] notes that the Waddell nonorganic signs are frequently used in FCEs. Scoring positively on the Waddell test should not allow one to conclude that the client is withholding full effort, and, conversely, demonstrating fewer than the necessary three of eight positive scores on the Waddell test is not necessarily indicative of "appropriate pain behavior," by which one could conclude that sincere effort has taken place. Dakos[4] speaks of multiple factors that should be considered in assessing genuine performance or effort and recommends that skilled functional capacity evaluators observe and report, but not analyze, performance-limiting behaviors. Analyzing performance-limiting data avoids the potential error in logic that a person who has conceivably set forth "genuine effort" during an FCE is necessarily a sincere and reliable examinee under all circumstances, including a return to work where conditions might be quite different from the controlled atmosphere of an FCE. See Chapter 11 for a discussion of this topic.

With respect to pain-related deficits, the results of FCEs are frequently described in reports with rather confusing language. Too frequently, the evaluation can be affected by a subjective complaint and, in some cases, less than maximal effort by the examinee. In cases involving litigation, the injured worker's effort in testing is often an issue, particularly if the person being evaluated anticipates financial gain by demonstrating weakness and/or dysfunction.

The FCE is also limited in its potential to discern between the results produced by pre-existing impairment (eg, osteoarthritis and degenerative joint disease) and traumatically induced, accident-related impairment. Vocational experts may be charged with the responsibility of determining residual employability and earning power following the accident, but, based on the medical history, the person may have had a pre-existing exertional impairment affecting strength and, of course, FCE outcomes. Consider, for example, a 56-year-old truck driver with a history of spinal complaints and radiographically documented severe spondylosis. He is examined with an FCE following a shoulder injury and is found to be physically capable of lifting no more than 20 lb and restricted to light work as defined by the US Department of Labor.[12] The government

; job is medium work, which is more demanding than his
ever, the question is: "What limits his measured functional
accident-related shoulder pathology or his pre-existing spinal
The FCE may be able to determine functional limitations attributable
to the shoulder injury and to the pre-existing back problems when evaluating
activities that predominantly stress the shoulder or the back. Nevertheless, the
FCE lacks the sophistication to apportion when evaluating complex activities
that require use of both areas. It is reasonable to point out that requiring an FCE
to provide this level of precision is inappropriate. Still, the question is one that
might have particular importance to an assessment of the person's preaccident
capacities to work and earn money, particularly in truck driving.

Functional testing has become an increasingly important aspect of the VE's
analysis of residual employability, but it is not beyond challenge. With the fabled
US Supreme Court decision in *Daubert v Merrell Dow Pharmaceuticals*,[6] the
American court system has increased the standards and refined its definition
of what constitutes relevance and reliability for expert testimony. According
to Dominick,[11] with the standards of expert testimony increasing, VEs should
be prepared to deal with cross-examination regarding measurement theories,
reliability, validity, test selection, testing methods, outside entity standards, and
FCE vulnerability.

Standardized FCEs would seem to hold substantial promise in providing accurate
and reliable data regarding a person's physical capacities for work, particularly
when compared with the conjecture of a health care professional who has been
asked to simply fill out a checklist or provide a generic statement (eg, "light
duty") of what he or she thinks a patient might be able to do in the workplace.
Unfortunately, FCE standardization seems far off. Lechner[9] identified 10 FCE
protocols, all proprietary, and noted an apparent lack of research supporting
the validity and reliability of the methods. King[8] encourages and challenges
FCE developers to conduct research and improve their assessments to levels of
reliability and validity that are scientifically sound and legally defensible.

Although FCEs hold the potential to be an invaluable tool for the VE, there is
a need to continue to refine the process, especially the precision and standardization of the report language. Vocational experts remain concerned about the
efficacy of FCEs. When the purpose of the FCE is to provide the VE with the
basis for case testimony, FCE validity, reliability, and language are critical.
Functional capacity evaluators and VEs will, for the foreseeable future, need to
continue a refinement dialogue.

References

1. Weed RO, Field TF. *Rehabilitation Consultant's Handbook*. Revised ed. Athens, GA: Elliott & Fitzpatrick, Inc; 2001:31–32.
2. Brandt EN Jr, Pope AM. *Enabling America: Assessing the Role of Rehabilitation Science and Engineering*. Washington, DC: National Academy Press; 1997. Quoted by: Cocchiarella L, Andersson GBJ, eds. *Guides to the Evaluation of Permanent Impairment*. 5th ed. Chicago, IL: American Medical Association; 2005:8.
3. Cocchiarella L, Andersson GBJ, eds. *Guides to the Evaluation of Permanent Impairment*. 5th ed. Chicago, IL: American Medical Association; 2005.
4. Dakos MS. The application of functional capacity evaluations in the provision of vocational expert services. *J Forensic Vocational Anal*. 2004;7:105–117.
5. ARTICLE VII. OPINIONS AND EXPERT. Rule 702. Testimony by Experts www.law.cornell.edu/rules/fre/rules.htm#Rule702. Accessed July 25, 2007.
6. Field TF, Choppa T, Dillman EG, et al. *A Resource for the Rehabilitation Consultant on the Daubert and Kumho Rulings*. Athens, GA: Elliott & Fitzpatrick, Inc; 2000:61–104.
7. Hale BL. From the editor's laptop [editorial]. *Vocational Expert*. Spring 2007;23(3):3.
8. King PM. Analysis of the reliability and validity supporting functional capacity evaluations. *J Forensic Vocational Anal*. 2004;7:75–82.
9. Lechner DE. The well-designed functional capacity evaluation: application in forensic vocational analysis. *J Forensic Vocational Anal*. 2004;7:83–96.
10. McDaniel RS, Tilton J, Philadelphia A. Use of the functional capacities evaluation in the vocational expert practice: help or hindrance. *J Forensic Vocational Anal*. 2004;7:97–104.
11. Dominick BK. Daubert & ADA decisions: will functional capacity evaluations hold up in court? *J Forensic Vocational Anal*. 2004;7:119–126.
12. *Dictionary of Occupational Titles, Revised*. 4th ed. Washington, DC: US Dept of Labor, Employment and Training Administration, US Employment Service; 1991:1013.
13. Geisser ME, Robinson M, Miller Q, Bade S. Psychosocial factors and functional capacity evaluation among persons with chronic pain. *J Occup Rehabil*. 2004; 13:259–276.

CHAPTER 19

CHAPTER 20

Legal Issues in Functional Capacity Evaluations

Gwen Simons, PT, JD, OCS, FAAOMPT

Functional capacity evaluation (FCE) providers have to be concerned about the legal issues surrounding the provision of FCE services. Every FCE has potential for legal controversy due to the nature of the issues FCE evidence seeks to resolve. The FCE provides presumably objective information about a person's physical abilities and tolerance for various work activities, allowing medical providers to determine whether a healthy person is fit for a new job or whether an injured person can return to work. If the worker is motivated to work, the FCE is given great weight in the return-to-work decision-making process. However, FCEs are frequently used as medical evidence in legal proceedings (such as disability determinations, personal injury civil suits, and workers' compensation cases) in which a person's abilities and motivation to work may be in question. In these cases, there is always an opponent to the FCE evidence, creating potential issues for the credibility of the FCE provider and the FCE method. When functional tests are used for pre-employment or postoffer employment screenings, the legal issues become even more complicated. Employers who use functional tests to select employees must comply with the Americans' with Disabilities Act and the Civil Rights Act of 1964. The standards judging the legality of the test in the employment context are completely different and sometimes misunderstood by FCE providers. In addition, FCEs pose a risk of causing a new injury, reinjury, or symptom exacerbation, exposing the evaluator to malpractice (negligence) claims.

This chapter looks at some of the legal issues surrounding FCEs, including the different standards among various courts for admitting expert testimony from the FCE provider and the credibility issues for FCEs. Workers' compensation decisions are available in some states, which provide some guidance on how FCE evidence may be challenged. A partial list of Web sites for workers' compensation decisions can be found in Table 20–1. However, these decisions do not set precedence until they are challenged on appeal, creating case law. Some case law will be presented for purposes of illustration, but case law only carries precedence in the jurisdiction from which it came and can be applied only to cases with similar facts. It is also important for readers to recognize that the outcome of a case is frequently contingent on the legal strategy and the skills of the attorneys. A case that was wrongly decided based on a faulty legal argument could be overturned in the future. At the time of this publication, the development of case law for FCEs was very limited. Therefore, to some extent, the discussion is academic. For purposes of stimulating interest in improving legal credibility of FCEs, I occasionally interject a personal opinion with the disclaimer that my opinion is subject to change as the scientific research and case law develop.

TABLE 20–1	Workers' Compensation Decision Web Sites in Selected States
State	**Web Site**
Alaska	http://labor.state.ak.us/wc/legaldir.htm
Arkansas	www.awcc.state.ar.us/opinionmain.html
California	www.dir.ca.gov/WCAB/wcab_dars.htm
Connecticut	http://wcc.state.ct.us/CRB/menus/crb-opin.htm
Idaho	www.iic.idaho.gov/legal/decisions/dec_main.htm
Iowa	www.iowaworkforce.com/wc/decisions.htm
Kansas	www.dol.ks.gov/wcboard/wcappeal_Res.html
Kentucky	www.comped.net/
Maine	www.maine.gov/wcb/Board_Decisions/
Michigan	www.michigan.gov/dleg/0,1607,7-154-10576_17495-58938—,00.html
Minnesota	www.workerscomp.state.mn.us/
Missouri	www.dolir.mo.gov/lirc/wcdecisions/index.htm
Montana	http://wcc.dli.mt.gov/
Nebraska	www.wcc.ne.gov/
New Jersey	http://lwd.dol.state.nj.us/labor/wc/legal/cases/
Rhode Island	www.courts.ri.gov/workers/appellatedecisions.htm
South Dakota	www.state.sd.us/dol/DLM/Decisions%20-%20Workers%20Compensation.htm
Tennessee	www.tsc.state.tn.us/OPINIONS/WORKCOMP/Oplstwc.htm
Utah	http://laborcommission.utah.gov/AdministrativeServices/Decisions/CommissionerDecisions/index.html Appeals: http://laborcommission.utah.gov/AdministrativeServices/Decisions/AppealsBoardDecisions/index.html
Vermont	www.labor.vermont.gov/Decisions/tabid/127/Default.aspx
Virginia	www.vwc.state.va.us/cgi-bin/GetSearchParms.cgi
Wisconsin	www.dwd.state.wi.us/lirc/wc_find.htm

CHAPTER 20

Informed Consent and Malpractice Risks

Obtaining informed consent is recommended, if not legally required, for all medical procedures, especially FCEs. Obtaining informed consent ensures that the evaluee has knowingly consented to the procedures after being informed of the potential risks. First, FCE recipients are frequently involved in legal claims or controversies. Second, the nature of the examination, asking someone to perform physical tasks to the limit of his or her maximum abilities, is risky even if the provider takes all safety precautions.

Informed consent for FCEs should be obtained in writing. The consent form should state the purpose of the FCE, explain the FCE procedure, and state the risks of harm from the procedure. Risks include, but are not limited to, soreness from using muscles the evaluee has not used in a long time, experiencing an exacerbation of pain and other symptoms, being reinjured, and experiencing a new injury. The consent form should explain the safety procedures that are followed to minimize these risks and inform the evaluee of his or her responsibility for communicating pain and symptoms to the evaluator, which shifts some of the responsibility for any harm done to the evaluee. Under the laws of many states, even if the FCE provider was negligent, the evaluee's damage award could be substantially reduced if he or she was found to have contributed to his or her own harm by not communicating symptoms to the provider as instructed.

In addition to informed consent, the FCE provider should have a procedure of informing evaluees about what to do if soreness, increased pain, or a change in symptoms occurs after they have left the FCE site. Most people will have some soreness following an FCE. It is not uncommon for a plaintiff to testify that he was in so much pain after the FCE he had to stay in bed for days. This kind of testimony can discredit an otherwise credible FCE. Providers who discount complaints of pain may increase their risk for a malpractice claim in addition to discrediting their FCE if they do not at least make an attempt to distinguish between the same pain and additional harm. At a minimum, the provider should tell evaluees to call the FCE site the day after the FCE if their condition is significantly worse or there is a change in symptoms. This instruction shifts the burden of proving pain or changed-symptoms back to the evaluee and provides a mechanism for the Defense to discredit the evaluee's testimony. If an evaluee calls with a report of a change in condition, the provider can document the complaints and determine whether a follow-up examination is required. If the symptoms are different in character or intensity, or symptoms are in a different location, providers should do a follow-up examination for their own malpractice protection.

The Functional Capacity Evaluation as Medicolegal Evidence

The FCE evidence, whether given through verbal testimony or a written report, must survive challenges directed at whether the evidence is relevant, the FCE witness is qualified to testify as an expert, the scientific methods used by the expert are reliable, and the expert's methods and opinions are relevantly applied to the facts of the case. These challenges may come: (1) before the evidence is admitted in the form of an objection to the expert's testimony, (2) during cross-examination if the expert is allowed to testify, and (3) on appeal if the trial court or adjudicator adopted the opinion of an expert that was insufficiently supported.

Before analyzing these issues, one must have an understanding of the rules courts and administrative agencies use in deciding cases and controversies.

The Role of the Fact-Finder in Determining Legal Issues and Liability

Legal causation, liability, and economic damages are all questions for the fact-finder in a legal case or controversy. The fact-finder will be a jury, judge, or administrative agency adjudicator, such as an administrative law judge (ALJ) or a hearing officer, depending on the court. Medical and FCE experts provide evidence and may offer an opinion on the legal issues, but it is the fact-finder who ultimately decides what evidence to believe. When evidence is not reliable or competent, the fact-finder can choose to disregard it or not give it much weight in the decision. As long as there is substantial evidence in the record to support the fact-finder's decision, despite the existence of contrary evidence, the decision will be upheld on appeal. In federal courts, *substantial evidence* is defined as "such relevant evidence that a reasonable mind might accept as adequate to support a conclusion."[1] State courts define substantial or sufficient evidence similarly.

The Court's Role as Gatekeeper for Reliable Evidence

All evidence in a legal proceeding is admitted subject to the rules of evidence of the court (or tribunal) hearing the case. Each jurisdiction will have rules about the admissibility of evidence and qualifications of experts. These rules are intended to ensure that the fact-finder (jury, judge, or agency adjudicator) hears or considers only evidence that is reliable and relevant. The court is responsible for keeping "unreliable and irrelevant information from the jury," because of its "inability to assist in factual determinations, its potential to create confusion, and its lack of probative value."[2] The gate-keeping role is important because "the expert's opinion can be both powerful and quite misleading because of the difficulty in evaluating it."[3] There is a delicate balance between the role of gatekeeper and the jury as ultimate fact-finder. The court may not "evaluate the credibility of opposing experts" or the "persuasiveness of competing scientific studies," but limits its duty to "ensur[ing] that the fact-finder weighs only sound and reliable evidence."[4]

In an administrative hearing, such as in a workers' compensation or Social Security hearing, there is no jury. An agency adjudicator, such as an ALJ or hearing officer, fulfills the role of both judge and jury as fact-finder. Evidence standards in agency hearings may, consequently, be less restrictive because there is no need to screen out unreliable evidence for the layperson jury. However, this does not mean that the FCE does not have to meet high standards. The FCE evidence is still subject to cross examination and appeal for being insufficient to support a conclusion.

Rules on Admissibility of Expert Testimony

Historically, federal and state courts admitted expert testimony if the expert's opinion was based on scientific evidence "generally accepted" as reliable in the relevant scientific community.[5] This is known as the *Frye* standard for admissibility of scientific expert opinions. Many state courts still use this standard.

In 1975, Congress adopted Federal Rules of Evidence (FRE) that changed the rule for admissibility of expert testimony in the federal courts. FRE 702 has become known as the *Daubert* standard. Rule 702 states: "If scientific, technical, or other specialized knowledge will assist the trier of fact to understand the evidence or to determine a fact in issue, a witness qualified as an expert by knowledge, skill, experience, training or education, may testify thereto in the form of an opinion or otherwise, if: 1) the testimony is based upon sufficient facts or data, 2) the testimony is the product of reliable principles and methods, and 3) the witness has applied the principles and methods reliably to the facts of the case."[6]

The rationale for changing from the *Frye* to the *Daubert* (Rule 702) standard was to provide a more flexible rule for new scientific methods so that expert testimony would be admissible as long as the method had scientific reliability, even though it may not have yet acquired broad-based acceptance in the relevant scientific community.

The Supreme Court interpreted rule 702 in *Daubert v. Merrell Dow Pharmaceuticals* to require the judge to consider the following: (1) whether the expert's underlying method or technique had been or could be tested; (2) whether it had been subjected to peer review; (3) whether it had a known or potential rate of error; and (4) whether and to what degree the method or technique had been accepted within the relevant scientific community.[7] These are the inquiries that will determine whether FCE evidence is admitted in a *Daubert* jurisdiction.

Some state courts have adopted something between the *Frye* and *Daubert* standards. In administrative agency hearings such as workers' compensation or Social Security disability hearings in which a judge or hearing officer is the fact-finder instead of a jury, a lower standard of admissibility of expert testimony may be the rule. For example, the "Rule of Privilege" allows evidence to be admitted if it is "the kind of evidence that reasonable persons are accustomed to rely on in the conduct of serious affairs."[8] Although more evidence gets in under these lower standards, the evidence may be assigned a lower weight if found to lack credibility after cross-examination.

Regardless of what scientific reliability standards the evidence is held to, the evidence must be relevant to the facts in the case. In addition, it is still subject to cross-examination and appeal, and even if admitted, must survive several challenges that are discussed below.

Relevancy Issues

As a threshold issue, evidence must be relevant and help the fact-finder determine an issue in the case to be admissible. Relevant evidence is defined as "evidence having any tendency to make the existence of any fact that is of consequence to the determination of the action more probable or less probable than it would be without the evidence."[9] The FCE evidence is used in legal controversies in which the plaintiff is seeking damages or compensation for an injury or illness. The threshold for liability or entitlement to a benefit or compensation depends on the applicable laws that govern the case. The proof required to determine eligibility for compensation may also vary by jurisdiction. The FCE provider must know the legal questions to provide evidence in the written documentation or testimony that will assist the fact-finder (judge or jury) in determining a fact at issue in the case. Some of the legal questions are common to each type of case and are discussed in the following sections.

Workers' Compensation

In most states, workers' compensation cases are decided through an administrative agency process, such as a hearing before an ALJ or a hearing officer. In a workers' compensation claim, entitlement to benefits depends on whether the injury arose out of and in connection with work.[10] Each state has specific statutes, regulations, and case law that will specifically define whether a work-related injury is compensable under the state's workers' compensation act. Causation is the most common controversy, which may involve the following: (1) whether the injury really occurred at work, (2) whether the injury was in connection with work activity vs non–work activity, and (3) whether the manifestation of symptoms or disability are a result of an injurious work activity or a pre-existing condition.

The FCE evidence does not assist the fact-finder in answering the first two questions because the FCE does not address causation per se. However, FCE evidence may assist the fact-finder in distinguishing the source of the work incapacities. Take the example of a worker with pre-existing chronic obstructive pulmonary disease and high blood pressure who sustains a work-related low back injury and is rehabilitated but still cannot return to work because he cannot repetitively lift the required 25 lb. The worker's continued entitlement to workers' compensation benefits depends on whether the work incapacity is due to the work-related injury or the pre-existing conditions. Documentation and/or testimony from the FCE expert indicating that lifting is safe but repetition is limited by shortness of breath or other cardiovascular signs can help the fact-finder decide that the residual work incapacity is not work-related, even though the work-related injury initially caused the incapacity. In this case, the FCE must collect and correlate the physical findings to the functional tests to substantiate any limitations.

Once it has been determined that the injury arose out of and in connection with work, the worker is entitled to workers' compensation benefits. The next legal question is whether or to what extent the employee has work capacity or is entitled to temporary or permanent indemnity benefits. Functional capacity evidence can help answer this question, but first the evaluator needs to know whether the statute requires the employer to make reasonable accommodations and whether the employee is required to do *any* suitable work. Answers to both of these questions help the provider know how to structure an FCE to collect relevant evidence about the worker's capacity to perform other available jobs with or without accommodations. If the state requires an employee to accept "reasonable employment," the provider must know what the definition of reasonable employment is to answer the legal question. For example, Maine's workers' compensation statute defines *reasonable employment* as "work that is within the employee's capacity to perform that *poses no clear and proximate threat to the employee's health and safety....*"[11] Under this definition, FCE evidence would answer the legal question only if the FCE data reported maximum performance in terms of what was *safe*, not in terms of what the claimant was willing to do if he or she were willing to exceed safety standards. If the FCE data reports performance levels that are *beyond* safety limits, the FCE does not answer the statutory question and overestimates what is reasonable employment.

Private Insurance Disability Claims

The legal issues in disability claims are quite different from workers' compensation. The extent of the disability, not causation, is the issue. To determine if the claimant is entitled to benefits, the insurance policy must be considered.

Private disability insurance policies are contracts between the insurance company and the individual. The policy will describe what proof of disability is required to receive benefits. In general, a disability policy will insure a person against being disabled from his or her "own occupation" or "any occupation." A person who has an "own occupation" insurance policy must only prove that he or she cannot perform the essential job functions of that occupation. The FCE may therefore be shortened significantly to include only the most physically challenging essential functions because failure on any essential function will entitle the claimant to benefits. Additional standardized FCE test items provide no additional relevant evidence to the claim and are, therefore, only an unnecessary expense.

When a person has an "any occupation" policy (most common among group disability policies), a standardized FCE is appropriate to identify a general level of work the claimant may be able to tolerate. Precautions and limitations should be identified if they narrow the scope of meaningful work that a claimant can do within a general work category.

Claimants have the burden of proving they are disabled and entitled to benefits under the policy. The insurer decides whether the burden of proof has been met under the contract with the insured and the laws governing the plan. Claimants must exhaust all internal appeals with an insurance company when their claims have been denied before filing suit against the insurer in the jurisdiction that governs the policy. Private insurance policies are regulated under state insurance law unless the plan is exempt from state regulation under the Employee Retirement Income Security Act (ERISA). Under ERISA, the plan administrator's disability determination is given great deference by the courts and will be overturned only for abuse of discretion.[12] The level of proof required to support the insurer's denial of disability benefits may be lower in an ERISA plan. Although ERISA law is complicated and beyond the scope of this chapter, FCE providers should be aware that, generally speaking, ERISA plans give great decision-making power to the plan administrator and have very little federal oversight.

Social Security Disability

The Social Security Act[13] provides disability insurance benefits to people who have a physical or mental disability. *Disability* is defined as an "inability to

CHAPTER 20

engage in any substantial gainful activity by reason of any medically determinable physical or mental impairment that has lasted or can be expected to last for a continuous period of not less than 12 months."[14] A claimant's disability must be so severe that he or she cannot, considering his or her age, education, and work experience, engage in *any* substantial gainful work that exists in the *national economy*, regardless of whether such work is available where the claimant lives or whether he or she would be hired if he or she applied for work.[15]

The Social Security disability claims are decided by an ALJ through a sequential five-step process. Social Security statutes and regulations set forth burdens of proof that must be met to prove or disprove entitlement to benefits under the Act. Social Security disability entitlement essentially involves the following: (1) a determination of the person's inability to perform work done in the past and (2) identification of transferable skills or residual work capacity to perform other work in the national economy. If the claimant is found to have a severe impairment or combination of impairments that meets or equals an impairment in the Listing of Impairments,[16] the claimant is presumed disabled with or without FCE evidence. If the claimant's impairments are not in the Listing of Impairments or equal to the Listing of Impairments, the claimant has the burden of proving that his or her residual functional capacity (RFC) is not sufficient to perform past relevant work to be entitled to benefits.[17] Past relevant work refers to any work the claimant has previously done. A job-specific FCE that tests the essential functions of all past jobs held by the claimant will provide the most reliable and valid evidence to meet the claimant's burden of proof. Additional standardized FCE data are not required at this stage. In fact, the claimant or the claimant's attorney may not want additional FCE data to be collected because proving that the claimant cannot do *any work* is the ALJ's burden. If a standardized FCE is done at this stage, the FCE provider's professional opinion should state specifically whether the claimant can perform past relevant work, not just the general category of work the claimant can perform.

Once the claimant proves he or she cannot perform past relevant work, the burden shifts to the ALJ to show that, despite the claimant's impairments and inability to perform past work, he or she has the RFC to perform other work that exists in the national economy.[18] A vocational expert must be consulted to identify other work in the national economy, but the claimant must have the transferable skills and RFC that match the proposed work. At this stage, the standardized FCE would provide the best evidence to meet the ALJ's burden. Therefore, the FCE provider must know who the referral source is so he or she will know whether to perform a standardized or job-specific test.

In a Social Security claim, the ALJ *must* consider the claimant's pain and symptoms together with other evidence.[19] The ALJ will consider the claimant's statements about the intensity, persistence, and limiting effects of pain and will evaluate those statements in relation to the objective medical evidence and other evidence in reaching a conclusion as to whether the claimant is disabled.[20] The ALJ may reject the claimant's testimony about the severity of pain and symptoms only if he or she provides "specific, clear, and convincing reasons for doing so."[21] Therefore, the FCE provider should report the claimant's subjective complaints of pain throughout the FCE. Lack of pain or no change in pain or symptoms during the FCE test is equally important because it may provide clear and convincing evidence that the claimant is not disabled despite pain and symptoms being considered. More important, monitoring of pain and symptoms throughout the FCE can be important to protect the FCE provider against malpractice claims should someone claim to have been further injured during the FCE.

Last, in Social Security cases, FCE evidence is considered only when provided by "acceptable medical sources." Non-physician FCE providers are not considered acceptable medical sources. Therefore, the FCE must be adopted and relied on by the testifying physician to carry weight.[22]

Personal Injury Cases (Civil Litigation)

Personal injury cases are civil lawsuits in state or federal court. A plaintiff in a personal injury lawsuit must prove that he or she has suffered damages from the negligent acts of a defendant. The plaintiff must first prove the defendant owed a duty of care and that the duty of care was breached. If there was no duty or if the duty of care (or standard of care in a malpractice claim) was not breached, there is no negligence, even if there are damages. Once the plaintiff proves that a duty of care was breached and the defendant was negligent, the plaintiff must prove that the defendant's negligence was the actual cause of the plaintiff's injuries or damages. At this point, the legal questions include causation, legitimacy and extent of the impairments and disabilities, the amount of damages from pain and suffering, loss of work, loss of consortium, and estimated future medical expenses. The FCE evidence may be used to answer these legal questions. Damages may be awarded to the plaintiff for any injury that causes impairment or pain whether it results in a functional disability or not if the defendant was negligent. Therefore, while the extent of the disability may increase the damage award, complete incapacity is not necessary to receive some compensation for damages. In these cases, measurements of musculoskeletal impairments (or lack thereof) and a thorough assessment of pain may be as important as the quantification of the functional disabilities.

Both plaintiff and defense attorneys use FCE experts in personal injury cases. The FCE provider must know which side he or she has been hired by, not to be able to function as a "hired gun," but to understand what evidence the referral source needs to meet their burden of proof. Contrary to popular belief, attorneys want medical professionals to provide an objective analysis of the strengths and weaknesses of the medical and FCE evidence. This analysis helps attorneys negotiate a settlement closer to the realistic value of the case or know when to push a case to trial if a settlement agreement cannot be reached.

Challenges to the Functional Capacity Evaluation Expert's Qualifications

An FCE provider may testify as a fact witness or an expert witness, but only an expert witness can offer a professional opinion about a fact at issue in the case. To testify as an expert witness, the FCE provider must be qualified as an expert before opinion testimony is offered. If there is an objection to the admission of the expert's testimony, the judge will review the expert's qualifications and hear arguments for and against admission of the testimony outside the presence of the jury. "There is no mechanical checklist for measuring whether an expert is qualified to offer opinion evidence in a particular field,"[1] but the courts consider the expert's skill, experience, training, and education.[23] The courts look for experts to use the "same level of intellectual rigor that characterizes the practice of an expert in the relevant field."[1] If the testimony is allowed (the objection overruled), the expert's qualifications must still be identified to the jury so the jury can weigh the expert's credibility. The expert's credentials will also be subject to cross-examination.

A physician can give the ultimate opinion from the FCE data. Physician experts are entitled to rely on data and tests performed by others in formulating opinions as long as that reliance is reasonable. This transfers the burden of showing the FCE evidence is admissible and credible to the physician. If the FCE survives the admissibility challenge, the physician will still be subject to cross-examination on the methods, so it behooves the physician to understand the FCE methods used and rely only on credible and qualified providers.

Professional opinions from FCE data may include the following: (1) what physical demand category of work from the *Dictionary of Occupational Titles* the claimant/plaintiff is predicted to be able to tolerate in an 8-hour work day, (2) whether a worker can return to a specific job or any job with or without accommodations, (3) whether the worker gave full effort on the test, and (4) whether the worker has potential to improve his or her tolerance for work demands with rehabilitation or has reached maximum functional improvement. The expert relies on a review of the medical records, physical examination findings, and the interpretation of the FCE data to formulate his or her opinion. Therefore, to be credible,

FCE providers must have the skills and statutory scope of practice to reach the conclusions formulated in their professional opinion.

The FCEs that have been performed by providers who are acting outside their legal scope of practice can be discredited if the opposing side knows what issues to raise in objection to the expert. A recent workers' compensation case in Delaware is a good example of how bad case law can develop when the attorneys do not assert the right basis for their objection to the expert's testimony. The Delaware Superior Court upheld on appeal the Industrial Accident Board's decision that a physical therapist assistant (PTA) was qualified to testify as an FCE expert.[24] Apparently, the issue that the PTA is prohibited by the regulations of the Examining Board of Physical Therapists and Athletic Trainers from performing evaluations was not raised.[25] Had the issue been raised that the PTA may have violated the Physical Therapy Practice Act by performing an evaluation, the outcome of the case may have been different. The North Carolina Board of Physical Therapy Examiners recently adopted the position that the PTA is qualified and permitted by the North Carolina Physical Therapy Practice Act to *assist* the physical therapist with the performance of an FCE on a *limited and restricted basis*. A PTA *may not* perform FCEs independently. After a thorough description of an FCE and a statement of the limited tasks a PTA can perform with regard to data collection in an FCE, the Board concluded that it must be the physical therapist who makes "all observations that require an evaluation or determination, including whether a task can be performed in the workplace, at what level a task can be performed, or how long the task can be performed."[26]

The North Carolina position statement provides evidence that the qualifications of persons opining to be FCE experts is a serious issue. Unqualified providers may erroneously be recognized as experts by the courts from time to time, but FCE providers should know that a smart attorney will use practice act statute and regulations, licensure board opinions, and practice guidelines from professional associations to discredit the FCE provider's testimony.[27]

Challenges to the General Acceptance of or Scientific Support for the Expert's Testimony

Once the witness is qualified as an expert and it is determined that his or her testimony is relevant and will assist the fact-finder, the witness may testify in the form of an opinion or otherwise, subject to the jurisdiction's admissibility rules regarding the reliability of the evidence supporting the opinion. When an expert's opinion is challenged, the court will evaluate the methods used to form the basis of the opinion. If the methods used to formulate the opinion meet the court's requirements, the certainty of a medical opinion must only be within a "reasonable degree of medical certainty" to meet the sufficiency requirement. This is a preponderance of the evidence standard, which means that the evidence to support the opinion just has to outweigh other possibilities.

Frye Jurisdictions

In courts that use the *Frye* standard (Table 20–2) to determine whether evidence is admissible, the judge must decide whether the evidence has gained sufficient "general acceptance" in the FCE community. Case law in various jurisdictions may provide more guidance on how general acceptance is determined, but it does not require the judge to separately analyze the scientific method. For example, the Florida Supreme Court held that general acceptance may be satisfied by establishing that the technique is supported by a "clear majority" of the members of that scientific community, not a unanimous view.[28] A clear majority may not be required for a specific FCE approach, but for the collective view that functional testing is a generally accepted method to determine work capacity. General acceptance would be established through testimony of the expert who is the proponent of the evidence, subject to the arguments from the opponent of the evidence that the method does not have general acceptance. The *Frye* standard may be easily met by using an FCE protocol that is well established in the market, whether it has been scientifically tested or not. This does not, however, mean that the expert's testimony will be admissible or carry weight. The FCE opinion will still be subject to scientific scrutiny on cross-examination and must still be relevant to facts in the case.[29] Therefore, although the FCE evidence may be more easily admitted under the *Frye* standard, it may not carry evidentiary weight if it is not found to be credible.

Daubert Jurisdictions

Federal courts and some state courts are *Daubert* jurisdictions (see Table 20–2). The Supreme Court held in *Kumho Tire v. Carmichael* that the judge's gate-keeping obligation in *Daubert* jurisdictions extended to all expert testimony, including opinions proffered by experts with technical or other specialized knowledge.[30] This leaves no doubt about whether the *Daubert* standards apply to FCE testimony in *Daubert* jurisdictions.

Once the expert is qualified, the *Daubert* analysis has two prongs. The first requires that the judge analyze the scientific reliability and validity forming the basis for the expert's opinion. The second is to determine whether the scientific methods used and conclusions generated were relevant to the facts in the case.[7]

TABLE 20–2	Standards of Admissibility of Expert Testimony in Workers' Compensation Cases in Selected States

State	Standard
Alaska	Daubert
California	Frye
Florida	Frye
Idaho	Daubert
Kentucky	Daubert
Louisiana	Daubert
Massachusetts	Daubert
Minnesota	Frye
Mississippi	Frye
Montana	Daubert
New Jersey	Frye
New Mexico	Daubert (with some exceptions)
North Dakota	Frye
Ohio	Daubert
Oklahoma	Daubert
Rhode Island	Daubert
South Dakota	Daubert
Texas	Daubert
Wyoming	Daubert

CHAPTER 20

The Scientific Reliability Prong The *Daubert* analysis cannot begin until the FCE methods used are known. The FCE methods that are not disclosed because they are proprietary secrets will not likely survive a *Daubert* challenge. Whether all four *Daubert* factors (previously mentioned) are pertinent may depend "on the nature of the issue, the expert's particular expertise, and the subject of his testimony."[30] The judge has broad discretion to determine admissibility[31] subject to a fundamental requirement of reliability, which, at minimum, requires that the expert use "the same level of intellectual rigor" he or she would use outside the courtroom when working in the relevant discipline.[30] The expert must account for "how and why" the proffered opinion was reached.[31]

The *Reference Manual on Scientific Evidence*[32] was written to assist judges in evaluating scientific evidence. It states that in law, the word *evidence* has a precise meaning, and rules govern what evidence is admissible in court. In science, evidence may be something less than *proof.*[32] The *Reference Manual* also distinguishes the meaning of *error* in science and law. In law, an error is synonymous with mistake, whereas in science, error and mistake have different meanings. The authors of Chapter 21, The Scientific Status of FCE, distinguish reliability from error, stating "reliability concerns the degree to which patients can be distinguished from each other, despite measurement error." Under the *Daubert* standards, the court is interested not only in reliability, but also in error rate. "A high confidence level [the confidence interval that measures standard error or the likelihood of random error alone] means very little, but a high confidence level for a small interval is impressive, indicating that random error in the sample estimate is low."[32] The magnitude of the error and its potential impact may be very important. In criminal cases in which a defendant may lose his or her freedom, the courts will expect the expert's opinion to have a very low error rate. With regard to FCEs, a high error rate could mean the difference between receiving long-term disability benefits or not.

Research studies on the BTE (BTE Technologies, Hanover, MD) are good examples of this issue. In one study, the test-retest reliability of handgrip and lifting was found to be reliable in healthy subjects,[33] but in another study comparing real and simulated lift tasks, the results suggested that the BTE may overestimate actual lifting abilities.[34] These two studies together suggest that an FCE opinion based on BTE tests may have a substantial potential for error in predicting lift ability even though the test results are repeatable.

The Relevancy Prong The second prong of the *Daubert* test addresses the relevancy of the scientific methods as applied to the facts in the case. The 11th Circuit Court assesses: "whether the reasoning or methodology underlying the testimony is ... valid and whether that reasoning or methodology properly can be applied to the facts at issue."[3] Testimony is not reliable when it fails to "fit" with the facts of the case.[35] Testimony lacks fit when "a large analytical leap must be made between the facts and the opinion."[31] Thus, testimony may be reliable but nevertheless excluded if it does not have "sufficient bearing on the issue at hand to warrant a determination that it [is 'helpful' to the trier of fact]."[36]

A common example of an FCE lacking fit is when a standardized FCE tries to answer the legal question of whether a claimant can perform a specific job. Even if the standardized FCE has good interrater or intrarater reliability for identifying safe maximum performance on standardized FCE tasks, the FCE results will be irrelevant if they lack fit with the specific job requirements.

It is important to distinguish between the test methods and the conclusions they generate. The methods themselves must be reliable and relevant to the legal question, but the professional does not have to be 100% certain to provide a credible opinion. The professional opinion need only be stated as a "more likely than not" conclusion. If the FCE provider's opinion is based on a rational analysis of reliable methods, the provider should not be afraid to make a definitive statement. Opinions that express possibilities (such as may, might, and could) instead of probabilities (such as more likely than not and within a reasonable degree of medical probability) do not carry legal weight and may not satisfy the relevancy rule for evidence.[37] However, when there is a large analytical gap between the provider's opinion and the data, the opinion can be characterized as speculative and unreliable.

This distinction can be seen in the FCE provider's ultimate opinion of the category of work to which a person can return. The FCE providers must be very careful about concluding what general level of work an evaluee can do without qualifying what activities might be limited within that category. Take the case of a plaintiff who can safely lift a maximum of 30 lb on a kinesiophysical lifting test. There is a growing body of evidence to support the interrater and intrarater reliability of determining a safe maximum lift using the kinesiophysical approach,[38–40] whereas the interrater reliability of identifying static position tolerance is not as good. If the legal question is what level of lifting can the plaintiff perform at work, the kinesiophysical FCE methods of determining maximum lifting ability at 30 lb would survive a *Daubert* analysis. The FCE provider's ultimate opinion that the plaintiff can more likely than not perform lifting activity in the medium category of work (20–50 lb occasionally) is supported by reliable methods. However, the legal question "Can the plaintiff tolerate sitting at a sedentary job 8 hours per day?" is not answered with this data, even though it is presumed that the plaintiff can do sedentary work if he or she can do medium-level work. The otherwise reliable lifting data lack "fit" with the legal question and, therefore, do not pass the relevancy prong of the *Daubert* analysis. The FCE methods that teach reliance on dynamic lifting data alone to assign a category of work would be unlikely to pass muster under *Daubert* or *Frye* because the data is irrelevant to the facts and legal questions in the case.

Many providers question the reliability of extrapolating from the FCE to predict an evaluee's ability to perform during an 8-hour day. Extrapolation methods have not been adequately studied, but the expert FCE provider can give an admissible professional opinion on this issue if the opinion is based on relevant and reliable data. At least the FCE is based on some objective data vs a physician's best guess.

CHAPTER 20

of Effort as an Ultimate Opinion

Most FCEs have some method of evaluating whether the evaluee is giving a full effort on the test. The FCE provider must understand that this ultimate opinion must be supported by a reliable method. The science behind these determinations is discussed in Chapters 11 and 21, but the misuse of the terminology in the legal context is worth discussing here. The term *validity* has been misused by FCE providers and is misunderstood by the legal profession. Validity, in scientific and legal terms, refers to "the extent to which an instrument measures what it is supposed to, rather than something else."[32] When the term *validity* is used to describe whether a claimant is giving full effort, it confuses lawyers and judges. Other terms, such as *malingering* and *symptom magnification,* imply intentional fraudulent behaviors. *Sincerity of effort* implies that the test measured some element of the claimant's psyche to determine whether he or she was "sincere." The use of the word *submaximal* or *inconsistent* to describe the level of effort or performance may be more factually accurate. These terms simply describe the performance without speculating as to the reason for it. The FCE provider should keep this in mind when deciding how to label an evaluee's effort. Because this label reflects the provider's ultimate opinion, the provider should choose the label carefully. The label should reflect only what can be reliably deduced from the test. If the test did not measure intent, the FCE provider should not label the effort as insincere or invalid. The FCE provider could come across as being biased by inappropriately assigning a speculative, inaccurate label. More important, the FCE provider should not overestimate the value of such tests. Such tests frequently do not answer the legal question (unless the question is whether the claimant is committing fraud) and, thus, do not always help resolve the case.

Cross-examination of the Functional Capacity Evaluation Witness

It is more likely that FCE providers will encounter credibility challenges on cross-examination than challenges to the admissibility of their testimony. The Advisory committee notes to rule 702 under the Federal Rules of Evidence gives further guidance on evaluating whether an expert's testimony is credible, suggesting an analysis of the following[41]: (1) whether the expert is proposing to testify about matters growing naturally and directly out of research he or she has conducted independent of litigation, or whether he or she has developed his or her opinion expressly for the purposes of testifying; (2) whether the expert has unjustifiably extrapolated from an accepted premise to an unfounded conclusion; (3) whether the expert has adequately accounted for obvious alternative explanations; (4) whether the expert is being as careful as he or she would be in his or her regular professional work outside paid litigation consulting; and (5) whether the field of expertise claimed by the expert is known to reach reliable results for the type of opinion the expert would give.[42] These are all appropriate inquiries for cross-examination if the expert is allowed to testify.

The opposing attorney will ask the expert about education, training in the provision of FCEs, years of experience performing FCEs, and number of FCEs performed. Even the most experienced FCE provider can be tripped up by the spin the attorney places on the question. For example, an attorney may ask what percentage of the provider's revenue comes from performing FCEs. If this service is a very small percentage of the provider's practice, the inference would be that he or she cannot possibly be an expert.

Provider bias will also be explored. The opposing attorney will ask the provider by whom he or she was hired, how many referrals come from plaintiff vs defense attorneys, and, perhaps, how much he or she was paid. Treating providers are expected to have a more intimate knowledge of their patient's condition but are also expected to be biased in favor of their patient. The treating provider may be permitted to testify as a fact or expert witness, ensuring that the witness gets to testify at least to the facts even if not to his or her expert opinion. Nontreating providers who see a claimant for a one-time consultation are expected to be more objective but to have less intimate knowledge of the patient's condition. However, experts hired only for litigation purposes and not to evaluate or treat the patient do not qualify as fact witnesses and, therefore, do not get to testify at all if not qualified as an expert.

In my experience, cross-examination of the methods and foundation for the expert's opinion are not directed so much at the scientific evidence as the *Daubert* analysis would suggest. A cross-examination of scientific methods may bore or overwhelm the jury. However, because juries are capable of rationale thought, the FCE provider can expect attacks on the most simple facts on which the opinion is based. For example, "Is overhead lifting safe when the arms begin to shake?" "The plaintiff told you that he had pain, didn't he?" "Is it your opinion that the plaintiff can work in a stooped position frequently even though he has a disk bulge and his pain increased from 5/10 to 7/10 on a 5-minute stooped standing test?" The attorney's job is to bring out inconsistencies in the expert's testimony by asking closed-ended questions. However, a good, objective FCE can actually help both sides (and the jury) reach middle ground, which is the best situation for the FCE expert because neither side wants to discredit the witness.

For example, take the case of a slip-and-fall injury in a parking lot in which the owner of the premises breaches a duty to keep the parking lot free of hazards, resulting in the plaintiff sustaining a fractured patella. The defense attorney refers the plaintiff to the FCE provider to quantify the damages right before trial.

By this time, the plaintiff has had successful rehabilitation and has returned to modified work activity. His range of motion impairments are minimal, strength is normal, and gait is essentially unimpaired. During the FCE, the plaintiff gives full effort and even overestimates his safe work abilities. He is able to perform medium-level work in general but is limited in kneeling on the bad knee, squatting repetitively, and sustaining a full-range squat. These limitations would not impair one's ability to perform many manual labor jobs, but this plaintiff happens to be a roofer. Although his impairments are minimal, he cannot assume or sustain a full-squat position for roofing work. The plaintiff also claims he is unable to play golf, which is not supported by the FCE. Although the FCE expert was hired by the defense, the objective FCE helps both sides. The defense attorney can make the most of the testimony that the impairments are minimal; the plaintiff is still functioning at a high level and can still play golf, which minimizes the damages. The plaintiff's attorney can make the most of the fact that the plaintiff gave full effort and is disabled from roofing work. Neither side wants to discredit the FCE provider for fear of losing an important piece of evidence for their case.

Legal Issues in Employment Screenings

In Chapter 13, the authors discuss the scientific evidence for the use of FCEs in preemployment or postoffer employment screenings. However, it is critical to note that employment laws drive this area of practice. There are significant legal risks for any organization that uses any type of physical performance test as a criterion in hiring or placement; therefore, health care providers who offer this service should be knowledgeable of the laws and seek legal counsel to ensure their procedures comply with the laws.

In the United States, the laws that govern the use of functional tests for employee selection are the Civil Rights Act of 1964, which prohibits discrimination based on gender, race, religion, and national origin, and the Americans with Disabilities Act (ADA), which prohibits discrimination against otherwise qualified persons with disabilities.[42] The antidiscrimination provisions in both Acts are essentially the same: to determine whether an applicant is qualified for a job, the selection criteria (or postoffer screening under the ADA) must be job-related and consistent with business necessity. The Equal Employment Opportunity Commission (EEOC) has regulations in place to help employers comply with both Acts. Under the ADA, the regulations specifically identify what examination procedures may be performed before and after an offer of employment is made and which procedures can be used to validate that the employee meets the job qualifications.

Under the Civil Rights Act, the EEOC has developed Uniform Guidelines on Employee Selection Procedures.[43] These guidelines tell employers how to determine if a selection procedure is legal and how to validate selection procedures that tend to screen out people in a protected class. Jobs with heavy physical demands may use selection procedures to legitimately screen out candidates with less physical strength. If the candidates who are screened out are disproportionately women or people with disabilities, the employer must be able to prove that the selection procedure was job-related with content, construct, or criterion validity data. These validity measures are scientifically defined in other sections of this book, but it is important to understand the government's definition as it relates to the legal use of functional tests in preplacement and postoffer examinations.

Content Validity

According to the EEOC guidelines, content validity is established by showing the selection procedure is representative of important aspects of performance on the job. The guidelines clearly link the analysis of the selection procedure's validity to the job analysis. Content validity cannot be established from job descriptions that are old, inaccurate, or have not been validated by incumbent workers or objective physical measurements. Therefore, a job-specific FCE or any physical tests that mimic the essential job demands could meet content validity requirements, whereas a standardized FCE may not.

Criterion Validity

Criterion-related validity is "demonstrated by empirical data showing that the selection procedure is predictive of or significantly correlated with important elements of work behavior."[43] If the selection procedure does not have content validity but still claims to test important job-related functions, it must have criterion validity. An example of a screening tool that claims to have criterion validity is isokinetic testing. While clinicians may agree in general that it is important to have good back strength for heavy-lifting jobs, it is more difficult to determine at what level the strength (or strength deficit) crosses the line from being a "potential risk" for injury (which cannot be used to deny employment) to a direct threat to the health and safety of the employee or others (which can be used to deny employment). More important, it is difficult to show the link between a test done on a machine and the actual job functions because there are too many variables.

Many selection procedures, including isokinetic tests, attempt to borrow criterion validity from published or nonpublished studies performed by others.

However, the EEOC makes it clear that such borrowed studies can be used only to prove the validity of the employer's test under three conditions: (1) when the population tested in the validity study has the same work demands as employees being screened; (2) when the validity study includes a study of test fairness for each racial, sex, and ethnic group relevant to a labor market; and (3) when there are no validity variables between the borrowed validity study and the employer's jobs. If variables are present, employers must complete an internal validity study, which can be costly and time-consuming.

Construct Validity

Construct validity is "demonstrated by data showing that the selection procedure measures the degree to which candidates have identifiable characteristics which have been determined to be important for successful job performance."[43] The guidelines caution that construct validity is a more complex way to prove the validity of the selection procedure.[43]

After validity is proven, the employer must prove that there were no suitable selection criteria that were less discriminatory as an alternative. This requirement can be satisfied by choosing appropriate cutoff scores or "exclusion criteria" at the level at which applicants pose a direct threat to the health and safety of themselves or others. A *direct threat* is defined as a "significant" and "imminent" threat, not a speculative or potential risk. Applicants who cannot perform the essential job functions with or without accommodations do not meet the job qualifications.

EEOC v Dial Corp

When a screening examination is not properly designed, the stakes can be quite high for the company. The *Dial* case is a good example of the legal risks a company assumes by using a poorly designed employment screening examination. In *EEOC v Dial*, the federal appeals court upheld a decision that Dial Corporation had discriminated against women by not offering jobs to female applicants who failed a "strength" test.[44] The company was hit with a judgment of $3.2 million, to be paid to 52 rejected female job applicants. The screening examination designed and used by health care professionals at Dial was not unlike examinations typically performed at a wide range of companies across the country.

In 2000, Dial began requiring employees to pass a work tolerance screen (WTS) in an effort to reduce workplace injuries. This test consisted of lifting and carrying a 35-lb bar and placing it between 2 frames at 30 in and 60 in off the floor, to simulate the essential job function of lifting and carrying 35 lb of sausage.

During a normal work shift, an employee would lift and carry approximately 18,000 lb and walk the equivalent of 4 mi.

The company's attempt to design a valid job-related test failed, however, because applicants worked faster during the screening test than they were required to work on the actual job. Workers on the job performed only 1.25 lifts per minute, with rests between lifts. Although applicants were told to go at their own pace during the test, they still performed 6 lifts per minute without breaks on the WTS.

The court determined that the screening examination did not have content validity because the frequency of lifting on the WTS did not match the job requirements. In addition, it appeared that the pass-fail criteria were subjective and inconsistently applied, exposing Dial to suspicion about their motives. *Dial* teaches that the risk of civil liability or EEOC fines is significant and real for employers who do not comply with EEOC regulations. It teaches providers of these tests the importance of validating their procedures and consulting legal counsel.

Summary

Functional capacity evaluations provide valuable medicolegal evidence when the provider is qualified and the FCE methods are reliable. When questionable methods are used, providers are not qualified, or opinions are not supported, FCEs as a whole come under scrutiny. Providers need to be aware of the legal issues and stay up-to-date on the research to support their methods and opinions. More important, FCE providers must obtain expert witness skills. Whether the science behind the opinion is reliable or not, the provider must be able to give written and/or verbal testimony that is persuasive and supported.

References

1. *Magallanes v Bowen*, 881 F2d 747, 750 (9th Cir 1989).
2. *Allison v McGhan Med Corp*, 184 F3d 1300, 1311–12 (11th Cir 1999).
3. *US v Frazier*, 387 F3d 1244, 1260 (11th Cir 2004).
4. *Quiet Tech DC-8, Inc v Hurel-Dubois UK, Ltd*, 326 F3d 1333, 1341 (11th Cir 2003); *Frazier*, 387 F3d at 1272.
5. *Frye v US*, 293 F 1013 (DC Cir 1923).
6. Fed. R. Evid. 702 (2007). Federal Rules of Evidence. No. 9. Washington, DC: US Government Printing Office; 2007. Rule 702.

CHAPTER 20

7. *Daubert v Merrell Dow Pharmaceuticals, Inc*, 509 US 579 (1993).
8. 39-A Me Rev Stat Ann §309(2) (2005). (Maine applies a "rule of privilege" in workers' compensation hearings under administrative agency rules.)
9. Federal Rules of Evidence. No. 9. Washington, DC: US Government Printing Office; 2007. Rule 401.
10. Larson A, Larson L. Larson's Workers' Compensation. Albany, NY:Matthew Bender: 1994.
11. 39-A Me Rev Stat Ann §214(5) (2005).
12. *Woo v Deluxe Corp*, 144 F3d 1157 (8th Cir 1998).
13. 42 USC §423 (2006).
14. 42 USC §423(d)(1)(A) (2006).
15. 42 USC §423(d)(2)(A) (2006).
16. 20 CFR §404.1520 (2008).
17. 20 CFR §404.1520(e) (2008).
18. See *Terry v Sullivan*, 903 F2d 1273, 1275 (9th Cir 1990).
19. 20 CFR §404, subpt P, app 2 §200.00(c) (2008).
20. 20 CFR §404.1529(c)(4) (2008).
21. *Smolen v Chater*, 80 F3d 1273, 1281 (9th Cir 1996).
22. 20 CFR §404.1513 and §404.1527 (2008).
23. *Poulis-Minott v Smith*, 388 F3d 354 (1st Cir 2004).
24. *Spencer v Air Liquide Am*, 2008 Del Super Lexis 166, (May 6, 2008).
25. 24 Del C §2602(3) (2008). (The Physical Therapist Assistant *shall not* perform interpretation of referrals, *physical therapy evaluation* [emphasis added] and reevaluation, major modification of the treatment plan, final discharge of the patient, or therapeutic techniques beyond the skill and knowledge of the Physical Therapist Assistant or without proper supervision.
26. North Carolina Board of Physical Therapy Examiners. The Scope of Authority of the Physical Therapist Assistant to Assist the Physical Therapist With Functional Capacity Evaluations: A Position Statement of the North Carolina Board of Physical Therapy Examiners. Durham, NC, North Carolina Board of Physical Therapy Examiners; December 2, 2004. www.ncptboard.org/Office/Positions/FCEPositionStatement12-06-04.htm. Accessed November 19, 2008.
27. American Physical Therapy Association. Occupational Health Physical Therapy: Evaluating Functional Capacity. Alexandria, VA. Available at: www.apta.org/AM/Template.cfm?Section=Policies_and_Bylaws&CONTENTID=29717&TEMPLATE=/CM/ContentDisplay.cfm. (These guidelines were in the process of being amended at the time of this publication.) Accessed November 19, 2008.
28. *US Sugar Corp v Henson*, 787 So 2d 3 (Fla 1st DCA 2001).
29. Federal Rules of Evidence. No. 9. Washington, DC: US Government Printing Office; 2007. Rule 402.
30. *Kumho Tire Co v Carmichael*, 118 S Ct 2339 (1998).
31. *Gen Elec Co v Joiner*, 522 US 136 (1997).
32. Federal Judicial Center. *Reference Manual on Scientific Evidence*. 2nd ed. 2000. www.fjc.gov/public/pdf.nsf/lookup/sciman00.pdf/$file/sciman00.pdf. Accessed November 19, 2008.
33. Lee GK, Chan CC, Hui-Chan CW. Consistency of performance on the functional capacity assessment: static strength and dynamic endurance. *Am J Phys Med Rehabil.* 2001;80:189–195.

34. Ting W, Wessel J, Brintnell S. Maikala R, Bhambhani Y. Validity of the Baltimore Therapeutic Equipment Work Simulator in the measurement of lifting endurance in healthy men. *Am J Occup Ther.* 2001;55:184–190.

35. *McDowell v Brown*, 392 F3d 1283, 1298 (11th Cir 2004).

36. *Bitler v A.O. Smith Corp*, 391 F3d 1114, 1121 (10th Cir 2004).

37. *Bowers v Norfolk S Corp*, 537 F Supp 2d 1343 (Middle D Ga 2007).

38. Lechner DE, Jackson JR, Roth DL, Straaton KV. Reliability and validity of a newly developed test of physical work performance. *J Occup Med.* 1994;36:997–1004.

39. Brouwer S, Reneman MF, Dijkstra PU, Groothoff JW, Schellekens JMH, Göeken LNH. Test-retest reliability of the Isernhagan Work Systems Functional Capacity Evaluation in patients with chronic low back pain. *J Occup Rehabil.* 2003;13:207–218.

40. Gross DL, Battié MC. Reliability of safe maximum lifting determinations of a functional capacity evaluation. *Phys Ther.* 2002;82:364–371.

41. Federal Rules of Evidence. No. 9. Washington, DC: US Government Printing Office; 2007. Rule 702 Advisory Committee Notes.

42. 42 USC §2000e (1964).

43. Section 60–3, Uniform Guidelines on Employee Selection Procedure (1978); 43 FR 38295 (August 25, 1978). www.access.gpo.gov/nara/cfr/waisidx_07/29cfr1607_07.html. Accessed July 11, 2008.

44. *EEOC v Dial Corp*, 49 F3d 735 (8th Cir 2006).

CHAPTER 20

21

The Scientific Status of Functional Capacity Evaluation

Michiel Reneman, PT, PhD, Harriët Wittink, PT, MS, PhD, and Douglas P. Gross, PT, PhD

Describing functional capacity evaluations (FCEs) and their components requires clarification of the terminology commonly used in this area. Confusion reigns regarding the vocabulary used when assessing a patient's capacity to perform a task. Terms such as FCE, functional capacity assessment, physical capacity evaluation, physical performance analysis, work capacity evaluation, work tolerance screening, functional ability evaluation, and many more have been and still are used interchangeably and, in some cases, mistakenly to describe assessments of a person's ability to perform work-related tasks. The International Classification of Functioning, Disability, and Health qualifiers for activities and participation classification make it possible to clearly separate a person's inherent capacity to perform actions within a domain from performance in his or her actual environmental context. *Capacity* refers to the environmentally adjusted inherent ability of the person or, in other words, the highest probable functioning of a person in a given domain at a given point in time in a standardized environment. *Performance*, on the other hand, describes what a person actually does in her or his current environment and, thus, describes the person's functioning as observed or reported in the person's real-life environment with the existing facilitators and barriers.

We use the term *functional capacity evaluation* in this chapter, realizing that the abbreviation FPE (for functional performance evaluation) may be more accurate because in its essence, the FCE is an evaluation of a person's ability to perform activities. As noted in Chapter 1, the FCE reflects not only the person's physical abilities, but also motivation and the degree to which the immediate environment of the evaluee (eg, evaluator and laboratory) tend to encourage greater degrees of demonstrated physical ability. Hence, the degree to which this environment is standardized may affect reproducibility of FCE results, as may the environment in which the FCE takes place, ie, the purpose of the FCE, as well as societal, financial, and cultural influences, to name a few. While the term *performance* may thus be better to describe the essence of the evaluation, the connotation 'FCE,' referring to capacity is more widely known in the field. For this reason, we have chosen to use the term *FCE* rather than *FPE* in this chapter. Placed into the context of work, an FCE becomes a test to measure the individual's ability to perform work-related activities.

This chapter is devoted to the scientific status of FCEs. The main question to address is whether an FCE fulfills the criteria of a useful measuring instrument. The American Physical Therapy Association has published professional practice standards for measurement. In these standards, five issues must be addressed in the selection and use of any test in a patient population. These issues, presented in hierarchical order and adapted for FCE,[1] are as follows:

- **Safety:** Given the known characteristics of the patient, the procedure should not be expected to lead to injury.

- **Reliability:** The test score should be reproducible across evaluators, patients, and the date or time of test administration.
- **Validity:** The interpretation of the test score should be able to predict or reflect the patient's performance in a target work setting.
- **Practicality:** The cost of the test procedure should be reasonable and customary. Cost is measured in terms of the direct expense of the test procedure plus the amount of time required of the patient plus the time required to provide the information derived from the procedure to the referral source.
- **Utility:** The usefulness of the procedure is the degree to which it meets the needs of the patient, referrer, and payer.

The current evidence concerning each of these is discussed in the remainder of this chapter. The status reflects the situation as of summer 2007*. The majority of this chapter is based on literature written in the English language and published

---

* Since this literature review was completed, the Editors are aware of at least two published articles investigating reliability that are not included in this chapter. These are:

1. Brubaker PN, Fearon FJ, Smith SM, et al. Sensitivity and specificity of the Blankenship FCE system's indicators of submaximal effort. Abstract. *J Orthop Sports Phys Ther.* Apr 2007; 37(4): 161–168.

Abstract:
STUDY DESIGN: Single-blinded, randomized, posttest only design.
OBJECTIVE: To help contribute to the body of evidence in defining the validity of functional capacity evaluations. **BACKGROUND:** Functional capacity evaluations (FCEs) are tests used to help determine an individual's readiness to return to work. Most FCEs incorporate indicators of effort within the evaluation. Published evidence validating the use of these indicators is limited. **METHODS AND MEASURES:** Forty-nine injured and noninjured individuals 18 to 65 years of age participated in this study. The participants were randomly assigned to 1 of 2 groups: 100% effort or 50% effort. Raters were blinded to participant group. The Blankenship Version 6.0 software was used to analyze the data and a Blankenship FCE validity profile was scored. A score of 70% or greater was deemed a valid FCE as adopted by the Blankenship protocol. **RESULTS**: The sensitivity of the FCE components tested was demonstrated to be 80% and specificity was 84.2%. The positive likelihood ratio was 5 and the negative likelihood ratio was 0.2. A receiver operating characteristic (ROC) curve demonstrated the 70% cut-off value for scoring the FCE was optimal. **CONCLUSION:** Four components of the

(footnote continued)

CHAPTER 21

in peer-reviewed journals. The literature was retrieved from the electronic data-bases PubMed and MEDLINE by using the following key words: functional OR physical capacity OR performance evaluation OR assessment AND safety OR reliability OR validity OR practicality OR utility. In certain cases, recent unpub-lished developments are mentioned and are identified as such. Only full-length articles were included. A discussion of FCEs designed and used for selection of workers (ie, pre-employment screening) is not included in this chapter. Reports of the psychometric properties of FCE for patients with specific systemic medi-cal diagnoses, such as rheumatoid arthritis, were also not included. Areas that need further scientific attention are identified. The last paragraph of this chapter is dedicated to future research. This chapter ends with a comprehensive list of the scientific literature available to date.

Blankenship FCE system demonstrated good sensitivity and specificity for detect-ing submaximal effort. However, clinicians should note that false positives (maxi-mum effort identified as submaximal effort) may occur and scores of "equivocal" are not scored in the "criteria passed" category. The rater should be aware that this method of scoring could potentially influence a client's overall FCE score.

2. Durand MJ, Brassard B, Hong QN, Lemaire J, Loisel P. Responsiveness of the physical work performance evaluation, a functional capacity evaluation, in patients with low back pain. Abstract. *J Occup Rehabil.* Mar 2008; 18(1): 58–67.

Abstract:
BACKGROUND AND PURPOSE: The Physical Work Performance Evaluation (PWPE) is a functional capacity evaluation. This study investigated the respon-siveness of the PWPE. **METHODS:** The internal and external responsiveness was tested. For the internal responsiveness, the change in the pre-/post-test PWPE scores of a group participating in a work rehabilitation program (n = 27) was compared to that of a comparison group of healthy subjects (n = 30). The external responsiveness was tested with the rehabilitation group, and the change in their PWPE scores was compared to concurrent and empirical criteria. **RESULTS:** The comparison of the change in pre-/post-test PWPE scores showed that the change for the rehabilitation group was significantly different from that for the comparison group, but only for one section of the PWPE. Changes in six criteria were seen after completion of the program, but there was no significant correlation between these changes and the change in the overall PWPE score. **DISCUSSION AND CONCLUSION:** The overall PWPE level of work score does not appear to have the ability to measure clinically significant changes achieved through a work rehabilitation program.

Safety

The term *safety* is often used in FCE literature but rarely defined. The American Physical Therapy Association task force on objective functional measurements defined safety as "given the known characteristics of the evaluee, the procedure should not be expected to lead to new injury."[1(p682)] This definition, however, cannot be tested because a definition for injury is absent, and because of the wording used ("...should not be expected to..."). If an FCE led to an injury but the injury was not expected, should the FCE still be considered safe?

Safety has been researched to determine whether operational definitions of safety could be applied reliably by evaluators during FCEs.[2] These operational definitions of safety include biomechanical, metabolic, and psychophysical aspects to ensure that evaluees remain within defined limits of strength and heart rate and that patients do not perform beyond the point that they feel unsafe or unwilling to proceed. However, whether applying these operational definitions of safety leads to a safe assessment of functional capacity has been investigated only once.[3] Safety was operationally defined as follows: "An FCE was considered safe when no formal complaints of injury were filed by the patients, and when increased symptoms returned to or below their pre-FCE level. A temporary increase in symptom intensity was not considered unsafe." In this study, a total of 92 patients with chronic low back pain (CLBP) underwent an FCE; however, no formal complaints were filed. In addition, although the majority of patients reported an increase in symptom intensity after the FCE, symptoms of all responders returned to the pre-FCE level within weeks. The authors concluded that a temporary increase in symptom intensity following FCEs is common in patients with CLBP; however, within the operational definitions of safety used in the study, FCEs appear safe. No criteria were available to interpret what constitutes a "temporary" increase or how to interpret its intensity and duration; determination of what intensity and duration of increased symptoms is acceptable remains a clinical decision. A temporary increase of symptoms was not considered unsafe. The results may not apply to other (implicit) definitions of injury or safety. However, we are unaware of definitions of safety and injury that are widely agreed on.

Other researchers have also reported findings of pain exacerbation after FCE. It has been reported that some patients refuse to undergo a second test session because they do not feel capable of participation in manual handling activities owing to pain.[4] In a study in which patients with CLBP were retested on the day following the FCE, patients lifted and carried on average 6% to 9% better than the day before.[5] However, 8% to 21% of patients performed worse on the second day. Whether these three observations are related to a large "normal" variation in patient performance or to lack of safety of the FCE is uncertain and should be the subject of future research. Future studies should also consider larger samples to enable multivariate analyses, for example, to predict symptom increase.

Some contradictory findings are reported as well. Biomechanical analyses have demonstrated that during lifting tests of an FCE, healthy subjects lifting 22.5 kg may endure spinal loads that are considered potentially hazardous compared with lifting guidelines.[6] Clinicians have also voiced their opinion that medium to heavy lifting is potentially unsafe.[7] Patients with CLBP, however, have demonstrated abilities to lift (far) beyond 22.5 kg, exceeding "safe" lifting guidelines derived from the National Institute for Occupational Safety and Health recommendations, without evidence of reinjury or other serious adverse effects.[3,8]

Discussion

From the preceding information, it is clear that safety research in FCE is scarce. Researchers have only scratched the surface of this important topic and learned that sound knowledge is lacking. More studies are needed, as are further conceptualization and definition of the constructs safety and injury. Future studies should use validated measures for repeated measurements of pain intensity (visual analog score or numeric rating scales), control for pain medication use, and consider large samples to enable multivariate analyses to predict symptom increase. Future studies should also differentiate between a normal nonspecific response to unusually high-intensity exertion and the onset of "specific" injuries.

Reliability

Introduction of Terms

Reliability involves the extent to which repeated measurements in stable persons provide similar results. The test score should be reproducible across evaluators, patients, and the date or time of test administration. A distinction should be made between reliability and agreement.[9] *Agreement* concerns the absolute measurement error, expressed as the standard error of measurement or by limits of agreement.[10] *Reliability* concerns the degree to which patients can be distinguished from each other, despite measurement error. This reproducibility may be over time (test-retest reliability); between different raters, observers, or evaluators (interrater reliability); between more than one identical session rated by the same evaluator (intrarater reliability); or between equivalent parts of the same test (internal consistency). Although all types of reliability are important, establishment of test-retest and interrater reliability are deemed most important in FCEs because they ensure that any change found in the assessment is the result of change in the person and not the result of measurement inconsistencies over time or between examiners.

The difference between reliability and validity is not always clear. An example of this is internal consistency, an area that may benefit from further development. By examining the correlation between test items, it may be possible to streamline evaluation batteries to include only the items that assess necessary activities, rather than duplicating items that assess the same or similar activities. On the other hand, there may be situations when duplicating items provides information about the consistency of demonstrated limitations that might otherwise not be easily available. This and other aspects of streamlining an FCE are discussed in the section of this chapter that discusses practicality. Another gray area between reliability and validity is responsiveness, which is discussed in the validity section of this chapter.

A number of factors may influence the reproducibility of results. These factors can be grouped into sources of variance: the evaluee, the evaluator, the evaluation, and the occasion. In addition, these sources of variance can interact with each other. A wide range of factors may influence an evaluee's performance. If these factors are known to consistently do so, they are described under validity because if (variance in) performances are consistently correlated with (variance in) other factors, they are then dependent on this factor. Thus, the validity question that should be asked is: "Are we measuring what we intend to measure?" For example, if pain intensity consistently correlates highly with performance, then we are in fact measuring pain intensity (in part), not capacity. A portion of the variance in performance can thus be attributed to variance in pain intensity. There is also a portion of variance that remains unexplained. This portion is called the "natural variation" of the measurement, or measurement error. For an instrument to be precise, the measurement error should be small. Articles that report on reliability should produce not only data on mean differences of gross reliability quotients, but also data on variances of performances and, preferably, on sources of variance.

Published Evidence on Reliability of Functional Capacity Evaluation

In a previous review of the scientific evidence of FCE reliability,[11] it was concluded that the evidence for reliability of a wide range of FCEs ranged from nonexistent to being investigated and reported in sufficient detail. There did not seem to be a single FCE that had been thoroughly and comprehensively investigated for all relevant aspects of reliability. The last review of the scientific evidence of the reliability of four FCEs used in the Netherlands was published in 2004.[12] Of the four FCEs reviewed, three had demonstrated little or no evidence of reliability (Ergos Work Simulator [Simwork Systems of Tucson Inc, Tucson AZ], Blankenship FCE [Quest Medical Group, Inc, West Jordan, UT], and Ergo Kit FCE [Ergo Control, Enschede, the Netherlands]). There was more published evidence on reliability of one FCE (WorkWell FCE [Duluth, MN], formerly known as the Isernhagen Work Systems FCE). Overall, developers and users of FCEs and researchers seem to have a growing understanding of the need to investigate and report on reliability. A number of articles reporting on the reliability of FCEs or tests of FCEs are now published in peer-reviewed journals. Reports containing data of different aspects of reliability were identified for the following FCEs:

- Baltimore Therapeutic Equipment Primus FCE (BTE [BTE Technologies, Hanover, MD]: Test-retest reliability of strength and endurance protocols for handgrip and lifting was evaluated for 30 healthy subjects and found to be good.[13] The reliability of three other tests (isolated wrist flexion and extension and elbow flexion) was also studied, with similar results, but it may be questioned whether these tests should be considered "functional." Apart from these findings, the authors discussed the observed changes in reliability coefficients of their study in that higher consistency was observed among subjects in the assessment of static strength than in the assessment of dynamic endurance strength. They concluded that greater control (standardization) of protocols, leading to lesser degrees of freedom, increased the consistency of performance, which was considered applicable and generalizable to other FCEs.

- Ergo Kit FCE: The reliability of seven items was tested on healthy people by using a within-subjects design with three test occasions and two evaluators (items: isometric back torso lift test, isometric shoulder lift test, forward manipulation test standing, lower manipulation test crouching, carrying lifting strength test, lower lifting strength test, and upper lifting strength test). The isometric and dynamic lifting tests demonstrated moderate to high levels of reliability, and the manipulation tests were found to have low reliability.[14] In 24 patients with CLBP, only the isometric and dynamic lifting protocols were tested, and all demonstrated good reliability with agreement between raters and occasions.[15]

- Ergos Work Simulator: The test-retest reliability of seven upper extremity items (sensibility of fingertips, keyboarding, fingering and handling, hand grip strength, functional pinch strength, strength of palmar and dorsal flexion of the wrist, and strength of wrist pronation and supination) were tested on 12 healthy subjects. A within-subjects counterbalanced design in which testing order and time of testing was varied indicated good reliability for all seven tests.[16] Because these tests all assessed specific upper extremity activities, the occupational relevance (in terms of applying the results of this study to functional assessment other than related to the upper extremities) is unclear.

- Gibson Approach to FCE (GAPP FCE): Findings of a preliminary study of 14 subjects suggested acceptable levels of interrater reliability for this FCE, as indicated by similarity in recommended return-to-work (RTW) levels.[17] In contrast with most other studies mentioned in this section, the consistency of therapist recommendations and not the consistency of test performances were analyzed.

- ErgoScience Physical Work Performance Evaluation (Birmingham, AL): Test-retest reliability of the nine main items of this FCE was evaluated for 24 subjects with stable physical injuries (mainly back disorders): lifting floor to waist, bilateral carrying, pushing, sitting, standing, kneeling, stair climbing, repetitive squatting, and walking. The results indicated moderate to substantial reliability of the items tested.[18] The interrater reliability of the level of work and subject participation was studied in a sample of 40 patients with back pain.[19] Results indicated high levels of agreement between raters for most of the 21 tasks evaluated. Some tasks, however, were more difficult to rate consistently, and the authors discussed possible reasons for this as being self-limiting behavior and alterations in pain scores, position adjustments, and movement deviations.

- WorkWell FCE: Several reports of interrater and intrarater and test-retest reliability of the material handling items have indicated good overall reliability in healthy subjects and patients.[5,20–25] Test-retest reliability of two tests measuring maximum holding times of static postures indicated good reliability in healthy young adults.[26] Test-retest reliability of almost all items of the FCE, tested on 30 patients with CLBP, indicated a wide range of reliability, varying from unacceptable to good.[20]

Discussion

Although many FCEs do not have demonstrated reliability evidence in peer-reviewed journals, ongoing developments seem positive. A number of studies have been performed with reasonable to good scientific scrutiny, using injured and uninjured subjects, by different independent researchers. Generally, these studies demonstrate that performance-based measurements, such as FCEs, can, at the very least, be used to reliably evaluate certain aspects of a person's functional capacity. They also demonstrate that, although reliable at a group level, the performance of symptomatic people (with CLBP) may vary substantially between occasions. It seems that this variance can in large part be attributed to variance in patient performance rather than to measurement inconsistencies over time or between raters. In other words, it seems that the instruments themselves are sufficient, but the construct being measured (which is the performance of a person) can vary. This, in turn, provides scores that may vary between occasions. Further research is needed, however, to evaluate this possibility and ascertain how to identify and, perhaps, correct for it. Given the variability between FCE protocols and approaches, it is unknown if or to what extent knowledge gained from research on one FCE can be generalized to other protocols.

CHAPTER 21

Validity

Introduction of Terms

Validity is generally defined as the degree to which an instrument measures what it is intended to measure and refers to the appropriateness, meaningfulness, and usefulness of the specific inferences made from the test results. Although there are many inferences that could be made from the data provided through an FCE, the validity of results applicable to the performance of work-related activities is clearly the most important. Validity depends on the purpose of the assessment and, therefore, the test objectives. It is not a universal overall characteristic of an assessment, and there is generally no single measure sufficient to determine an assessment's validity. There are also multiple forms of validity, each of which must be evaluated within the context of the test's intended purpose and a specific population. Several forms of validity are relevant to FCEs: face, content, criterion-related (concurrent and predictive), and construct; responsiveness is also important (Table 21–1). In this section, predictive validity and responsiveness are described separately from other forms of validity.

Published Evidence on the Validity of Functional Capacity Evaluation

The contextual relationship of FCEs with work can easily be explained from their original purpose. Most FCEs have been inspired by the taxonomy described in the US Department of Labor *Dictionary of Occupational Titles* (DOT).[28] This taxonomy, although never formally tested for its validity, has gained sup-

TABLE 21–1	Definitions of Validity[27]
Term	**Definition**
Face validity	The apparent ability of an assessment to measure what it intends to measure via a seemingly plausible method of doing so
Content validity	The degree to which test items represent the performance domain (such as ability to work) the test is intended to measure; usually determined by a panel of experts who examine the relationship between test objectives and test items or by knowledge of the usual practices used

(continued)

TABLE 21-1 Definitions of Validity[27] (continued)

Term	Definition
Construct validity	The extent to which a test can be shown to measure a hypothetical construct. For example, a work-related assessment may be considered to have some support for construct validity if it is able to differentiate between clients who are able to lift safely and clients who are unable to do so, when the construct being measured is safe lifting ability (also called discriminant validity). The "known groups method" is the most general type of construct validity and involves the ability of the test results to discriminate between groups known to be different (eg, different diagnostic groups, different age groups, and different occupational groups) in a theoretically appropriate manner. Correlation with other tests involves the examination of the degree of convergence and/or divergence with other tests that are presumed to measure the same or different constructs or traits.
Criterion validity	The systematic demonstration of the extent to which test performance is related to some other valued measure of performance or external criterion; composed of concurrent and predictive validity and is considered the most practical approach to validity testing and the most objective
■ **Concurrent validity**	The correlation between two or more measures given to the same subject at approximately the same time, with both presumably reflecting the same ability or behavior
■ **Predictive validity**	The degree to which a subject's performance at the initial time of testing accurately predicts performance obtained at a future date as measured by another highly valued measure or "gold standard." For work-related FCEs, the ability to predict a client's success in returning to work is a highly valued criterion.
Responsiveness	The ability of a test to detect clinically important changes in the ability to perform the activities evaluated (work or work-related activities)

port in many countries around the world. The DOT classification is similar to selected domains of the International Classification of Functioning, Disability, and Health and classifications such as a back-specific classification called the Functional Assessment Taxonomy.[29] Among others, the DOT provides information about the work characteristics of most jobs in the United States in terms of the physical demands the jobs place on workers. The demand classification is based on certain principles assumed or demonstrated to be key elements in the nature of work. These key elements are defined in the DOT as the physical demands of a specific job and are called *job factors*. There are 20 job factors, with some broken into subfactors: standing, sitting, walking, lifting, carrying, pushing, pulling, climbing, balancing, stooping, kneeling, crouching, crawling, reaching, handling, fingering, feeling, talking, hearing, and seeing. These job factors express the requirements of the job and the capacities a worker must have to meet or exceed the demands. It has been stated that the content validity of FCEs based on the DOT is sufficient and that most of the commercially available FCEs cover many to all of these work characteristics.[27]

In their systematic review of FCEs, King et al[30] found little evidence in the literature of the inclusion of physical fitness assessments in FCEs. This lack is in contrast with the finding that the development of most FCEs is inspired by the DOT, in which the energy requirements of jobs are defined. The level of aerobic fitness directly affects the amount and intensity of physical activity a person is able to perform. Most physical activities are described in terms of their energy or metabolic cost. It would consequently seem that the failure of many FCEs to include physical fitness (aerobic) assessment as part of the testing protocol may be inappropriate when the primary goal is to ascertain whether the evaluee is capable of returning to a given level of work. Chapter 10 provides an in-depth elaboration on assessing aerobic capacity.

Historically, assessment of functional capacity was performed by asking patients about their activity levels. A large variety of questionnaires have been developed to measure patients' perception of their physical activity levels and disabilities. Studies of patients with chronic pain, however, have identified discrepancies between self-reports and actual levels of physical activity. When comparing the results of FCE with the results of questionnaires, it has been shown that the outcomes are substantially different and correlate moderately at best.[31-36] Typically, the physical activity level reported via questionnaire is lower than levels observed during FCE. It seems that instruments based on self-report or based on performance measure different dimensions of the same construct.

The last reviews of the scientific evidence of the validity of FCEs were published in 1999[11] and in 2004.[12] The authors demonstrated that the evidence for validity of a wide range of FCEs ranged from nonexistent to having been investigated and reported in sufficient detail. Few FCEs demonstrated adequate validity in more than one area or in more than one study. As was the case with reliability, developers and users of FCEs now seem to better appreciate the need to investigate and report validity evidence, which will presumably lead to future studies of this important construct. Although the current status of the literature is, consequently, far from optimal, reports containing data about different aspects of validity were identified for the following FCEs:

- Baltimore Therapeutic Equipment Work Simulator (BTE): Real and simulated lifting tasks were compared. The results suggest the BTE may overestimate real lifting endurance performance in healthy men. Lower physiologic stresses during the simulated task suggested a significant difference between the real and simulated loads.[37]
- Dictionary of Occupational Titles Residual Functional Capacity battery: Stooping, climbing, balancing, crouching, feeling shapes, handling left and right, lifting, and carrying seemed to have construct validity in patients with chronic pain.[28]
- Ergos Work Simulator: In comparing different ways of assessing functional capacity, the authors found that a 4-hour Ergos evaluation yielded similar information on strength and endurance for industrial physical capacity compared with information obtained from a 2-week VALPAR (Valpar International Corporation, Tuscon, AZ) work sample evaluation.[38] In a different study, it was found that patients with higher pain behaviors, operationally defined by Waddell scores, performed at lower levels compared with patients with low or no pain behaviors.[39]
- Functional Assessment Screening Test: An evaluation of this short FCE found some evidence to confirm criterion validity because performance of patients with CLBP was inversely related to self-reported depression, disability, and different dimensions of pain experience.[40] The strength of the relationships, however, was not reported. Of particular interest was the strong relationship between psychosocial variables and physical test performance, suggesting that extensive FCEs may not be necessary or valid in assessing the physical performance of patients with chronic back pain. Although it is unknown to what degree self-report measures are commonly used as integral parts of or in conjunction with most FCEs, this study supported the use of standardized measures to assess self-reported disability and psychological constructs in conjunction with FCE. The section "Determinants of Performance" in this chapter and the section on psychometric testing in Chapter 5 provide more information.
- GAPP FCE: The authors described a study in which five expert occupational therapists reviewed content validity, technical adequacy, and how the FCE met established test criteria of safety, reliability, validity (primarily face and content validity), sensitivity, practicality, and utility. Support for most criteria was demonstrated, and points for improvements were identified.[41]
- WorkWell FCE: *Disability* is a multidimensional construct with no consented "gold standard" instrument to measure it. Studies have demonstrated that performance-based disability, measured with the WorkWell FCE, was related to different forms of self-reported disability that were measured with questionnaires.[35,36] The strength of these relationships,

however, was poor to moderate. The observation that these two measures correlate poorly to moderately indicates that the measures are related but different. This finding means that performance-based measures of disability are different from self-reported measures of disability, indicating that different dimensions of the disability construct are being assessed. A strong correlation between self-reports and performance-based testing would indicate that they were measuring the same or similar constructs. Absence of a relation would indicate that the measures were independent from each other. The presence of a moderate relationship suggests that they are indeed related, although not identical, hence confirming construct validity.

Self-reports of function or prediction of function were also poorly related to actual function on tests measuring maximum holding times of sustained postures.[26] As seen in other performance tests,[42] differences in material handling performance between males and females were observed. One study found preliminary evidence in support of the ecological validity of this FCE because test results were not relevantly influenced by differences in test conditions.[43] A direct comparison between FCE performance and the ability to perform work demands could be made in 7 of 11 activities studied.[44] In patients with CLBP, relationships of moderate strength between FCE performance and pain intensity were found in 1 study,[36] but weak or nonexistent relationships were found in two other studies.[45,46] The relation between FCE performance and fear-avoidance beliefs was found to be nonexistent in patients with CLBP,[45,46] which is counter to what some would expect. On the other hand, self-efficacy beliefs were moderately related to results on the lifting tests in patients with CLBP.[47] A comparison of FCE results of 3 groups of similar patients with CLBP among three different countries and settings revealed differences in performance between the Dutch group on the one hand and the Canadian and the Swiss groups on the other hand.[48] The authors controlled for several potential confounding variables, such as differences in sex, age, pain intensity, and self-reported disability, but were not able to explain the differences. As suggested by others,[49] the authors recommend further research to study potential influences of evaluator characteristics and beliefs and environmental factors, such as the purpose of the FCE (for entry into rehabilitation, disability claim determination, RTW, or other) on test results.

Determinants of Performance

An important aspect of the construct validity of FCE is referred to as *determinants of performance*. In other words, even though testing procedures may be reliable, the test results for a person can and do fluctuate. In all test-retest reliability studies described in this chapter, wide ranges of individual variance, referred to as the *normal* or *natural variation* of the measurement, and the limits of agreement were found. It was demonstrated that of all potential sources of variance, the largest amount must be attributed to the evaluee. This means that human performance in an FCE varies between occasions. Although these variances may be quite large, they should not be considered abnormal when they stay within the ranges of normal variation. One of the challenges for future research is understanding the relative contribution of potential sources of variance between and within individuals and determining how to account for this variance when interpreting the results of an FCE.

In addition, confusing and inappropriate use of the term validity occurs in some work-related assessments. The terms *validity profile, valid, conditionally valid, conditionally invalid,* and *invalid effort* are used in some FCEs. These terms do not refer to the measurement concept of validity as it pertains to the instrument or test battery results, but rather the level of effort exerted by the evaluee. Because the term validity profile has not been defined and no evidence has been found defining validity in this context in the peer-reviewed literature, there is no scientific justification for the use of this and similar terminology in relation to functional testing.

The term *capacity* also connotes the maximum physical ability of the evaluee, which at times is beyond the level of performance or tolerance that is being measured. Capacity is the evaluee's potential, determined by biological and physiologic factors. The use of the term capacity is somewhat misleading because capacity is rarely measured in a performance task, unless the evaluee is highly motivated and trained to perform that particular task. Examples of maximum task performance are found when experienced athletes compete. When the evaluee is an injured worker, the functional capacity is usually inferred from evaluation of task performance. The maximum level of performance that can be measured is the portion of capacity the evaluee is willing to produce. Thus, the performance of the person depends on his or her physical abilities to perform and his or her motivation to perform, which leads to two critical questions: (1) How can capacity and performance be differentiated when evaluating a person (ie, are the results reflective of maximal or submaximal physical abilities)? (2) What factors determine the motivation of a patient to perform? Neither question has been answered with scientific certainty.

Methods used to differentiate between maximal and submaximal performance (also referred to as sincerity of effort) include the following: Waddell nonorganic signs,[50] descriptions of pain behavior and symptom magnification, coefficients of variation, correlations between musculoskeletal evaluation and demonstrated function, grip measurements, and the relations between heart rate and pain intensity.[51] Despite the widespread use of these methods, little has been published either to address their reliability and validity specific to the FCE setting or to describe the theoretical justifications for these methods. Nevertheless, studies that tested strategies to differentiate between maximal and submaximal performance in a lifting test have been published. These studies have shown promising results vis-á-vis the sensitivity and specificity of their methods in differentiating between maximal and submaximal effort levels.[52–54] However, some studies used healthy subjects, which may not be representative of patients with musculoskeletal conditions. In addition, the studies dichotomized maximal and submaximal effort, suggesting a greater distinction than is present in daily practice. Typically, a range or continuum of effort levels ranging from very low to maximum is observed in subjects who are seen clinically. The challenge for future developments in this area is to develop and test methods to differentiate between levels (ie, from minimal to maximum physical effort), not only in healthy subjects but also in relevant patient groups. Nevertheless, a published study has indicated that in healthy subjects and in patients with CLBP, a trained observer can differentiate maximal from submaximal effort on lifting tasks using visual observations only.[55] Until further studies are performed, generalizations beyond the patient groups and the specifically tested items cannot be made. In addition, the reasons why some subjects exert submaximal effort are unknown, but could be attributed to factors such as depression, fear, or lack of understanding of test instructions (especially in nonnative language speakers). Until a better understanding of how to identify and interpret subject's effort levels is gained, clinicians should remain cautious in classifying and inferring meaning from an evaluee's performance levels. Chapter 15 provides more discourse on the differences between performance and capacity.

The second question deals with factors determining the motivation of a patient to perform during an FCE. Watson[56] developed a model in which task performance during a performance evaluation of patients with chronic pain is explained. Other than physiologic factors, the following nonphysiologic factors are postulated in the model: task familiarity and learning, functional self-efficacy, pain self-efficacy, fear-avoidance beliefs, current pain level, and outcome expectancy. Based on these factors and, perhaps other factors not in the model,[57] a patient may be motivated to perform to maximum capacity or to terminate an activity before reaching maximum. It is important to assess not only the extent to which a patient is willing to perform to his or her physical maximum, but also the reason(s) why he or she performs as such. This assessment may require knowledge beyond the professional capabilities of functional capacity evaluators, often physical or occupational therapists. Consistent with major standards and guidelines of chronic pain and work injury management, it is advocated that the services of a clinical psychologist or a behavioral therapist be used to assess these aspects in conjunction with the evaluation of functional capacity or, at the very least, use some psychometric or psychological testing in addition to tests that focus purely on the measurement of physical function. Psychological assessments, however, should meet the same criteria of reliability and validity as any other assessment and should preferably not rely only on self-reports or clinical expertise.

Predictive Validity

A few studies were found that studied the predictive validity of FCE. Each study had slightly different purposes for the FCE and outcomes that the FCE was predicting.

In a study on functional capacity and psychological measures, it was concluded that psychological variables were related to measures of functional capacity measured at the admission stage of a rehabilitation program, but that psychological measures at admission were not good predictors of later functional capacity measures. In addition, some functional capacity measures were identified as important predictors of follow-up employment outcome, but RTW could not be predicted without considering pain intensity.[58] In another prospective cohort with 185 patients with chronic pain who underwent an FCE following a pain management program, future employment status and levels (in terms of DOT categories) were evaluated 30 months later. Employment levels could not be predicted, but employment status could be predicted with reasonable accuracy (75% sensitivity and specificity) by using pain intensity levels and the number of FCE tasks completed.[59]

A study of another large cohort of patients (n = 650; diagnoses not specified) evaluated retrospectively found sex and time off work to be the strongest predictors of whether the patients returned to work, with performance on a lifting task adding little (r or r^2) but statistically significantly (P) to the prediction. Of patients who returned to work, performance on the floor-to-waist lift and horizontal lift were related to the level of work (higher performance was related to higher levels of work).[60]

Authors of a study examining the ability of the Isernhagen FCE to predict a timely RTW in workers' compensation claimants with low back pain found that better performance on the FCE was weakly associated with faster recovery; however, the amount of variation explained was small.[61-63] Similar findings were reported by others,[64] with one task in the FCE (lifting floor to waist height) as predictive as the entire protocol. This predictive ability was replicated in another study focusing on claimants with upper extremity diagnoses with regard to the ability of the protocol to predict future work status (better performance on the FCE was weakly associated with faster recovery; small amount of variation explained) and one task (lifting overhead) being as predictive as the rest of the protocol.[65] Another study examined the ability of an FCE to predict sustained recovery in workers' compensation claimants with low back pain and found that better FCE performance, as indicated by a lower number of failed tasks, was associated with higher risk of recurrence.[62] The validity of the FCE's purported ability to identify claimants who are "safe" to RTW may, thus, be suspect.

It may be questioned whether FCEs will ever be found valid for the prediction of a safe and lasting RTW or whether FCE should be considered a predictor for any type of RTW.[66] The construct of "workability" is widely regarded as a multidimensional construct. Whether a patient successfully returns to work depends on more than functional capacity by itself. It is critical to understand that an instrument measuring a single dimension cannot be expected to assess a multidimensional construct. It is, therefore, by definition incorrect to suggest or to claim that the results of an FCE should be able to predict a person's work ability or, an even more complex factor, a *successful* RTW. At best, one may expect an FCE, in conjunction with endurance testing, to measure a person's immediate functional ability to perform work-related activities. This ability should be seen as *one* of the prerequisites for a successful RTW. Seen in this light, the role of the physical domain may prove to be a modest one. Indeed, in recent literature, evidence was found that the proposed dominance of the physical domain might not be as valid as commonly suggested.[33,67,68] For these and other reasons, efforts have been made to streamline current testing protocols (see the section "Practicality").

Responsiveness

The term *responsiveness* refers to the ability of a test to detect clinically important change in the construct of measure (ability to perform work-related activities in the case of FCE). Responsiveness is a critical metric for FCE because these tests are frequently used as indicators of outcome following rehabilitation programs. We were unable to locate any studies in the peer-reviewed literature in which FCE responsiveness was studied.[69,70]

Two major challenges are apparent that may account for the dearth of studies evaluating the responsiveness of FCE. These challenges were illustrated in a sample of patients with CLBP who underwent an FCE before and after a pain management program.[71] On average, while differences in FCE performances before and after treatment were observed, the authors were unable to determine whether these differences represented clinically important changes in observed functional performance. The reasons were the absence of a valid external criterion to which to compare the changes and a substantial natural variation of "normal" performance, as presented in the "Reliability" section of this chapter, making it almost impossible for patients to improve their performance beyond these natural variations. These issues remain unresolved and present a future research challenge.

Discussion

Although many FCE protocols still do not have demonstrated evidence of validity in peer-reviewed journals, some developments have been made. A number of studies concerning different aspects of validity on different FCE protocols have been published. As was the case with reliability, it is unknown whether the knowledge gained from studying one protocol can be generalized to other protocols. Indeed, one study in which upper lifting performance was tested according to two FCE protocols revealed significant differences in results.[72] Similar findings were found by others testing different tests on different patient groups.[25,73] This indicates that differences in operational definitions of the activity tested, for example lifting height and repetitions, really matter. Even though the amount of evidence is limited, it suggests that generalization across FCEs is not recommended.

In summary, it has been demonstrated clearly that the results of functional capacity measurements differ fairly substantially from results of self-report questionnaires. Furthermore, psychological factors seem to influence FCE results. Although the extent to which they do so remains unclear and warrants future research, the need to devote a substantial period during an FCE to the evaluation of physical abilities in the context of significant psychosocial overlay remains unclear. The predictive power of FCEs with regard to predicting safe and lasting RTW has not been clearly demonstrated, and the results of different studies seem conflicting. Potentially, the useful information gained from FCEs relevant to RTW could be obtained from a less expensive short-form assessment. This requires identification of which factors are relevant to RTW and amenable to evaluation by functional testing.

Practicality

Full-length FCEs are lengthy clinical measures, typically requiring hours of the patient's and the evaluator's time. However, great variability is seen across protocols, with some FCEs requiring a few hours on one day while other FCEs can take many hours to perform divided over multiple days. Some developers have recommended dividing assessment over consecutive days to allow clinicians to evaluate the effects of evaluation across occasions. It has also been suggested that FCEs should shorten the time needed to collect data to meet consumer demand.[30] It would certainly seem that the length or comprehensiveness of the FCE should be tailored to the purpose of the evaluation and evidence of its validity.

As discussed in the section on predictive validity (one or a few tests being as predictive as a full FCE), the results of recent studies suggest that it may be possible to reduce testing time without affecting clinical outcomes. It has been suggested that full-length testing is not needed when psychosocial issues are dominant, as can be the case in chronic pain syndromes.[40] Potentially, the useful functional and predictive information obtained from current protocols could be gained in a shorter, less expensive version. A shortened version has been shown to be a useful screen for filtering out people who self-limit their performance owing to pain behaviors.[40] A randomized, controlled trial has also been conducted providing evidence in support of a short-form FCE protocol[74] to predict RTW. Similar RTW outcomes were seen in subjects with a wide range of compensable musculoskeletal conditions undergoing traditional and short-form assessments. In addition, subject satisfaction with the assessment process was reported as comparable between the short and long protocols. Other researchers have tested the need for a 2-day evaluation in patients with CLBP. They found that on average, patients perform similarly on the second day, leading to the conclusion that the need for a standard 2-day evaluation procedure for patients with CLBP could not be confirmed. Overall, no published evidence was found demonstrating that long, full-length, multiple-hour FCEs are superior to short FCEs.

Although there are valid arguments to decrease testing time, the important question remaining is how to do so. Different approaches are described in the literature:

- Based on job characteristics[75]: A strategy has been described to develop a job-specific FCE derived from a full-length protocol. Mainly by elimination of irrelevant tests, evaluation time was reduced from 6 to 1.5 hours.[76]
- Based on epidemiology or validity evidence: Research has demonstrated that only a few tests were needed to explain most of the variance of the total FCE.[74] These tests differed based on the affected body parts, for example, CLBP or upper extremity disorders,[61,65] but it may seem possible to apply this research toward designing FCEs that provide useful (and predictive) answers to discreet clinical questions.
- Based on risk factors: Based on published physical risk factors for work-related upper extremity disorders[77] and neck pain,[78] two 1-hour protocols were developed to ascertain whether these risk factors would potentially affect RTW.

Continued ongoing research of this nature is needed to focus current FCE protocols, with the goal of maximizing the amount of useful information obtained in a cost-effective manner.

Utility

To be of value, an FCE should assist all parties involved in making RTW decisions to determine subjects' abilities to perform work-related activities. The most important method to ensure the utility of an FCE is a clear, consistent, and brief written report, which can be interpreted clearly by all parties.[79]

Obviously, there are alternatives to FCE; other instruments also aim to determine ability to perform work-related activities. The two most well-known alternatives are self-report questionnaires and expert assessments, most often performed by a physician who bases the determination on a medical history and a clinical evaluation. Questionnaires measure a person's self-reported ability to perform activities, which have been shown to be related to but different from actual performance. With regard to expert assessments, although they are commonly used, few studies have been performed to analyze the reliability and validity of a physician's assessment of (aspects of) disability. When studied, the reliability seems poor[80] and the results of physicians' assessments relate weakly to moderately to performance and are also, in absolute terms, different from performance in FCEs.[80-82]

An expert review of the GAPP FCE provided support for the utility of this FCE in Australia.[41] Gibson et al[17] and Strong et al[83] reported that most study participants (representatives of workers' compensation, employees, referrers, employers, and patients in Canada) perceived FCEs as useful for the purposes the FCEs were used. Recommendations to improve the utility of FCEs were provided, indicating aspects ranging from referral, cooperation of parties involved, and reporting style and language, to the provision of service to the evaluee. In the Netherlands, Wind et al[84] found that physicians and other experts in the field of RTW and disability claims had a very diverse range of opinions about the utility of FCE, ranging from useless to very useful, leading to recommendations for further research investigating the validity of arguments presented by clinicians for or against the utility of FCE. A study performed in Switzerland indicated that FCEs seemed to positively contribute to the quality and content of medical fitness-for-work certificates,[85] with a trend reported toward a higher attested work capacity in medical reports that used FCE vs medical reports that did not. However, without a single criterion gold-standard measure to compare FCE outcomes, it is not possible to state which approach is most accurate.

Discussion

Functional capacity evaluations are used frequently to measure a person's ability to perform a work-related activity. Questionnaires can be used to measure a person's self-reported ability to perform an activity and to measure the psychosocial factors that might influence self-report and performance. It is advocated to use performance-based and self-report measures to obtain a more comprehensive picture of a person's disability.

Conclusion and Future Research

During the past decade, a growing scientific literature has emerged related to the clinimetric or measurement properties of FCE, as several reports about different aspects of safety, reliability, validity, practicality, and utility have been published. Overall, FCEs appear to be reliable indicators of overall functional work ability. Conflicting evidence has emerged, however, related to their construct and predictive validity, which has important implications for their clinical use. FCEs seem to provide some important information for guiding RTW decision making, yet they should be viewed as only one piece of a multidimensional puzzle. Efforts to streamline current assessment protocols have been made, potentially leading to improved cost-effectiveness and clinical utility. In addition to the topics mentioned throughout this chapter, many other very important topics still need to be studied.

Specifically, more studies are needed to further conceptualize and define the constructs safety and injury. Future studies should use validated measures for repeated measurements of pain intensity (visual analog score or numeric rating scales), control for pain medication use, and consider larger samples to enable multivariate analyses to predict symptom increase. Future studies should also differentiate between a normal nonspecific response to unusually high-intensity exertion and the onset of specific injuries.

The results of FCEs are, by definition, compared with the anticipated physical workload of the evaluee for making RTW decisions. The same psychometric criteria apply for the assessment of workload as to the FCE. Until now, little effort has been made to systematically analyze the psychometrics of the workload assessments performed routinely in conjunction with FCEs. Until this research is performed, results of workload assessments as performed routinely by clinicians should be interpreted with care. Relying on patient self-reports as a means to assess workloads seems to be inaccurate when compared with measured workloads,[86–89] just as using only self-report for the assessment of functional capacity seems to result in an underestimation of functional capacities.

Many differences exist between FCE protocols in the choice of activities, the operational definitions of the activities tested, and test termination criteria. Consequently, if performance of the same person would be tested using different FCE protocols, differences in results are likely to be observed. The underlying issue is the lack of consensus of the definition of FCE or its underlying construct, resulting in differences in operational definitions and, thus, in heterogeneity of tests included in each FCE. This is of great importance and needs to be addressed. The proprietary nature of most protocols poses a challenge to resolving these differences, but as long as differences in operational definitions exist, generalizations of research outcomes from one FCE to another should be made with great caution.

Often, FCEs are criticized because the claim that they evaluate "objective functional capacity" may not be correct. Performance, not capacity, is evaluated. Further research is needed to evaluate strategies developed to differentiate between performance and capacity or more specifically between maximal and submaximal FCE performance in different patient groups and among different tests. It is also important to assess not only the extent to which an evaluee is willing to perform to his or her physical maximum, but also the reason(s) he or she performs as such. In addition, research is needed to unravel variability of patient performance. As demonstrated in the section on reliability in this chapter, natural variations between performances are quite large and, for the most part, unexplained. Previous research on determinants of FCE performance has been performed on relatively small patient samples (< 100 patients), which makes large multivariable prediction models unstable. In addition, this previous research has focused on biological and psychological variables as predictors for functional capacity, whereas social variables have been underresearched. Only one study was found evaluating subject performance across settings and countries. Further methodologically sound research is needed evaluating determinants of FCE performance from the social domain, including such variables as compensation status.

Last, an important area of FCE research relates to efficacy and cost-effectiveness. It is currently unknown whether FCE is effective for guiding decisions and facilitating sustained RTW, especially in relation to self-report measures and physician expert evaluation.

CHAPTER 21

References

1. Hart DL, Isernhagen SJ, Matheson LN. Guidelines for functional capacity evaluation of people with medical conditions. *J Orthop Sports Phys Ther.* 1993;18:682–686.
2. Gibson L, Strong J. Safety issues in functional capacity evaluation: findings from a trial of a new approach for evaluating clients with chronic back pain. *J Occup Rehabil.* 2005;15:237–251.
3. Reneman MF, Kuijer W, Brouwer S, Preuper HR, Groothoff JW, Geertzen JHB. Symptom increase following a functional capacity evaluation in patients with chronic low back pain: an explorative study of safety. *J Occup Rehabil.* 2006;16:192–200.
4. Gross DP, Battie MC. Reliability of safe maximum lifting determinations of a functional capacity evaluation. *Phys Ther.* 2002;82:364–371.
5. Reneman MF, Dijkstra PU, Westmaas M, Goeken LN. Test-retest reliability of lifting and carrying in a 2-day functional capacity evaluation. *J Occup Rehabil.* 2002;12:269–275.

6. Cole MH, Grimshaw PN, Burden AM. Loads on the lumbar spine during a work capacity assessment test. *Work.* 2004;23:169–178.

7. Kersnovske S, Gibson L, Strong J. Item validity of the physical demands from the *Dictionary of Occupational Titles* for functional capacity evaluation of clients with chronic back pain. *Work.* 2005;24:157–169.

8. Kuijer W, Dijkstra PU, Brouwer S, Reneman MF, Groothoff JW, Geertzen JH. Safe lifting in patients with chronic low back pain: comparing FCE lifting task and NIOSH lifting guideline. *J Occup Rehabil.* 2006;16(4):579–589.

9. Terwee CB, Bot SD, de Boer MR, van der Windt DA, Knol DL, Dekker J, et al. Quality criteria were proposed for measurement properties of health status questionnaires. *J Clin Epidemiol.* 2007;60:34–42.

10. Bland JM, Altman DG. Statistical methods for assessing agreement between two methods of clinical measurement. *Lancet.* 1986;1:307–310.

11. Innes E, Straker L. Reliability of work-related assessments. *Work.* 1999;13:107–124.

12. Gouttebarge V, Wind H, Kuijer PP, Frings-Dresen MH. Reliability and validity of functional capacity evaluation methods: a systematic review with reference to Blankenship system, Ergos Work Simulator, Ergo-Kit and Isernhagen Work System. *Int Arch Occup Environ Health.* 2004;77:527–537.

13. Lee GK, Chan CC, Hui-Chan CW. Consistency of performance on the functional capacity assessment: static strength and dynamic endurance. *Am J Phys Med Rehabil.* 2001;80:189–195.

14. Gouttebarge V, Wind H, Kuijer PP, Sluiter JK, Frings-Dresen MH. Intra- and interrater reliability of the Ergo-Kit functional capacity evaluation method in adults without musculoskeletal complaints. *Arch Phys Med Rehabil.* 2005;86:2354–2360.

15. Gouttebarge V, Wind H, Kuijer PP, Sluiter JK, Frings-Dresen MH. Reliability and agreement of 5 Ergo-Kit functional capacity evaluation lifting tests in subjects with low back pain. *Arch Phys Med Rehabil.* 2006;87:1365–1370.

16. Boadella JM, Sluiter JK, Frings-Dresen MH. Reliability of upper extremity tests measured by the Ergos work simulator: a pilot study. *J Occup Rehabil.* 2003;13:219–232.

17. Gibson L, Strong J, Wallace A. Functional capacity evaluation as a performance measure: evidence for a new approach for clients with chronic back pain. *Clin J Pain.* 2005;21:207–215.

18. Tuckwell NL, Straker L, Barrett TE. Test-retest reliability on nine tasks of the Physical Work Performance Evaluation. *Work.* 2002;19:243–253.

19. Durand MJ, Loisel P, Poitras S, Mercier R, Stock SR, Lemaire J. The interrater reliability of a functional capacity evaluation: the Physical Work Performance Evaluation. *J Occup Rehabil.* 2004;14:119–129.

20. Brouwer S, Reneman MF, Dijkstra PU, Groothoff JW, Schellekens JM, Goeken LN. Test-retest reliability of the Isernhagen Work Systems Functional Capacity Evaluation in patients with chronic low back pain. *J Occup Rehabil.* 2003;13:207–218.

21. Isernhagen SJ, Hart DL, Matheson LM. Reliability of independent observer judgments of level of lift effort in a kinesiophysical functional capacity evaluation. *Work.* 1999;12:145–150.

22. Smith RL. Therapists' ability to identify safe maximum lifting in low back pain patients during functional capacity evaluation. *J Orthop Sports Phys Ther.* 1994;19:277–281.

23. Reneman MF, Jaegers SM, Westmaas M, Goeken LN. The reliability of determining effort level of lifting and carrying in a functional capacity evaluation. *Work.* 2002;18:23–27.

24. Gardener L, McKenna K. Reliability of occupational therapists in determining safe, maximal lifting capacity. *Aust Occup Ther J.* 1999;46:110–119.

25. Soer R, Poels BJ, Geertzen JH, Reneman MF. A comparison of two lifting assessment approaches in patients with chronic low back pain. *J Occup Rehabil.* 2006;16:639–646.

26. Reneman MF, Bults MM, Engbers LH, Mulders KK, Goeken LN. Measuring maximum holding times and perception of static elevated work and forward bending in healthy young adults. *J Occup Rehabil.* 2001;11:87–97.

27. Innes E, Straker L. Validity of work-related assessments. *Work.* 1999;13:125–152.

28. Fishbain DA, Abdel-Moty E, Cutler R, Khalil TM, Sadek S, Rosomoff RS, et al. Measuring residual functional capacity in chronic low back pain patients based on the *Dictionary of Occupational Titles. Spine.* 1994;19:872–880.

29. Gaudino EA, Matheson LN, Mael FA. Development of the functional assessment taxonomy. *J Occup Rehabil.* 2001;11:155–175.

30. King PM, Tuckwell N, Barrett TE. A critical review of functional capacity evaluations. *Phys Ther.* 1998;78:852–866.

31. Lee CE, Simmonds MJ, Novy DM, Jones S. Self-reports and clinician-measured physical function among patients with low back pain: a comparison. *Arch Phys Med Rehabil.* 2001;82:227–231.

32. Wittink H, Rogers W, Sukiennik A, Carr DB. Physical functioning: self-report and performance measures are related but distinct. *Spine.* 2003;28:2407–2413.

33. Wittink H, Hoskins MT, Wagner A, Sukiennik A, Rogers W. Deconditioning in patients with chronic low back pain: fact or fiction? *Spine.* 2000;25:2221–2228.

34. Smeets RJ, van Geel AC, Kester AD, Knottnerus JA. Physical capacity tasks in chronic low back pain: what is the contributing role of cardiovascular capacity, pain and psychological factors? *Disabil Rehabil.* 2007;29:577–586.

35. Reneman MF, Jorritsma W, Schellekens JM, Goeken LN. Concurrent validity of questionnaire and performance-based disability measurements in patients with chronic nonspecific low back pain. *J Occup Rehabil.* 2002;12:119–129.

36. Gross DP, Battie MC. Construct validity of a kinesiophysical functional capacity evaluation administered within a worker's compensation environment. *J Occup Rehabil.* 2003;13:287–295.

37. Ting W, Wessel J, Brintnell S, Maikala R, Bhambhani Y. Validity of the Baltimore Therapeutic Equipment Work Simulator in the measurement of lifting endurance in healthy men. *Am J Occup Ther.* 2001;55:184–190.

38. Dusik LA, Menard MR, Cooke C, Fairburn SM, Beach GN. Concurrent validity of the ERGOS Work Simulator versus conventional functional capacity evaluation techniques in a workers' compensation population. *J Occup Med.* 1993;35:759–767.

39. Cooke C, Dusik LA, Menard MR, Fairburn SM, Beach GN. Relationship of performance on the ERGOS Work Simulator to illness behavior in a workers' compensation population with low back versus limb injury. *J Occup Med.* 1994;36:757–762.

40. Ruan CM, Haig AJ, Geisser ME, Yamakawa K, Buchholz RL. Functional capacity evaluations in persons with spinal disorders: predicting poor outcomes on the Functional Assessment Screening Test (FAST). *J Occup Rehabil.* 2001;11:119–132.

CHAPTER 21

41. Gibson L, Strong J. Expert review of an approach to functional capacity evaluation. *Work.* 2002;19:231–242.

42. Novy DM, Simmonds MJ, Olson SL, Lee CE, Jones SC. Physical performance: differences in men and women with and without low back pain. *Arch Phys Med Rehabil.* 1999;80:195–198.

43. Reneman MF, Joling CI, Soer EL, Goeken LN. Functional capacity evaluation: ecological validity of three static endurance tests. *Work.* 2001;16:227–234.

44. Kuijer W, Brouwer S, Reneman MF, Dijkstra PU, Groothoff JW, Schellekens JM, et al. Matching FCE activities and work demands: an explorative study. *J Occup Rehabil.* 2006;16:459–473.

45. Reneman MF, Jorritsma W, Dijkstra SJ, Dijkstra PU. Relationship between kinesiophobia and performance in a functional capacity evaluation. *J Occup Rehabil.* 2003;13:277–285.

46. Reneman MF, Schiphorts Preuper HR, Kleen M, Geertzen JH, Dijkstra PU. Are pain intensity and pain related fear related to functional capacity evaluation performances of patients with chronic low back pain? *J Occup Rehabil.* 2007;17:247–258.

47. Asante AK, Brintnell ES, Gross DP. Functional self-efficacy beliefs influence functional capacity evaluation. *J Occup Rehabil.* 2007;17:73–82.

48. Reneman MF, Kool J, Oesch P, Geertzen JH, Battie MC, Gross DP. Material handling performance of patients with chronic low back pain during functional capacity evaluation: a comparison between three countries. *Disabil Rehabil.* 2006;28:1143–1149.

49. Rudy TE, Lieber SJ, Boston JR. Functional capacity assessment: influence of behavioral and environmental factors. *J Back Musculoskeletal Rehabil.* 1996;6:277–288.

50. Menard MR, Cooke C, Locke SR, Beach GN, Butler TB. Pattern of performance in workers with low back pain during a comprehensive motor performance evaluation. *Spine.* 1994;19:1359–1366.

51. Lechner DE, Bradbury SF, Bradley LA. Detecting sincerity of effort: a summary of methods and approaches. *Phys Ther.* 1998;78:867–888.

52. Brubaker PN, Fearon FJ, Smith SM, McKibben RJ, Alday J, Andrews SS, et al. Sensitivity and specificity of the Blankenship FCE system's indicators of submaximal effort. *J Orthop Sports Phys Ther.* 2007;37:161–168.

53. Fishbain DA, Abdel-Moty E, Cutler RB, Rosomoff HL, Steele-Rosomoff R. Detection of a "faked" strength task effort in volunteers using a computerized exercise testing system. *Am J Phys Med Rehabil.* 1999;78:222–227.

54. Lemstra M, Olszynski WP, Enright W. The sensitivity and specificity of functional capacity evaluations in determining maximal effort: a randomized trial. *Spine.* 2004;29:953–959.

55. Reneman MF, Fokkens AS, Dijkstra PU, Geertzen JH, Groothoff JW. Testing lifting capacity: validity of determining effort level by means of observation. *Spine.* 2005;30:E40–E46.

56. Watson P. Non-physiological determinants of physical performance in musculoskeletal pain. Refresher course on pain management held in conjunction with the 9th World Congress on Pain. Vienna, Austria: International Association for the Study of Pain; 1999.

57. Kaplan GM, Wurtele SK, Gillis D. Maximal effort during functional capacity evaluations: an examination of psychological factors. *Arch Phys Med Rehabil.* 1996;77:161–164.

58. Cutler RB, Fishbain DA, Steele-Rosomoff R, Rosomoff HL. Relationships between functional capacity measures and baseline psychological measures in chronic pain patients. *J Occup Rehabil.* 2003;13:249–258.

59. Fishbain DA, Cutler RB, Rosomoff H, Khalil T, Abdel-Moty E, Steele-Rosomoff R. Validity of the *Dictionary of Occupational Titles* residual functional capacity battery. *Clin J Pain.* 1999;15:102–110.

60. Matheson LN, Isernhagen SJ, Hart DL. Relationships among lifting ability, grip force, and return to work. *Phys Ther.* 2002;82:249–256.

61. Gross DP, Battie MC, Cassidy JD. The prognostic value of functional capacity evaluation in patients with chronic low back pain, part 1: timely return to work. *Spine.* 2004;29:914–919.

62. Gross DP, Battie MC. The prognostic value of functional capacity evaluation in patients with chronic low back pain, part 2: sustained recovery. *Spine.* 2004;29:920–924.

63. Gross DP, Battie MC. Functional capacity evaluation performance does not predict sustained return to work in claimants with chronic back pain. *J Occup Rehabil.* 2005;15:285–294.

64. Kuijer W, Brouwer S, Reneman MF, Dijkstra PU, Groothoff JW, Schellekens JM, et al. Matching FCE activities and work demands: an explorative study. *J Occup Rehabil.* 2006;16:459–473.

65. Gross DP, Battie MC. Does functional capacity evaluation predict recovery in workers' compensation claimants with upper extremity disorders? *Occup Environ Med.* 2006;63:404–410.

66. Oliveri M, Jansen T, Oesch P, Kool J. The prognostic value of functional capacity evaluation in patients with chronic low back pain, part 1: timely return to work. And part 2: sustained recovery. *Spine.* 2005;30:1232–1233.

67. Smeets RJ, Wittink H. The deconditioning paradigm for chronic low back pain unmasked? *Pain.* 2007;130:201–202.

68. Verbunt JA, Westerterp KR, van der Heijden GJ, Seelen HA, Vlaeyen JW, Knottnerus JA. Physical activity in daily life in patients with chronic low back pain. *Arch Phys Med Rehabil.* 2001;82:726–730.

69. Wittink H. Functional capacity testing in patients with chronic pain. *Clin J Pain.* 2005;21:197–199.

70. Reneman MF, Dijkstra PU. Introduction to the special issue on functional capacity evaluations: from expert based to evidence based. *J Occup Rehabil.* 2003;13: 203–206.

71. Kuijer W, Brouwer S, Reneman MF. Determining responsiveness of FCEs, mission impossible? *Clin J Pain.* 2006;22:664–665.

72. IJmker S, Gerrits EH, Reneman MF. Upper lifting performance of healthy young adults in functional capacity evaluations: a comparison of two protocols. *J Occup Rehabil.* 2003;13:297–305.

73. Rustenburg G, Kuijer PP, Frings-Dresen MH. The concurrent validity of the ERGOS Work Simulator and the Ergo-Kit with respect to maximum lifting capacity. *J Occup Rehabil.* 2004;14:107–118.

74. Gross DP, Battie MC, Asante AK. Evaluation of a short-form functional capacity evaluation: less may be best. *J Occup Rehabil.* 2007, 17(3):422–435.

75. Pransky GS, Dempsey PG. Practical aspects of functional capacity evaluations. *J Occup Rehabil.* 2004;14:217–229.

76. Frings-Dresen MH, Sluiter JK. Development of a job-specific FCE protocol: the work demands of hospital nurses as an example. *J Occup Rehabil.* 2003;13: 233–248.

77. Reneman MF, Soer R, Gerrits EH. Basis for an FCE methodology for patients with work-related upper limb disorders. *J Occup Rehabil.* 2005;15:353–363.

78. Reesink DD, Jorritsma W, Reneman MF. Basis for a functional capacity evaluation methodology for patients with work-related neck disorders. *J Occup Rehabil.* 2007; 17:436–449.

79. Allen S, Rainwater A, Newbold A, Deacon N, Slatter K. Functional capacity evaluation reports for clients with personal injury claims: a content analysis. *Occup Ther Int.* 2004;11:82–95.

80. Brouwer S, Dijkstra PU, Stewart RE, Goeken LN, Groothoff JW, Geertzen JH. Comparing self-report, clinical examination and functional testing in the assessment of work-related limitations in patients with chronic low back pain. *Disabil Rehabil.* 2005;27:999–1005.

81. Walker WC, Cifu DX, Gardner M, Keyser-Marcus L. Functional assessment in patients with chronic pain: can physicians predict performance? *Am J Phys Med Rehabil.* 2001;80:162–168.

82. Brokaw JP, Walker WC, Cifu DX, Gardner M. Sitting and standing tolerance in patients with chronic back pain: comparison between physician prediction and covert observation. *Arch Phys Med Rehabil.* 2004;85:837–839.

83. Strong S, Baptiste S, Clarke J, Cole D, Costa M. Use of functional capacity evaluations in workplaces and the compensation system: a report on workers' and report users' perceptions. *Work.* 2004;23:67–77.

84. Wind H, Gouttebarge V, Kuijer PP, Sluiter JK, Frings-Dresen MH. The utility of functional capacity evaluation: the opinion of physicians and other experts in the field of return to work and disability claims. *Int Arch Occup Environ Health.* 2006;79:528–534.

85. Oesch PR, Kool JP, Bachmann S, Devereux J. The influence of a functional capacity evaluation on fitness for work certificates in patients with non-specific chronic low back pain. *Work.* 2006;26:259–271.

86. Hoozemans MJ, van der Beek AJ, Frings-Dresen MH, van der Molen HF. Evaluation of methods to assess push/pull forces in a construction task. *Appl Ergon.* 2001;32:509–516.

87. Hansson GA, Balogh I, Bystrom JU, Ohlsson K, Nordander C, Asterland P, et al. Questionnaire versus direct technical measurements in assessing postures and movements of the head, upper back, arms and hands. *Scand J Work Environ Health.* 2001;27:30–40.

88. Balogh I, Orbaek P, Ohlsson K, Nordander C, Unge J, Winkel J, et al. Self-assessed and directly measured occupational physical activities: influence of musculoskeletal complaints, age and gender. *Appl Ergon.* 2004;35:49–56.

89. Unge J, Hansson GA, Ohlsson K, Nordander C, Axmon A, Winkel J, et al. Validity of self-assessed reports of occurrence and duration of occupational tasks. *Ergonomics.* 2005;48:12–24.

22

Conclusions and Agenda for the Future

Elizabeth Genovese, MD, MBA, and Jill S. Galper, PT, MEd

This book has established a framework through which people who request or apply functional testing can do the following:

- Better match the general content and scope of the functional tests they request to the medical and functional issues that need to be addressed;
- Choose evaluators and functional capacity evaluation (FCE) systems that are most likely to address their unique concerns;
- Understand the principles that an evaluator should adhere to when performing and interpreting data from tests done as part of a functional assessment;
- Know how these principles should be used in preparing the final report;
- Apply the results of functional testing to specific clinical and work situations, even when the quality of the study is suboptimal; and
- Understand the meaning of the raw data from functional testing.

Chapters 1 through 4 and 14 through 20 primarily focused on providing practical information; Chapters 5 through 13 described FCE test components and outlined the evidence basis for their use; and Chapter 21 provided an overall assessment of the literature regarding the safety, reliability, validity, and practicality of FCE as a whole. The literature indicates that although FCEs have generally been shown to be safe, with a substantive amount of literature supporting reliability and content validity of at least some protocols, there is less evidence of predictive validity for outcomes such as return to work. As discussed in prior chapters (Introduction, 16, 21) and, in particular, as illustrated by the International Classification of Functioning, Disability, and Health model (Introduction), this difference, at least in part, reflects the impact of a multitude of personal, environmental, and societal factors on disablement.

General problems with FCE as a whole can be described as falling into one of two (or both) categories, namely, lack of standardization and lack of evidence supporting validity. Different types of validity have been investigated in different contexts, including construct and criterion validity as they relate to the ability of FCEs to predict successful return to work, determine risk of injury, assess ability to safely perform job-related activities, and discriminate between people who can and cannot perform a given task when effort is inconsistent or submaximal.

There is a lack of standardization with regard to terminology; test length and components; the method and analytic framework used for material handling, movement and positional tolerance determinations; frequency projections and level of effort; report content and format (including the estimated physical capacities form); and evaluator qualifications. Given this lack of standardization, it is not surprising to find a lack of consensus about the usefulness and predictive value of functional testing. However, the lack of standardization does not account for the poor predictive validity of individual models for outcomes of interest, such as return to work and risk of injury. This lack of predictive validity may be due to problems with test design, but may also, as stated previously, indicate that it is inappropriate to expect the results of functional testing to predict outcomes that have been shown to primarily relate to factors other than physical ability per se.

Terminology

Problems with terminology begin with the name of the test itself. As noted in Chapters 1 and 21, although FCE is the default terminology used to describe functional assessment tests, the nomenclature varies substantially. It is also unclear whether FCE is the appropriate terminology because *performance,* rather than *capacity,* is what is being evaluated in most cases. It is not clear that the identification of capacity is relevant or necessary when establishing an evaluee's ability to sustain activity on a safe and dependable basis. Chapter 2 proposed alternative nomenclatures for describing functional testing that is primarily based upon the reason one is ordering the evaluation, but many other options would be acceptable.

Clarification of the terminology used to describe evaluee effort would also be useful. Descriptors such as valid or invalid, consistent or inconsistent, and even maximal or submaximal are widely used to characterize effort; however, the definitions are often unique to a given protocol or even a given evaluator. The meanings of descriptors such as conditionally valid, conditionally invalid, and marginal are even less clear.

Perhaps the most important issue regarding terminology, however, has to do with the characterization of specific test activities. For example, some frequently encountered activities such as balancing and climbing are commonly rated by using a frequency or work tolerance rating, when an aptitude or skill level rating may be more relevant. Does balancing refer to the ability of a person to have the balance required for ordinary activities or the higher degree of balance that might be required to work on scaffolding or walk a tightrope? Does climbing refer to the ability to climb stairs or ascend ladders? And does reaching overhead (or elevated reaching) mean reaching forward to a point that is just above one's head or working with one's arm fully extended upward (and, in some cases, one's neck in extension). The biomechanical ramifications of these differences are clearly large but rarely, if ever, discussed. A 2006 article by Kuijer et al[1] relied on an appendix providing specific operational definitions of activities when assessing the match between FCE activities and work demands. Reneman indicated, via e-mail correspondence, that these definitions were then applied toward a recent Delphi study that attempted to obtain consensus for the FCE framework and terminology

(R. Soer, C. P. van der Schans, J.W. Groothoff, J.H.B. Geertzen, and M.F. Reneman, PT, PhD, unpublished data, 2008). It may be possible to use the results to develop a widespread consensus about terminology among all relevant stakeholders.

Test Length and Components

Functional tests vary in length. Test length depends on the reason the test is being performed and on the model used. Two-day and multiday models have been justified by the need to assess functional abilities over time, the evaluee's clinical condition the day after the functional test, and/or the degree to which an evaluee experienced a deterioration in performance. Yet, there has been no overall determination about the value of longer tests or when they would be indicated. Variations in length of "1-day" models are due to the number of component tests and whether they are repeated during the protocol, the inclusion of a history and physical examination, and the use of items such as activities of daily living (ADL) and psychological questionnaires. Even if one assumes the inclusion of a history and physical examination and the overall test components, there is little consistency among FCEs in the specific test methods and scoring criteria used. Furthermore, some models allow the report recipient to review the raw data from the FCE (and, consequently, see what components were used), whereas other models do not provide this option. Even when the raw data are available, the scoring criteria on which determinations were made are often unknown because this "proprietary" information is not available. Considering the controversy about the predictive validity of FCE, an open discussion about test components and the rationale for their use would seem indicated. Psychometrically validated self-report questionnaires and/or psychological tests are not routinely used in many functional tests but may be valuable to help identify complicated cases that might benefit from a multidisciplinary assessment or other interventions. Furthermore, given the impact of psychological and socioenvironmental factors on the results of FCE, further investigation into the use of shortened tests such as the Functional Assessment Screening Test or Short-Form FCE[2-4] is needed to determine the critical test elements that should be used when the effect of these factors on results is such that a shortened test version is appropriate.

Determination of Material Handling

A number of different protocols used to assess dynamic lifting such as the PILE (developed at the University of Texas Southwestern Medical Center at Dallas), EPIC (BTE Technologies, Baltimore, MD), WorkWell (WorkWell Systems

Inc, Laguna Hills, CA), and DSI (DSI Work Solutions Inc, Duluth, MN) protocols have been thoroughly described in research and study literature (see Chapter 6). However, other protocols used in commercial models have not been described, even though the protocol developers have claimed that they are supported by internal data.

The first relevant question has to do with predictive validity. The results of one lifting protocol have not been shown to be generalizable to another.[5-7] Even more disconcerting is a study indicating that that one protocol (presumably performed the same way) led to different results in three different countries.[8] Although some models (WorkWell, DSI, and EPIC) determine constant (WorkWell and DSI) and frequent (EPIC) abilities through the test protocol, most other methods use an extrapolation. This extrapolation has not been validated. Furthermore, there is no consistency among job analysts and FCE protocols about how many repetitions correspond to materials handling terms such as occasionally, frequently, and constantly.

Agreement as to what constitutes a "safe" lift might help improve consistency between protocols. As noted in Chapter 6, the criteria defining safe or appropriate lifting technique are not standardized and potentially affect the test end point. Obtaining consensus about lifting technique and instructions to evaluees is needed.

Determination of Movement and Positional Tolerance Ability

This area can be viewed as a virtual "black hole." As noted previously, there are no fixed terminology or agreed-on operational definitions. Assuming that there were, commercial models have vendor-specific protocols for determining whether evaluees can perform these activities and the frequency with which they can be performed. These protocols, the scoring criteria, and the studies in support of them are not available for review because the protocols are proprietary. Comparison studies of movement ability have not been performed, but given the differences in test methods, poor agreement between methods is probable. It is unlikely that progress can be made in this arena unless some agreement about whether and how to share the results of these studies is made. Although the proponents of the methods-time measurement method in functional testing claim its applicability to repetitive movement testing, it was not originally intended for this purpose (see Chapter 9). Whether it is valid to use the rate of task completion as the basis for determining an evaluee's ability to tolerate a given activity over time has not been studied, and the basis for these determinations is unclear.

The terms *occasional, frequent,* and *constant* are used to describe physical abilities, but their definitions are vague, and it can be difficult for an FCE evaluator to apply them. As discussed in Chapters 9 and 16, these terms describe an overall percentage of the workday and do not allow for situations when intensive work tasks may be performed for extended periods only during certain parts of the day. For example, is it appropriate to consider a job that requires heavy lifting done for 45 consecutive minutes twice a day (which would meet criteria for occasional lifting) as equivalent to one that requires only 10 to 15 minutes of lifting per hour?

An ancillary issue relates to the extent to which frequency determinations are made in a test protocol and what to do when a model does *not* include a protocol for doing so. Some evaluators refuse to provide any guidance to the FCE requestors in these situations; others will do so reluctantly. When one considers that these projections are used by physicians who routinely make similar estimates without the benefit of having done **any** functional testing, one cannot help but question why a presumably skilled evaluator would be unable to do so. This is particularly relevant in regard to the term *constantly* as applied to sitting. Although many jobs ostensibly require constant sitting, most allow workers to get up or shift position at will. There is no literature regarding how to assess sitting. For an evaluator to provide a physical capacities assessment that clears the evaluee only for the occassional sitting in the absence of any clinical reason for the limitation, and base this determination on the excuse that "my model does not have a protocol for assessing sitting at more than an occasional level" seems unreasonable.

The lack of consistency in the recommendations (adjusted for anthropomorphic factors, medical history, and physical examination) among models that use proprietary methods is of concern. Consequently, given the absence of published models to use when formally assessing whether someone can sit, stand, or crouch constantly and the absence of specific guidance about the meaning of terms such as occasionally, frequently, and constantly, should evaluators be asked to base their projections about these activities primarily on the clinical examination and the presence of historical or physical contraindications for performing them? If this option is a possibility, it would be appropriate for there to be some consensus reached for when one could use terminology such as *no activity limitation* to address issues of positional tolerance that are not otherwise addressed by functional testing protocols.

Determination of Level of Effort

Functional testing reports generally comment on and quantify the level of effort (Chapters 11 and 16), yet the literature in support of individual components is mixed, and there is no consensus about how to integrate this information in a report.

There is, as yet, no consensus about the most valid processes for making determinations of the level of effort. A number of questions about existing processes have not been adequately addressed, such as the following:

- What is the relationship between heart rate and static testing results?
- How does one best assess effort during lifting protocols? In particular, can evaluation of a lifting task by a skilled observer adequately discriminate between evaluees who are and are not exerting maximal effort? An ancillary question is whether evaluators can adequately classify evaluees exerting submaximal effort (ie, effort that is so far below maximal as to be clearly identifiable as such)? The literature does not provide adequate guidance on this issue. For example:
    - Jay et al,[9] in their study of a nonpatient population using the EPIC, indicated that subjective evaluation of evaluee exertion could differentiate between evaluees who were asked to exert maximal and 50% of maximal effort.
    - The study by Lemstra et al[10] of the PILE test found that using this procedure (evaluation of accessory muscle recruitment, slower speed of movement, and whether a box was slid onto a shelf or pushed onto it with one's body) did not allow sufficient sensitivity or specificity to differentiate between evaluees exerting maximal and 60% of maximal effort.
    - The 2005 study by Reneman et al[11] using observation suggested that evaluators could accurately identify subjects with chronic low back pain who were clearly exerting submaximal effort, but were less able to assess whether they were exerting maximal effort.
- There also needs to be further investigation of the relationship between static and dynamic performance suggested by the Blankenship System[12] and whether this system can be used as an effort indicator. Can fewer tests be used to reflect effort than are currently used in this protocol because shortening the test procedure would undoubtedly facilitate its use?
- There are a number of older tests that seemed inherently logical and/or were supported in early literature but have not been adequately studied. These include the following:
    - Horizontal strength change (Chapters 8 and 11)
    - The implications of real-time force/time curves of force production of isometric tests (particularly the slope of the force curve) (Chapter 8)
    - Methods that evaluate muscle activation using surface electromyography. It has been suggested that these could provide a more accurate method than clinical substantiation, which would be reasonable; however, further studies are needed (Chapter 11).
- There are also newer tests that, used in combination with clinical examination and other functional test findings, hold promise, such as the following:
    - The bilateral simultaneous grip testing by Schapmire et al (Chapters 11 and 12);

CHAPTER 22

- The Visual Target Grip Test by Shechtman: Is this procedure safe for patient populations? Can a lesser grip target be used? (Chapters 11 and 12)
- Motion parameters: trunk velocity and acceleration monitored during functional activity (Chapter 11)
- Studies by Dvir and others of DEC (difference between eccentric/concentric ratios) with a modified Kin-Com hold promise, but how do we make this technology more available to clinicians? (Chapters 7 and 11)
- Combined methods, such as use of the BTE and Jamar hand dynamometer, as used in the study by King and Berryhill,[13] need to be tested on patient populations. In addition, as discussed in Chapter 11, cross-validation of these tests is needed.

Functional Testing (and Physical Capacities) Report Format

Chapter 16 discussed criteria that should be used as a framework when analyzing data from functional test components to make determinations. Although this chapter and others in this book have provided recommendations about how best to approach data analysis, there are no uniformly agreed-on methods about how to best do so or even about what information does and does not belong in a final report. Although commercial models have this advantage (ie, use of a consistent report format), there are few, if any, situations in which a referral source will use only one provider. Development of a formal quality assurance review process to compare one report with another, especially in terms of applying the information provided to specific clinical situations, seems warranted.

The format of physical capacity estimate (PCE) forms also needs to be addressed. The PCE forms virtually all require evaluators who complete them to indicate whether evaluees can perform a task or maintain a position at frequency levels ranging from occasional to constant. Physicians were initially asked to complete these forms and used a combination of patient interview and reasoned assessment about the probable functional implications of active medical diagnoses and abnormalities found during the physical examination or through diagnostic testing to do so. This is, incidentally, the reason the information on these forms was always considered an *estimate*. Functional testing provides evaluators with a more objective basis on which to make some of these decisions, yet, as noted previously, there is still no validated information (except that said to exist in the method behind various commercial models) to use in determining certain aspects of material handling (eg, frequent or constant lifting or the performance of tasks using the upper extremities) or positional tolerance. Recommendations about how to manage this dilemma were made previously, but if basing estimates of physical capacities on the results of a clinical evaluation is in excess of what evaluators can routinely be expected to perform, it may be better to decide to restructure PCE forms in a manner that is more consistent with what can truly be based, at least to some degree, on observed physical capacities. One way of doing so would be to eliminate frequency projections, at least in part, for some activities and substitute statements such as "no apparent evidence of limitation," with the report then clarifying the context in which such statements are made. Certainly this is a topic that needs to be discussed because the current situation, in which information on PCEs is almost as dependent on the FCE model and comfort level of the evaluator in making extrapolations as it is on the actual demonstrated physical attributes and abilities of evaluees, is clearly suboptimal.

Evaluator Qualifications

Consensus about how to best handle issues of standardization of report format and the basis on which PCE forms are completed is also relevant in terms of addressing another open question, that is "Who is most qualified to perform FCEs and functional tests?" It is the overall belief of the editors and chapter authors that FCE reports, in all but the most limited circumstances (preoffer skills assessment), are most useful and applicable to the needs of referral sources when evaluations are performed by skilled clinicians who integrate information obtained from the history, medical records, physical examination, and ongoing observation of the evaluee with data from individual test component impressions. Does this preclude potential evaluators who do not have the requisite clinical skills from performing functional testing, or can they be used in models that allow for a team approach? If the latter, there needs to be formal investigation of whether teams of evaluators can effectively perform FCEs and, in particular, the optimal process to ensure communication of all relevant information among team members. Regardless of who is doing testing, there should be a formal educational process and/or certification to ensure that all evaluators share a set of core competencies (see Chapter 17).

CHAPTER 22

Special Protocols

Even if we eventually reach some consensus about how to handle "routine" functional assessments, there are no data about how to best use them in the evaluation of people with chronic pain or fatigue. Chapter 15 provided recommendations regarding an overall approach to evaluating the former and then applying the data one obtains to the person's treatment and/or decisions about return to work. Chapters 16 and 18 discussed how to apply information obtained from the evaluation of evaluees who exert submaximal effort. Even so, it may be best to develop an entirely different model of testing, one that relies more heavily on the results of psychometrically validated self-report questionnaires or psychological testing, to evaluate people with chronic pain. This would also be applicable to the assessment of functional limitations of people with chronic fatigue (which is associated with many disease states), although endurance during testing from one day to the next also seems to be something that should be evaluated in cases of chronic fatigue. A uniform means of doing so should be developed.

Predictive Validity

Problems with predictive validity are undoubtedly responsible for some of the lack of enthusiasm for the use of FCE among many case managers, claims adjustors, employers, vocational rehabilitation specialists, physicians, and others who would presumably find reliable and valid information about functional abilities and limitations useful. For example, a qualitative study of Dutch case managers involved in return-to-work or disability claims management were asked to indicate, on a scale of 1 to 10, the degree to which they found FCE to be useful.[14] The mean valuation of the return-to-work managers was 6.5 (SD 1.5), while that of the disability claims managers was 4.8 (SD 2.2). Arguments in favor of FCE were its "ability to confirm one's own opinions" and the "objectivity of its measurement method." It is interesting to note that arguments against the FCE were that the information was "redundant" and "not objective." It was not clear whether this huge variation in opinion was due to dissimilarities in the FCEs reviewed by managers who found them to be objective vs nonobjective or in the knowledge base or overall orientation of managers who found them redundant as opposed to welcoming confirmation of their opinions. Regardless, the majority of case managers indicated that musculoskeletal disorders, a positive patient self-perception of ability to work, and the presence of an actual job were all indications for FCE, with FCE contraindicated in the presence of medically unexplained disorders, a negative patient self-perception of ability to work, and the existence of disputes and legal procedures. Another review of the use of functional capacity assessment in the evaluation of manual materials handlers with back injuries indicated that "the predictive value of tools used to evaluate functional capacity in manual materials handlers remains in question."[15] Yet, a third review,[16] discussing the "practical aspects of functional capacities evaluations," indicated that although limitations associated with FCEs have, in a few cases, been "overcome through thorough job analysis and careful work simulation, with protocols that closely parallel work activities, directed by expert evaluators, resulting in findings of reasonable certainty," FCE will "not be very helpful for practicing clinicians involved in return to work decisions." It was recommended that the majority of FCEs not conducted in relation to a specific job be viewed as "primarily administrative exercises, allowing for a demonstration of a range of performance that is acceptable to the worker." Potential therapeutic value in this setting was described in terms of the ability of an observer-based functional evaluation to "chart improvements, specify functional disparities with respect to job demands, and identify nonmedical factors influencing the ability to work" with results then contributing to "resolving issue of compensability, disability and employability."[16]

Lack of standardization in terminology, test length and components, determination of material handling, determination of movement and positional tolerance ability, determination of level of effort, functional testing (and physical capacities) report format, evaluator qualifications, and how to handle the evaluation of evaluees with pain or fatigue are undoubtedly some of the reasons for the low predictive validity of FCE for outcomes of interest such as the ability to perform specific job functions (especially on a sustained basis), risk of injury or reinjury, and ability to return to (and stay at) work. However, even if these were standardized, the previously noted (see Introduction and Chapters 15, 18, and 21) impact of psychological, job-related, and other socioenvironmental factors on worker performance will always have as much of a role as do actual physical abilities in determining the degree to which evaluees are able to initiate and sustain work-related (and even non–work-related) activities. In many circumstances, they may be the primary determinants. The precise impact of these factors cannot be quantified—all that can be said is that they have an impact and that people who request and apply functional testing must be aware of their potential contribution to ultimate outcomes because, in many cases, their role may be so great as to make the question "What is this person's true physical capacity" of limited, if any, relevance. Indeed, as stated by Gross[17] (and mirrored by Reneman et al in Chapter 21), FCEs do not "appear to be purely tests of physical capacity as performance during assessment is influenced by multiple personal and environmental contextual factors. FCEs are more accurately considered behavioral tests influenced by multiple factors, including physical ability, beliefs, and perceptions, and should be interpreted within the subject's broader personal and environmental context."

The value of tests is generally assessed by the degree to which they can affect the course of treatment, by confirming a clinical impression (which, in turn, will warrant use of a specific treatment option), or, rarely, by revealing evidence of unsuspected pathology that will in and of itself warrant some form of treatment. Despite questions about the overall predictive validity of FCEs, the information they provide about physical function is not directly available from other forms of testing and is certainly better than an educated guess.

CHAPTER 22

The studies by Brouwer et al[18] and Brokaw et al[19] demonstrated that physicians' predictions underpredicted patients' abilities, whereas Oesch et al[20] demonstrated that the quality of "work certificates" from physicians was improved when the physician used an FCE. Regardless, indiscriminate use of functional testing in all circumstances when the extent of a person's physical abilities needs to be quantified is not recommended. The application of FCE to address clearly articulated questions related to physical ability in the context of specific clinical scenarios is, however, reasonable.[21,22] In particular, the use of appropriately selected combinations of individual physical test components has been shown to be of value in the preoffer setting and seems to provide data that can be a viable basis for limited statements about function, especially by establishing a safe minimum and, with motivated evaluees, a safe maximum. Judiciously chosen combinations of tests, including the use of psychometric testing and self-report questionnaires, when integrated with information obtained from a thorough clinical evaluation of the evaluee, can also provide information about the impact of factors other than actual physical ability on perceived functional limitations and even can help clarify the extent to which these factors are under volitional control. There has been literature suggesting that a combination of a questionnaire and a functional test would seem to be the best instrument to assess functional capacity of the musculoskeletal system[23]; this suggestion needs to be further examined, as does use of existing forms of FCE that place less emphasis on the measurement of the physical domain[3] (R. Soer, C. P. van der Schans, J.W. Groothoff, J.H.B. Geertzen, and M.F. Reneman, PT, PhD, unpublished data, 2008; Chapter 21).

Although the literature does not demonstrate FCEs to be "objective" tests that are as sensitive, specific, reliable, or valid as many (but certainly not all) other commonly accepted medical tests, the latter are most useful when the method is standardized, clinical information is provided in conjunction with use, and they are applied to clinical situations in which their predictive value will be optimized. Improvements in the methods and standardization of functional testing; development of guidelines for the use of functional testing to address specific clinical, legal, or administrative questions; and determination (by professionals who have been most involved in the development or application of this testing) of the competencies that must be demonstrated by evaluators who perform FCE are mandatory. There should be concurrent research done to identify the factors that are relevant to return to work or risk of injury and amenable to evaluation by functional testing. In particular, the impact of psychological factors on the results of testing needs to be better defined and quantified because the "need to devote a substantial period during an FCE to the evaluation of physical abilities in the context of significant psychosocial overlay remains unclear" (Chapter 21).

The application of research about the aspects of the physical, psychological, and socioenvironmental domains that are most relevant to return to work to the design of FCE, in conjunction with efforts to improve methods and standardization, will give functional testing its "best chance" of being transformed from an amorphous, highly provider-dependent evaluation with unpredictable clinical value to a tool that can be used whenever objective assessments of physical function (and the factors that contribute to decreased function) are required. And, assuming it can reach this level, the development of more valid and reliable functional testing may also allow its regular and, perhaps, mandated application to scenarios when quantification of the impact of impairment on disability is required. Indeed, it is possible that at one point we will be able to develop a system of rating disability that is predominantly based on our ability to link specific deficits in functional testing to the ability (or inability) to perform specific ADLs, define the ADLs potentially affected by given objective anatomic or physiologic abnormalities, and use the results of functional testing to determine which ADLs have indeed been affected by a disease process as a guide to providing a more holistic and functionally based determination of disability consistent with the principles of the International Classification of Functioning, Disability, and Health.

Functional capacity evaluations have the potential to "bridge the gap" between the impairment rating and disability assessment. However, it is unlikely that the potential of FCE will be realized unless all stakeholders decide that the time has come to rectify the significant problems that have been identified in this book and in the literature as a whole.

Summary

The value of FCEs is limited by lack of standardization in terminology, test length and components, determination of material handling, determination of movement and positional tolerance ability, determination of level of effort, functional testing report format, evaluator qualifications, and how to handle the evaluation of evaluees with pain or fatigue. These limitations all contribute to the low predictive validity and frequent lack of usefulness of FCE in addressing outcomes of interest such as the ability to perform specific job functions (especially on a sustained basis), risk of injury or reinjury, and ability to return to work.

FCEs should be clinical evaluations in which qualified health care providers analyze and apply results of specific objective components in the context of the

CHAPTER 22

history, physical examination, and ongoing observations of the evaluee's subjective and objective response to testing to provide estimates of function. The degree to which evaluees' decisions to cooperate or not cooperate with testing affects FCE results to a larger extent than might be seen in tests such as X-rays and magnetic resonance imaging. Therefore, the use of FCEs in many clinical scenarios may include the use of self-report and psychological questionnaires. It must also mandate that a well-trained, qualified, and clinically observant evaluator weigh the contribution of subjective and objective factors to component test results individually and as part of an analysis of the overall pattern of findings in the context of why the FCE was requested.

When done well, FCEs are tools that can be used to characterize the effect of health status on work and non–work-related activities of daily living and, hence, bridge the gap between the impairment rating and disability assessment. Evaluators and users of FCE reports who must apply this information to determinations about ability and disability could routinely use this tool to assist in their decision making if it were reliable and valid.

Achieving this goal should begin with the assembly of expert panels to address problems with standardization, including how to best interpret tests results in the context of the evaluee's clinical condition. The study working toward standardization of terminology that was underway at the time this book was submitted for publication is an important step in the process. In addition, the American Physical Therapy Association has recently updated its guidelines on evaluating functional capacity, which represents another step toward standardization of terminology and improved quality in the functional test process.[24] Concurrent research should be performed to determine the result to which findings in functional testing, including findings related to psychological and socioenvironmental factors, are predictors of injury, recovery, and disability. These should all be integrated to develop models for FCE application to specific clinical situations that can be requested by referral sources whenever questions about physical abilities and limitations are germane to clinical, administrative, or legal determinations. Stakeholders who will benefit from improved functional assessment methods should consider funding some of these efforts.

This chapter was not submitted for final publication until all chapter-authors had reviewed and indicated their approval of its content.

References

1. Kuijer W, Brouwer S, Reneman M, et al. Matching FCE activities and work demands: an explorative study. *J Occup Rehabil.* Sep 2006;16(3):469–483.
2. Ruan CM, Haig AJ, Geisser ME, Yamakawa K, Buchholz RL. Functional capacity evaluations in persons with spinal disorders: predicting poor outcomes on the Functional Assessment Screening Test (FAST). *J Occup Rehabil.* 2001;11:119–132.
3. Gross DP, Battie MC, Asante A. Development and validation of a short-form functional capacity evaluation for use in claimants with low back disorders. *J Occup Rehabil.* 2006;16:53–62.
4. Gross DP, Battie MC, Asante AK. Evaluation of a short-form functional capacity evaluation: less may be best. *J Occup Rehabil.* 2007;17:422–435.
5. Ijmker S, Gerrits EH, Reneman MF. Upper lifting performance of healthy young adults in functional capacity evaluations: a comparison of two protocols. *J Occup Rehabil.* 2003;13:297–305.
6. Soer R, Poels BJ, Geertzen JH, Reneman MF. A comparison of two lifting assessment approaches in patients with chronic low back pain. *J Occup Rehabil.* 2006;16:639–646.
7. Rustenburg G, Kuijer PP, Frings-Dresen MH. The concurrent validity of the ERGOS Work Simulator and the Ergo-Kit with respect to maximum lifting capacity. *J Occup Rehabil.* 2004;14:107–118.
8. Reneman MF, Kool J, Oesch P, Geertzen JH, Battie MC, Gross DP. Material handling performance of patients with chronic low back pain during functional capacity evaluation: a comparison between three countries. *Disabil Rehabil.* 2006;28:1143–1149.
9. Jay MA, Lamb JM, Watson RL, et al. Sensitivity and specificity of the indicators of sincere effort of the EPIC lift capacity test on a previously injured population. *Spine.* 2000;25:1405–1412.
10. Lemstra M, Olszynski WP, Enright W. The sensitivity and specificity of functional capacity evaluations in determining maximal effort: a randomized trial. *Spine.* 2004;29:953–959.
11. Reneman MF, Fokkens AS, Dijkstra PU, Geertzen JH, Groothoff JW. Testing lifting capacity: validity of determining effort level by means of observation. *Spine.* 2005;30:E40–E46.
12. Brubaker PN, Fearon FJ, Smith SM, et al. Sensitivity and specificity of the Blankenship FCE system's indicators of submaximal effort. *J Orthop Sports Phys Ther.* 2007;37:161–168.
13. King JW, Berryhill BH. Assessing maximum effort in upper-extremity functional testing. *Work.* 1991;1:65–76.
14. Wind H, Gouttebarge V, Kuijer PP, Sluiter JK, Frings-Dresen MH. The utility of functional capacity evaluation: the opinion of physicians and other experts in the field of return to work and disability claims. *Int Arch Occup Environ Health.* January 14, 2006:1–7.
15. Jones T, Kumar S. Functional capacity evaluation of manual materials handlers: a review. *Disabil Rehabil.* 2003;25:179–191.

CHAPTER 22

16. Pransky GS, Dempsey PG. Practical aspects of functional capacity evaluations. *J Occup Rehabil.* 2004;14:217–229.

17. Gross DP. Measurement properties of performance-based assessment of functional capacity. *J Occup Rehabil.* 2004;14:165–174.

18. Brouwer S, Dijkstra PU, Stewart RE, Goeken LN, Groothoff JW, Geertzen JH. Comparing self-report, clinical examination and functional testing in the assessment of work-related limitations in patients with chronic low back pain. *Disabil Rehabil.* 2005;27:999–1005.

19. Brokaw JP, Walker WC, Cifu DX, Gardner M. Sitting and standing tolerance in patients with chronic back pain: comparison between physician prediction and covert observation. *Arch Phys Med Rehabil.* 2004;85:837–839.

20. Oesch PR, Kool JP, Bachmann S, Devereux J. The influence of a functional capacity evaluation on fitness for work certificates in patients with non-specific chronic low back pain. *Work.* 2006;26:259–271.

21. Hegmann KT. Evidence-based Practice Spine Panel. Low back disorders. In: Glass LS, ed. *Occupational Medicine Practice Guidelines: Evaluation and Management of Common Health Problems and Functional Recovery in Workers.* 2nd ed. Elk Grove Village, IL: American College of Occupational & Environmental Medicine; 2007.

22. Hegmann KT, ed. Evidence-based Practice Chronic Pain Panel. Chronic pain. In: Glass LS, ed. *Occupational Medicine Practice Guidelines: Evaluation and Management of Common Health Problems and Functional Recovery in Workers.* 2nd ed. American College of Occupational & Environmental Medicine. Beverly Farms, MA: OEM Press; 2004.

23. Wind H, Gouttebarge V, Kuijer PP, Frings-Dresen MH. Assessment of functional capacity of the musculoskeletal system in the context of work, daily living, and sport: a systematic review. *J Occup Rehabil.* 2005;15:253–272.

24. American Physical Therapy Association. *Occupational Health Guidelines: Evaluating Functional Capacity.* Alexandria, VA: American Physical Therapy Association; 1999.

Functional Capacity Evaluation Model Descriptions

Representatives from the most commonly used, commercially available functional capacity evaluation (FCE) models in the United States, Australia, and the Netherlands were contacted and invited to complete a "Model Description Table" about their FCE model. The editors of this book did not verify the information in the descriptions. The purpose of this information is to provide readers with information about the models that can be used as a starting point for further inquiry.

The following FCE vendors chose not to participate or did not respond to our invitation to provide information:

Did not respond
- Key FCA
- Digital Video FCE, formerly PhysioMetrics
- Kinematic Consultants
- WorkHab FCE System

Declined the invitation to participate
- Ergos Work Simulator

FCE Model: BTE Technologies

Contact Information:	**Corporate & Products Group** **7455-L New Ridge Rd** **Hanover, MD 21076** **Telephone: (410) 850-0333; Toll-free: (800) 331-8845**
What are the qualifications of the FCE evaluator (eg, PT, OT)?	Licensed physical or occupational therapist, chiropractor, physician.
Training: How long; what is the process; is continuing education in your FCE method required (please describe)?	There are 3 levels of training for therapists utilizing the BTE proprietary equipment. The first 2 levels provide an introduction to technology-based FCEs with basic competency using the equipment and software. Level 3 focuses on the applications of testing and critical thinking in FCEs. Providers performing BTE-referred FCEs are graded by our quality assurance program and continue to receive education/critique on reports and testing.
What is the FCE test length?	From 3 to 5 hours.
Is a history included as part of the FCE?	Yes.
Is a musculoskeletal examination included as part of the FCE?	Yes. Objective isometric strength testing is performed on the BTE system and range of motion testing of the spinal region or extremity with comparison of injured vs noninjured side.
What psychometric tests, if any, do evaluees complete? How are they used?	Oswestry Low Back Pain Questionnaire; Neck Disability Index; Waddell Signs; Dallas pain questionnaire may be included as well as other standardized self-report questionnaires.
Is aerobic testing performed? Which protocol? If not, how is aerobic endurance addressed?	MCAFT step test Single stage treadmill test Submaximal treadmill test Any 1 of 3 may be administered.

FCE Model: BTE Technologies (continued)

How is material handling tested? How is lifting frequency determined?	Material handling is performed during a lifting evaluation and a carrying evaluation. *Occasional* lifting is defined as 1 repetition per weight level in 10-lb increments. *Frequent* is defined as 4 repetitions per weight level.
What size box is used for lifting? Does the box have cutouts or handles?	12 × 12 × 12-in standard NIOSH size, weight 10 lb; there are 2 different crates, one has cutouts and the other handles. For the EPIC lift capacity, the handles are used per protocol.
How are non–material handling abilities determined, including movement and sustained positional tolerance? How is frequency determined?	Positional tolerances are tested using the BTE FROM (functional range of motion) board, which uses the internationally recognized MTM standard to assign a percentile ranking to the performance of work performed within a specific posture. Testing performed to establish occasional, frequent, and/or constant frequencies per the Department of Labor classification system.
What hand-related testing is performed in non–hand-specific FCEs (eg, grip, pinch, dexterity)?	The standard handgrip test The rapid exchange grip test Maximum voluntary effort grip (MVE) Universal Task Master isometric testing provides right and left forces independently and combined using various hand holds, forearm rotations, and angles in push and pulling. The software contains numerous preloaded description/ instructions of clinical tests for detecting symptoms associated with UE impairment including the Tinel sign; Phalen Test; Allen Test; Brachial Plexus Stretch Test; Finkelstein Test; etc. Standardized gross and fine motor testing including Minnesota Rate of Manipulation and Purdue Peg Board and/or other appropriate tools can be easily used as nonintegrated testing in the software producing the results in the final report details.
How flexible is your model? Can an evaluator vary the length and breadth of the test protocol?	Extremely flexible: The evaluator can vary the length and breadth depending on the referral questions and diagnosis. Custom tests can be created in order to simulate real work activities.

FCE Model: BTE Technologies (continued)

Do you offer "special" protocols (eg, upper extremity FCE, fatigue-related)? What are they, and how do they differ from your "routine" FCE?	FCE protocols are based on the referral questions, diagnosis, and/or employer/job-specific testing. The BTE system allows the use of real-time heart rate monitoring for improved safety and accurate interpretation of physiological response to activity. Computer integrated testing enhances validity with calculated CVs and strength curves making it easier to interpret effort and fatigue.
Does your model use specialized equipment, meaning items most therapists would not routinely have in the clinic?	Yes, our FCE model involves testing on BTE's proprietary functional testing equipment and software.
What research supports the test-retest and interrater reliability of your FCE system?	All of the standardized protocols used in the BTE system are backed by peer-edited, scientific research. Since the system is adjustable, it is very easy to set up the tests for position, height, and body placement, providing good interrater reliability.
What research supports the construct and/or predictive validity of your FCE system?	As referenced in Reneman and Dijkstra (2003), "taking into account the multidimensional construct of work no FCE has good predictive validity when using it to predict a safe and lasting return to work." Therefore, it is important that the FCE be performed by trained, qualified medical professionals using state-of-the-science tools.
What separates your FCE system from the rest? In other words, why should a clinician choose and use your system?	BTE's EvalTech/ER System sets a higher standard in FCE and the application of capacity assessment in managing recovery and return to work. Our longevity in providing advancements in computer integrated testing, our experience with national employers and insurers, and our in-house quality assurance process sets us apart from other FCE system/methods.
What is the cost to purchase your system? Are there any ongoing fees?	Variable.

FCE Model: BTE Technologies (continued)

Is the system "mobile" to allow testing in multiple locations?	BTE has a portable solution to help a provider get started in objective strength testing and impairment ratings. Complete with a powerful laptop computer running our state-of-the-art software, it comes in a mobile carrying case so you can perform on-site functional testing.
Is there Web access to the report?	Referrals and reports are transmitted via BTE's proprietary Web portal: OscarLink. This provides a secure communication platform for all network providers and referral sources to maintain HIPAA compliance and to expedite service and report delivery.
Is there certification of the FCE evaluator, and, if so, at what cost?	Yes, included with equipment purchase or rental.

Abbreviations: FCE indicates functional capacity evaluation; PT, physical therapist; OT, occupational therapist; NIOSH, National Institute for Occupational Safety and Health; MTM, method-time management; CV, coefficient of variation; and HIPAA, Health Information Portability and Accountability Act.

FCE Model: DSI Work Solutions Functional Capacity Assessment
Copyright 2004

Contact Information:	**Susan J. Isernhagen, PT; sisernhagen@dsiworksolutions.com (218) 625-1051**
What are the qualifications of the FCE evaluator (eg, PT, OT)?	PT or OT
Training: How long; what is the process; is continuing education in your FCE method required (please describe)?	The FCA is one 9-hour day and required to be a DSI FCA provider. It is generally part of a 3-day training of DSI program, which includes job-related training on job analysis, postoffer testing, and early return-to-work testing. The FCA training includes performing and writing a full 1-day, 3-hour FCA.
	Continuing education is not required; however, DSI provides advanced training and also a yearly DSI conference for advanced education.

FCE Model: DSI Work Solutions Functional Capacity
Assessment Copyright 2004 (continued)

What is the FCE test length?	The 1-day is 3 hours. The 2-day is 5.5 hours.
Is a history included as part of the FCE?	Yes
Is a musculoskeletal examination included as part of the FCE?	Yes
What psychometric tests, if any, do evaluees complete? How are they used?	There are no psychometric tests per se. The levels of effort and the reliability of performance are both evaluated according to evidence and content validity. Also, refusals or self-limitations are noted clearly, but no labels or judgments are put on these issues. DSI often finds that persons may limit themselves during one or a few tests, but they complete the rest of the test with full effort.
	Note: Many other FCE tests begin with symptom magnification or psychological tests to determine behavioral/psychological issues before the test even starts. All therapists who have reported to DSI that they formerly used this method also indicate that any negative issues arising during this pretesting did color their interaction with the client. DSI believes that all therapists should be neutral during the test and that any inference from any source that could color this neutral interaction is detrimental to the testing situation. All therapists who have had this experience also agree that they prefer not to begin a test by already having labeled a client.
	DSI recommends that if compliance/psych/symptom magnification testing is to be done at all (and DSI always allows a clinic to customize its test), then this testing should be done *after* the FCA, when the client has had a positive experience with the evaluator during test performance.
Is aerobic testing performed? Which protocol? If not, how is aerobic endurance addressed?	No specific aerobic testing is performed, but blood pressure and heart rate are monitored before and during the tests. This includes observing heart rate and other needed vital signs during and after tests. Heart rate is taken after every test to identify recovery rates and when a new test can be started. The information on these physiological processes is considered in each performance item's inclusion in the final FCA performance grid and report.

FCE Model: DSI Work Solutions Functional Capacity
Assessment Copyright 2004 (continued)

How is material handling tested? How is lifting frequency determined?	There are three categories of lifts: a lift/carry, a lift from floor to center of gravity, and a lift from center of gravity to shoulder level. In a 1-day test, these are replicated twice. In the 2-day test (used for anyone with endurance issues), the material handling tests are evaluated 4 times. This has given a great scope of observation. The highest weight is recommended for the lowest frequency and the lightest weight for the highest frequency, unless there are mitigating circumstances such as physical or physiological reaction to test items objectively observed. Examples of mitigating circumstances are discussed if they are not observed in the test given during training.
What size box is used for lifting? Does the box have cutouts or handles?	A 12 × 12 × 12 box is used. It has a handle, which is padded for best grip. The box has similarity to most jobs. The handles are padded to insure that discomfort from the handles is not a limiting factor. We are looking for lift ability, not reaction to poor ergonomic boxes.
How are non–material handling abilities determined, including movement and sustained positional tolerance? How is frequency determined?	Each movement or position test is replicated twice in a 1-day test and 4 times in the 2-day test. Frequency is determined by the ability to tolerate position or movement in addition to any dysfunctional patterns noted. Each movement and position evaluation item has a specific set of observational criteria.
What hand-related testing is performed in non–hand-specific FCEs (eg, grip, pinch, dexterity)?	Grip, bilateral, for maximum force and best position Pinch, bilateral, for maximum force Hand coordination tests using pegboard and nut/bolt tests In addition, hand activity is noted in each activity in which it is involved (which is the majority of other tests). The FCA looks for observations of whole body activity so that any body activity (like hand coordination or strength) is noted every time it is used. There are places in each test item to note hand issues if they are present.
How flexible is your model? Can an evaluator vary the length and breadth of the test protocol?	The DSI test is standardized but also can be customized by referrer need. We do not recommend changing the test items if full information is needed. The 1- or 2-day test is chosen based on the type of problem the evaluee has. Job-specific tests are encouraged if the FCA does not replicate critical elements requested.

FCE Model: DSI Work Solutions Functional Capacity
Assessment Copyright 2004 (continued)

Do you offer "special" protocols (eg, upper extremity FCE, fatigue-related)? What are they, and how do they differ from your "routine" FCE?	We encourage the FCA evaluator to ask referral questions up-front. The evaluator then can specialize the protocols as needed. We train the DSI evaluators to be aware of what the outcome report should contain and plan accordingly. This is covered in discussion on the FCA day. However, if the evaluators have taken the full 3-day DSI course, they already know how to determine job specificity and that FCAs are mostly generic. This has added understanding to the strengths and the limitations of FCAs.
Does your model use specialized equipment, meaning items most therapists would not routinely have in the clinic?	If the clinic is an occupational rehabilitation clinic, it would have the equipment. If it is not, it may need to obtain a lifting station, dynamometers, etc. Equipment is all useful in job-specific testing and in work rehabilitation also. Total cost if it is a fully new clinic with no equipment would be $2000 to $3000.
What research supports the test-retest and interrater reliability of your FCE system?	See the FCA list following this table.
What research supports the construct and/or predictive validity of your FCE system?	The FCA is meant to be part of a larger decision system. Physicians, employers, case managers, insurers, and attorneys need objective functional information to determine return-to-work decisions and placement. To this end, the FCA is a critical part meant to facilitate a team making the employment decisions. Because of this required team effort (physician, case manger, employer, insurer), FCA in context with *the team that uses it* for return-to-work needs to be studied for validity. Gross/Battie's studies pointed that out, but they drew the weak conclusion that FCA could not predict employment without realizing that the study design was flawed and FCA is only part of the process.
	DSI has also created job function testing, which is specific to jobs. This has demonstrated validity, although written outcomes studies are just coming in and have not been published. It differs from FCA in that it is job-specific, short, and much less expensive.
	An FCA is a generic test, so it is best used when a referrer needs information on global physical ability.

FCE Model: DSI Work Solutions Functional Capacity
Assessment Copyright 2004 (continued)

What separates your FCE system from the rest? In other words, why should a clinician choose and use your system?	First, the kinesiophysical observation method has been researched multiple times and found to be reliable. This is mostly Reneman-contributed research, but parts are also from Gross/Battie and Isernhagen/Matheson and Hart. Objective scoring of an FCA is important in evidence-based medicine. Kinesiophysical includes discussing the tests with the patient, but it also means the therapist determines the scoring, sometimes using evaluee input in conjunction with the observations. But, it is far preferable to the psychophysical method in which the evaluee says what the limits are. In this method, there is a negativity as the examiner has to prove if the evaluee is "lying," etc.

The DSI approach encourages respect and honest interaction with the client combined with objective observation criteria. This sets DSI apart and is why people use it or are drawn to it. It is a true medical model.

Second, the new DSI format is far superior to any past formats, as considerable focus group work was done to solicit information on what report format physicians, case managers, employers, etc, wanted. The outcome is a very comprehensive, yet clear and concise report. Nothing asked for is left out. There is an option to customize. The referral questions are asked and answered. And, the FCA items are clearly work-related as they have been grouped from thousands of job descriptions rather than from old state/federal forms. They meet the actual needs of being compared with real jobs.

Level of effort and reliability are scored separately, not together as in most other tests. (In those other tests, it is surmised that if a person has an inconsistent result, he or she must be faking). In the DSI model, we recognize that a person could put forth full effort, and yet the ability level could be increased on the second day (due to the client getting used to moving again), or could be reduced the second day (often due to a mild exacerbation of symptoms or fatigue). In each of these cases, the positives of full effort are important, and the inconsistencies between performances become important information on which to make final determinations of ability.

APPENDIX

FCE Model: DSI Work Solutions Functional Capacity
Assessment Copyright 2004 (continued)

A person could be consistent in giving submaximal effort. Here, it is the level of effort that is important, and the consistency of this observation is included in documentation.

DSI has excellent standards for level of effort and consistency.
a. Level of effort uses kinesiophysical criteria noted in researched items.
b. Consistency of effort uses the exact test data from the evaluee's own FCA scores. As mentioned earlier, the tests are given twice in a 1-day test. If a 2-day test is used, the first- and second-day scores are compared as the test is identical from the first to second day.

Because of the repetition of items noted above, the DSI FCA designers put in considerable points of observation of repeated items. For the evaluee, it has the result of far more intensely measuring endurance and consistency. Those trained in DSI FCA have also noted the significant improvement in test design without creating a need for a longer test.

The DSI team has an excellent reputation among insurers, employers, physicians, and therapists for FCA. Referrers are confident. Also, for the therapist users of DSI FCA, the ability to call and directly talk to an expert on FCA assists with production of quality FCAs.

The ease of interpretation and writing of the DSI FCA has been a hallmark of this new model. After training, there are few questions on writing the FCA as all the information and scoring criteria are very clear and designed so that, if these criteria are followed, there are no mistakes or gray areas.

Last, the DSI FCA combines evidence-based testing, real-world test categories useful for employment, and ease of use for trained therapists and meets requirements of referrers: physicians, employers, case managers, insurers, and lawyers.

APPENDIX

FCE Model: DSI Work Solutions Functional Capacity
Assessment Copyright 2004 (continued)

What is the cost to purchase your system? Are there any ongoing fees?	The cost is dependent on how many therapists are in the group to be trained, whether the faculty member has to travel to a site, whether the clinic is being trained in the other 2 DSI job function matching programs, and how many sites will be trained during the training session. The range starts at $4900.
Is the system "mobile" to allow testing in multiple locations?	Yes, equipment can be purchased that is "mobile." If shelving for lifts can be found, then all the other FCA equipment is mobile without purchasing a separate mobile unit.
Is there Web access to the report?	No. We chose not to do this due to past problems with other systems and the Internet issues that come with Web reports.
Is there certification of the FCE evaluator, and if so, at what cost?	Yes, certificates of completion are given to each therapist who is formally trained in DSI FCA. No informal training is allowed or backed. There is not an additional or separate fee.

Abbreviations: FCE indicates functional capacity evaluation; FCA, functional capacity assessment; PT, physical therapist; and OT, occupational therapist

DSI FCE Research List

Brouwer S, Dijkstra PU, Stewart RE, Göeken LNH, Groothoff JW, Geertzen JHB. Comparing self-report, clinical examination and functional testing to measure work limitations in chronic low back pain. *Disabil Rehabil.* In press.

Brouwer S, Reneman MF, Dijkstra PU, Groothoff JW, Schellekens JMH, Göeken LNH. Test-retest reliability of the Isernhagen Work Systems functional capacity evaluation in patients with chronic low back pain. *J Occup Rehabil.* 2003;13:207–218.

Gross DP, Battie MC. The construct validity of a kinesiophysical functional capacity evaluation administered within a workers' compensation environment. *J Occup Rehabil.* 2003;13:287–295.

Gross DP, Battie MC. The prognostic value of functional capacity evaluation in patients with chronic low back pain, part 1: timely return to work. *Spine.* 2004;29:914–919.

Gross DP, Battie MC. The prognostic value of functional capacity evaluation in patients with chronic low back pain, part 2: sustained recovery. *Spine.* 2004;29:920–924.

Gross DP, Battie MC. Reliability of safe maximum lifting determinations of a functional capacity evaluation. *Phys Ther.* 2002;82:364–371.*

Isernhagen SJ, Hart DL, Matheson LM. Reliability of independent observer judgments of level of lift effort in a kinesiophysical functional capacity evaluation. *Work.* 1999;12:145–150.†

APPENDIX

Matheson LN, Isernhagen SJ, Hart DL. Relationships among lifting ability, grip force, and return to work. *Phys Ther.* 2002;82:249–256.[†]

Reneman MF. *Functional Capacity Evaluation in Patients With Chronic Low Back Pain: Reliability and Validity* [dissertation]. Rijksuniversiteit Groningen, the Netherlands; 2004.

Reneman MF, Brouwer S, Speelman-Meinema A, Dijkstra PU, Geertzen JHB, Groothoff JW. Test-retest reliability of the Isernhagen Work Systems functional capacity evaluation in healthy adults. *J Occup Rehabil.* 2004;14:295–305.[*]

Reneman MF, Bults MMWE, Engbers LH, Mulders KKG, Göeken LNH. Measuring maximum holding times and perception of static elevated work and forward bending in healthy young adults. *J Occup Rehabil.* 2001;11:87–97.[*]

Reneman MF, Dijkstra PU, Westmaas M, Göeken LNH. Test-retest reliability of lifting and carrying in a 2-day functional capacity evaluation *J Occup Rehabil.* 2002;12:269–276.[*]

Reneman MF, Fokkens AS, Dijkstra PU, Geertzen JHB, Groothoff JW. Testing lifting capacity: validity of determining effort level by means of observation. *Spine.* 2005;30:E40–E46.[*]

Reneman MF, Jaegers SMHJ, Westmaas M, Göeken LNH. The reliability of determining effort level of lifting and carrying in a functional capacity evaluation. *Work.* 2002;18:23–27.[*]

Reneman MF, Joling CI, Soer EL, Göeken LNH. Functional capacity evaluation: ecological validity of three static endurance tests. *Work.* 2001;16:227–235.

Reneman MF, Jorritsma W, Dijkstra SJ, Dijkstra PU. The relationship between kinesiophobia and performance in a functional capacity evaluation. *J Occup Rehabil.* 2003;13:277–285.

Reneman MF, Jorritsma W, Schellekens JMH, Göeken LNH. Concurrent validity of questionnaire and performance-based disability measurements in patients with chronic non–specific low back pain. *J Occup Rehabil.* 2002;12:119–130.

Reneman MF, Kuijer W, Brouwer S, Dijkstra PU, Geertzen JHB, Groothoff JW. Safety of a functional capacity evaluation in patients with chronic low back pain. Submitted.

Reneman MF, Soer R, Gerrits EHJ. Test-retest reliability of an RSI functional capacity evaluation in healthy adults. *Work.* In press.

Smith RL. Therapists' ability to identify safe maximum lifting in low back pain patients during functional capacity evaluation. *J Orthop Sports Phys Ther.* 1994;19:277–281.[*]

[*] Research used directly in development of DSI FCA
[†] Research performed directly by Susan Isernhagen, PT.

APPENDIX

FCE Model: Ergo Kit

Contact Information:	**Ergo Control**
	Buurserstraat 214-216
	7544 RG Enschede
	The Netherlands
	info@ergocontrol.nl

Ask for: Laurent van der Kraats, Marike van Kalken, or Jan Plat
Laurent.vanderKraats@ergocontrol.nl; Marike.vanKalken@ergocontrol. nl; Jan.Plat@Ergocontrol.nl

---

FCE Model: Ergo Kit (continued)

What are the qualifications of the FCE evaluator (eg, PT, OT)?	PT (physiotherapist), Mensendieck therapist (practical training therapist, same degree of education as physio-therapists), human movement scientist.
Training: How long; what is the process; is continuing education in your FCE method required (please describe)?	The training for FCE evaluators is 4 contact days and (on average) 4 days of self-study. The contact days are aimed at the basic program: the test protocol (how to perform the test), how to interpret the results, and how to make the report. The self-study is aimed at practicing with the tests (on volunteers) and with the reports. They have to deliver 2 approved reports before being qualified. When certified, the evaluators have to attend 2 days of reeducation each year.
What is the FCE test length?	Depending on the question and on whether a FBO (job demands [physical demands] interview) is also performed; 2–6 hours. The standard procedure (with no specific question, only the question of an overall view of physical abilities, and no FBO) is 4 hours.
Is a history included as part of the FCE?	The history of the participant's complaints/limitations is part of the interview.
Is a musculoskeletal examination included as part of the FCE?	No, but in the interview, perceived physical limitations are asked.
What psychometric tests, if any, do evaluees complete? How are they used?	Oswestry questionnaire, consistency (evaluation of scores on comparable tests to determine whether the participant was consistent in performing the test: performing at his/her maximum as asked) and if necessary (to be determined by evaluator through, among other things, the consistency); Tampa questionnaire; and the Waddell tests.
Is aerobic testing performed? Which protocol? If not, how is aerobic endurance addressed?	Yes, but indirect. There are a number of lengthy tests, which provide information about the (perceived) cardio-respiratory possibilities (through, among other things, the perceived hindrance and heart rate).

FCE Model: Ergo Kit (continued)

How is material handling tested? How is lifting frequency determined?	Material handling is tested with a number of short and longer tests, where the materials are handled by the participant. Lifting frequency is tested only in global duration: rare ($< 33x$), frequent ($33–66x$), or constant ($66–100x$) per day. Apart from frequency, the maximum weight that can be safely lifted/carried is determined.
	All tests are ended/determined by an acceptable performance (safe performance), the degree of hindrance the participants report, the maximum to reach break-off point, and, for some tests, the heart rate. All the rules that determine break-off point and level (duration, weight, etc) are defined by a protocol. It is the evaluator who has to interpret this protocol, which endorses on the test a human value. At all times, the participant can break off/not start a specific test.
What size box is used for lifting? Does the box have cutouts or handles?	The box has handles. Size: $36 \times 26 \times 16$ (l × b × d).
How are non–material handling abilities determined, including movement and sustained positional tolerance? How is frequency determined?	Non–material handling is tested throughout the test. Some of these abilities are tested on their own, others are tested simultaneously with other (handling) abilities. The whole test/evaluation can be divided into parts where specific non–material handling abilities are tested. In each part, a number of tests are performed (short and long duration). The protocol describes how and why to determine the duration for which the participant can safely perform these abilities (during testing and afterwards in judging). The result is a judgment in duration in percentage of an 8-hour working day: rare ($< 33\%$), frequent ($33\%–66\%$), and constant ($66\%–100\%$); within each category, there is a 2-way division (eg, $< 10\%$ or $< 33\%$).

FCE Model: Ergo Kit (continued)

What hand-related testing is performed in non–hand-specific FCEs (eg, grip, pinch, dexterity)?	The protocol involves judging 2 kinds of hand-related abilities: – handling (eg, with whole hand handling materials) – fine-tuning motor movements of fingers/finger abilities To judge these 2 abilities, there are grip tests (handling) and finer motor finger tests (eg, putting small bars into small holes or working with screws). There is no prescribed way of performing: it is up to the participant to determine how exactly to handle the test in question.
How flexible is your model? Can an evaluator vary the length and breadth of the test protocol?	There are 55 tests that can be performed. The evaluator can vary length and breadth of the protocol, depending on the specific question, the specific job demands (as determined in the FBO: physical demands on the job interview), or the specific complaints.
Do you offer "special" protocols (eg, upper extremity FCE, fatigue-related)? What are they, and how do they differ from your "routine" FCE?	Yes, there is a "back" protocol, and we are working on a number of other special protocols (depending on specific complaints or on specific body regions). They mainly differ in number of tests (duration). But we have one protocol that differs in the terminology, description of abilities (and limitations), to coincide with the terminology of the purchaser.
Does your model use specialized equipment, meaning items most therapists would not routinely have in the clinic?	Yes.
What research supports the test-retest and interrater reliability of your FCE system?	Gouttebarge V, Wind H, Kuijer PP, Sluiter JK, Frings-Dresen MH. Intra- and interrater reliability of the Ergo-Kit Functional Capacity Evaluation method in adults without musculoskeletal complaints. *Arch Phys Med Rehabil.* 2005;86:2354–2360.

FCE Model: Ergo Kit (continued)

	Gouttebarge V, Wind H, Kuijer PPFM, Frings-Dresen MHW. Reliability and validity of functional capacity evaluation methods: a systematic review with reference to Blankenship system, Ergos work simulation, Ergo-Kit and Isernhagen work system. *Int Arch Occup Environ Health.* 2004;77:527–537.
	Ijmker S, Gerrits EHJ, Reneman MF. Upper lifting performance of healthy young adults in functional capacity evaluations: a comparison of two protocols. *J Occup Rehabil.* 2003;13:297–305.
	Gouttebarge V, Wind H, Kuijer PP, Sluiter JK, Frings-Dresen MH. Reliability and agreement of 5 Ergo-Kit functional capacity evaluation lifting tests in subjects with low back pain. *Arch Phys Med Rehabil.* 2006;87:1365–1370.
	There is more research on reliability and validity, but it is in Dutch. Most will be in the references of the articles listed herein. For more information, contact Ergo Control for relevant articles.
What research supports the construct and/or predictive validity of your FCE system?	Gouttebarge V, Wind H, Kuijer PPFM, Frings-Dresen MHW. Reliability and validity of functional capacity evaluation methods: a systematic review with reference to Blankenship system, Ergos work simulation, Ergo-Kit and Isernhagen work system. *Arch Occup Environ Health.* 2004;77:527–537.
	Rustenburg G, Kuijer PPFM, Frings-Dresen MHW. The concurrent validity of the ERGOSTM Work Simulator and the Ergo-Kit with respect to maximum lifting capacity. *J Occup Rehabil.* 2004;14:107–118.
	Dr AS Jackson, Houston University, has validated a number of used tests: hand dynamometer and back and leg dynamometer. Booklet: Preemployment isometric strength testing methods; Medical and ergonomic values and issues. June 1990. His theories are based on those of DB Chaffin.

FCE Model: Ergo Kit (continued)

What separates your FCE system from the rest? In other words, why should a clinician choose and use your system?	The research that supports the reliability and validity. The combination of the FBO (job demands interview) and the FCE (the combination makes the test and way to perform tests [more] job-specific). The report that can be described in job-specific abilities (and limitations). The combination of objectively determined rules/protocol and the human value (of participant and evaluator), which makes it tailor-made.
What is the cost to purchase your system? Are there any ongoing fees?	The costs are the initial cost of buying the test-unit + the cost of the initial education: € 696 (excluding taxes) + a fee (5%) for each performed test. Price per test is about € 1000 (FCE-FBO).
Is the system "mobile" to allow testing in multiple locations?	Yes.
Is there Web access to the report?	Yes, but only for the evaluator and supervisor (from our company).
Is there certification of the FCE evaluator, and, if so, at what cost?	Yes, the total of the training (with certificate after 2 approved test reports) is € 696 (excluding taxes).

Abbreviations: FCE indicates functional capacity evaluation; and OT, occupational therapist.

FCE Model: ErgoScience Physical Work Performance
Evaluation (PWPE)

Contact Information:	**www.ergoscience.com; phone: (866) 779-6447; email: Info@ergoscience.com**
What are the qualifications of the FCE evaluator (eg, PT, OT)?	PT, OT, exercise physiologist, athletic trainer.

APPENDIX

FCE Model: ErgoScience Physical Work Performance
Evaluation (PWPE) (continued)

Training: How long; what is the process; is continuing education in your FCE method required (please describe)?	Training is 3 days. Course participants must pass a written and practical examination to achieve certification. Recertification in development.
What is the FCE test length?	3–5 hours (average, 4 hours) for a comprehensive, "Any Occupation" FCE. Shorter tests can be performed. See below.
Is a history included as part of the FCE?	Yes.
Is a musculoskeletal examination included as part of the FCE?	Musculoskeletal screen is included.
What psychometric tests, if any, do evaluees complete? How are they used?	None.
Is aerobic testing performed? Which protocol? If not, how is aerobic endurance addressed?	Aerobic testing not performed.
How is material handling tested? How is lifting frequency determined?	Materials handling is tested dynamically using lift boxes and weights. Occasional lifting is tested. Frequent and constant lifting are extrapolated from occasional.
What size box is used for lifting? Does the box have cutouts or handles?	10 × 10, 12 × 12, and 14 × 14 boxes have cutouts or handles, but client does not use them unless required by job in job-specific FCE.
How are non–material handling abilities determined, including movement and sustained positional tolerance? How is frequency determined?	Non–materials handling abilities are observed, a variety of variables are measured, and frequency is determined using research-based algorithms. Frequency is reported according to the Department of Labor classification system (constant, frequent, occasional, never).

APPENDIX

FCE Model: ErgoScience Physical Work Performance
Evaluation (PWPE) (continued)

What hand-related testing is performed in non–hand-specific FCEs (eg, grip, pinch, dexterity)?	Grip tested for consistency of effort. Pinch and dexterity are added in hand-related FCE.
How flexible is your model? Can an evaluator vary the length and breadth of the test protocol?	Model is extremely flexible in length and breadth. Can be used for everything from a brief postoffer or postinjury screen up to a full 3- to 5-hour FCE. Research supports each individual task so that validity is not sacrificed with abbreviated testing.
Do you offer "special" protocols (eg, upper extremity FCE, fatigue-related)? What are they, and how do they differ from your "routine" FCE?	Upper extremity protocol adds additional items related to reaching, handling, fingering, and manual and finger dexterity.
Does your model use specialized equipment, meaning items most therapists would not routinely have in the clinic?	Our FCE uses generic equipment, ie, lift boxes, tool chest, adjustable-height shelving, push-pull sled, disk weights, heart rate monitor with upper-limit alarm, blood pressure cuff, ladder, access to stairs or clinic stairs, balance beam, force gauge, grip strength dynamometer, nuts, washers, and bolts.
What research supports the test-retest and interrater reliability of your FCE system?	Lechner DE, Jackson JR, Roth DL, Straaton KV. Reliability and validity of a newly developed test of physical work performance. *J Occup Med.* 1994;36:997–1004.
	Tuckwell NL, Straker L, Barrett TE. Test-retest reliability on nine tasks of the Physical Work Performance Evaluation. *Work.* 2002;19:243–253.
	Durand MJ, Loisel P, Poitras S, Mercier R, Stock SR, Lemaire J. The interrater reliability of a functional capacity evaluation: the physical work performance evaluation. *J Occup Rehabil.* 2004;14:119–129.

APPENDIX

FCE Model: ErgoScience Physical Work Performance
Evaluation (PWPE) (continued)

What research supports the construct and/or predictive validity of your FCE system?	Lechner DE, Jackson JR, Roth DL, Straaton KV. Reliability and validity of a newly developed test of physical work performance. *J Occup Med.* 1994;36:997–1004.
What separates your FCE system from the rest? In other words, why should a clinician choose and use your system?	The ErgoScience FCE was developed through university-based research. We use objective algorithms for making our 8-hour-day projections. The reliability and accuracy of our entire test—not just portions of it—are supported through research. We provide scoring and report-generating software that make report writing easy and efficient. ErgoScience has a referral center that sends FCEs, postoffer screens, job analysis, and ergonomic assessment referrals your way.
What is the cost to purchase your system? Are there any ongoing fees?	The cost to purchase our system varies widely. As of this writing, pricing models are available ranging from a monthly charge to an up-front purchase of our system. Clinics should call ErgoScience or submit questions to info.ergoscience.com to obtain a current pricing model that fits their needs.
Is the system "mobile" to allow testing in multiple locations?	Yes, equipment can be transported to a variety of locations. Approximately 10–30 minutes of setup time is required, depending on the number and type of tasks tested.
Is there Web access to the report?	No, there is no Web access to report.
Is there certification of the FCE evaluator, and, if so, at what cost?	Certification to perform the ErgoScience FCE is required. Pricing is combined with the cost for license and software purchase. For current prices, go to info@ergoscience.com

Abbreviations: FCE indicates functional capacity evaluation; PT, physical therapist; and OT, occupational therapist.

FCE Model: Global Services-Functional Abilities &
Capacity Test FCE

Contact Information:	**Global Services Group** **473 McLaws Circle, Williamsburg, VA, 23185** **Telephone: (757) 220-8282; fax: (757) 220-8823** **Insurance Services: www.global-services-group.com** **Technology: www.factsfce.com**
What are the qualifications of the FCE evaluator (eg, PT, OT)?	PT or OT.
Training: How long; what is the process; is continuing education in your FCE method required (please describe)?	Standard operator training, 1 day; advanced VCU-supported course, 3 full days, CEU-based program. Annual program updates are available but not mandatory.
What is the FCE test length?	3 hours plus additional 1 hour for report completion.
Is a history included as part of the FCE?	Yes.
Is a musculoskeletal examination included as part of the FCE?	Yes.
What psychometric tests, if any, do evaluees complete? How are they used?	Although there are a number available, clinicians primarily use the standardized pain illustration and abilities questionnaires. Ransford, McGill, Oswestry, Waddell, Zung, and Neck pain are available as well.
Is aerobic testing performed? Which protocol? If not, how is aerobic endurance addressed?	MTM-based activities include walk, carry, dynamic push/pull, Dynamic Lift-Met levels, ACFT step test, Kasch (step test), treadmill test.
How is material handling tested? How is lifting frequency determined?	We use the SPOT and PILE protocol for most tasks, but clinicians are able to also use MTM-supported tasks or can create their own.

FCE Model: Global Services-Functional Abilities &
Capacity Test FCE (continued)

What size box is used for lifting? Does the box have cutouts or handles?	Box is actually round/circular with 3 handle cutouts at 2, 4, and 6 in with top cover to hide weights and ability to use dual handles or single handle; also converts to push/pull cart with sliders or wheels.
How are non–material handling abilities determined, including movement and sustained positional tolerance? How is frequency determined?	MTM and SPOT protocols include carrying and walking protocols, which aid in movement determination. Our whole person ROM device provides sustained work tolerance testing through timed work samples in low, medium, high, and overhead activities.
What hand-related testing is performed in non–hand-specific FCEs (eg, grip, pinch, dexterity)?	Pinch (key, tip, palmar), grip (standard, rapid exchange, MVE), MTM-based handling, fingering, feeling, ROM with goniometry and muscle testing. Also available with the same tools are 5-position grasp strength evaluations.
How flexible is your model? Can an evaluator vary the length and breadth of the test protocol?	We provide standard protocol formats, but evaluators are able to customize tests and protocols. All subtests are based on peer-reviewed published research.
Do you offer "special" protocols (eg, upper extremity FCE, fatigue-related)? What are they, and how do they differ from your "routine" FCE?	Yes. 1. Upper extremity FCE includes specialized MTM tests, including work sample tests 2. Chronic pain protocol includes cognitive tests, exercise capacity, and fatigue monitoring; 3-day examination 3. Injury-specific–joint-specific testing with ROM, strength, and, if needed, cardio
Does your model use specialized equipment, meaning items most therapists would not routinely have in the clinic?	Yes. The clinician has the choice to use manual tools and enter data into software or to use our fully computerized technology to accurately evaluate strength, ROM, and cardiovascular abilities.

FCE Model: Global Services-Functional Abilities &
Capacity Test FCE (continued)

What research supports the test-retest and interrater reliability of your FCE system?	WCBBC/Price Waterhouse independent study documented less than 2% difference in results submitted by multiple clinicians, same client.
What research supports the construct and/or predictive validity of your FCE system?	MTM analysis, standardized peer-reviewed published literature, test, and protocol.
What separates your FCE system from the rest? In other words, why should a clinician choose and use your system?	Versatility, no ongoing costs, upgradable, market-accepted, advanced education through university affiliation, reliable, most advanced tool technology on the market.
What is the cost to purchase your system? Are there any ongoing fees?	Ranges from rental-only programs to a full porta-ble system at $19,995 to $29,995 for a full clinical package.
Is the system "mobile" to allow testing in multiple locations?	Yes, fully portable technology that can be transported to remote locations; full setup in less than 15 minutes.
Is there Web access to the report?	Yes, the report can be transferred electronically.
Is there certification of the FCE evaluator, and, if so, at what cost?	Yes, a CFE (certified functional evaluator) designation is available after completion of all 3 levels of training; aver-age cost of training is $795 for a nonuser and zero for a new user.

Abbreviations: FCE indicates functional capacity evaluation; PT, physical therapist; OT, occupational therapist; VCU, Virginia Commonwealth University; CEU, continuing education unit; MTM, Methods-Time Measurement; MVE, maximal voluntary effort; and ROM, range of motion.

APPENDIX

FCE Model: Joule FCE by Valpar

Contact Information:	**Neal Gunderson, President** **Valpar, Int. Telephone: (800) 633-3321**
What are the qualifications of the FCE evaluator (eg, PT, OT)?	OTs and PTs are qualified to perform Joule FCEs. Other professionals may also be qualified if they provide proof that they meet specific educational criteria, have musculo-skeletal evaluation and treatment skills, and the administration of the FCE is within the scope of practice according to their professional association.
Training: How long; what is the process; is continuing education in your FCE method required (please describe)?	The Joule FCE training is conducted over 3 days at the provider's site. The first day of training includes policies, procedures, test philosophies, report formats, a thorough demonstration of all equipment and FCE protocols, and a thorough demonstration of software functions. The attendees also analyze a video of the weighted tasks in Joule and discuss the determination of safe maximum end points. The second day of training is entirely devoted to practice. Teams of 2 participants administer a full FCE using all equipment and software. The third day of training is devoted to the specialty features of Joule: postoffer, prehire screen, upper extremity FCE, custom plans and protocol development, and job analysis.
What is the FCE test length?	The length of Joule FCE administration varies because of several factors: First, Joule can be administered over a 1- to 5-day period (although a 1-day FCE is the most common). Joule has a standard FCE format and also 20 job-specific FCEs (such as health care worker, construction, manu-facturing, food service). In addition, Joule purchasers can customize FCE plans and protocols. All of these elements affect the length of the FCE. In general, however, the stan-dard 1-day FCE format is approximately 3.5 hours. In a 2-day FCE, the second day is approximately 90 minutes.
Is a history included as part of the FCE?	Yes. Data collection screens in the software guide the evaluator through in-depth medical, functional, and work histories. These data appear in the FCE report under the heading "History and Mechanism of Injury."
Is a musculoskeletal examination included as part of the FCE?	Yes. Joule has 2 musculoskeletal evaluations: a general evaluation and a detailed upper extremity evaluation. Both contain "blank" evaluation sections, so an evaluator can add other appropriate tests as needed. Both can be printed and included in the FCE report at the evaluator's discretion.

FCE Model: Joule FCE by Valpar (continued)

What psychometric tests, if any, do evaluees complete? How are they used?	No strictly psychometric tests are included. A functional history questionnaire is given to identify the client's perceived level of function, and a pain scale is used pre-FCE and post-FCE.
Is aerobic testing performed? Which protocol? If not, how is aerobic endurance addressed?	Aerobic conditioning is assessed in protocols such as repetitive squatting, stair climbing, walking, and lifting. In addition, Joule's customizing features can be used to create more strenuous aerobic protocols, such as running, for clients returning to very strenuous occupations.
How is material handling tested? How is lifting frequency determined?	First, a client is placed into 1 of 3 weight-progression categories based on diagnosis, functional history, and results of the musculoskeletal evaluation. This is done so that strong clients can avoid very small weight progressions, which unnecessarily fatigue them, and client's with lesser lifting abilities can progress by smaller increments, which is safer and allows the evaluator to assess repetitive lifting even when end points may be low.

Lifts of different heights are not conducted separately. Joule lifts are done in a sequence referred to as the "core lifting sequence": waist-to-waist lift, then waist-to-floor lift, followed by waist-to-above shoulder lift. The next weight in the progression is added, and the sequence is repeated until a maximum is determined for each lifting level. This method is advantageous because fatigue is distributed evenly among the different lifts. It is also a more complex movement pattern than isolated lifts. This is more representative of lifting in real work situations and is more difficult for clients to manipulate their performance.

Software automatically breaks down the weights placing the last safe lift amount in the "rare" category, and lesser weight amounts are distributed throughout the categories of "occasional," "frequent," and "constant." The evaluator can make adjustments to the breakdown based on diagnosis, functional performance, and professional expertise.

FCE Model: Joule FCE by Valpar (continued)

What size box is used for lifting? Does the box have cutouts or handles?	All Joule systems come with 3 standardized lifting containers: heavy lifting tub with cutout hand holds (16 in L, 12 in W, 10 in H), light lifting tub with cutout hand holds (16 in L, 12 in W, 8 in H), and unilateral carry container with toolbox-type handle (15 in L, 9 in W, 6 in H plus height of handle). All 3 lifting containers in Joule have an interior grid for placement of color-coded steel bar T-handled weights. This prevents weights from sliding within the containers or pinching fingers. Lifts with custom tubs or lifting of objects with no tubs (such as cardboard boxes, sheetrock, or salt bags) can be done via Joule's customizing system.
How are non–material handling abilities determined, including movement and sustained positional tolerance? How is frequency determined?	To determine the frequency and duration of non–material handling work tasks, the evaluator gathers and analyzes data according to specific Joule procedures. This includes data from objective and subjective findings, heart rates (when appropriate), duration and completion of test, functional abilities demonstrated in similar protocols, functional history, and diagnosis.
What hand-related testing is performed in non–hand-specific FCEs (eg, grip, pinch, dexterity)?	In FCEs administered to non–upper extremity (UE)-injured clients, 5-setting grip strength and fine motor coordination are formally tested. In addition, UE function is casually observed in materials handling tasks and work tasks performed during positional tolerance tests.
How flexible is your model? Can an evaluator vary the length and breadth of the test protocol?	Joule is very flexible. Custom protocols and custom plans can be made and stored in the Joule software. Valpar standardizes this process by training evaluators to use a specific method when customizing FCEs. This ensures continuity and interrater reliability will be maintained through the customizing process. Evaluators can also customize "on the fly" by repeating protocols that represent essential job functions and modifying repetitions and durations to replicate job demands.
Do you offer "special" protocols (eg, upper extremity FCE, fatigue-related)? What are they, and how do they differ from your "routine" FCE?	Joule has many specialized features: upper extremity FCE, postoffer, prehire screen, progress notes, work conditioning documentation system, and job analysis software that can be used as a freestanding tool and/or imported into the FCE. All special features are included at no additional cost.

FCE Model: Joule FCE by Valpar (continued)

Does your model use specialized equipment, meaning items most therapists would not routinely have in the clinic?	The only equipment that must be purchased from Valpar are the 3 lifting containers, a set of color-coded T-handled weights, and the Joule fine motor coordination test (the Value Package). A more comprehensive, optional equipment package includes all items in the Value Package plus a materials-handling shelving system, push/pull plates, functional task attachments (eg, foot pedal, bolt box, forceful tool box), and notebook computer. All equipment packages include software, support, certification, training, and trainers' expenses. Other equipment used in the Joule FCE is frequently found in most clinics: eg, dynamometers, force gauge, sensory tests, balance beams, ladder.
What research supports the test-retest and interrater reliability of your FCE system?	Interrater reliability data are available on the Valpar Web site at www.valparint.com.
What research supports the construct and/or predictive validity of your FCE system?	Outcome study data are available on the Valpar Web site at www.valparint.com.
What separates your FCE system from the rest? In other words, why should a clinician choose and use your system?	Although Joule is an exceptional FCE in multiple ways, the following elements are truly unique: 1. Joule is all-inclusive-FCE, UE FCE, work conditioning, job analysis, postoffer, prehire screens all integrated in 1 software and 1 training for 1 price. 2. Joule is extremely functional and flexible. 3. Absolutely no documentation time required following the FCE. Evaluators make decisions as the evaluation progresses and use features such as point-and-click comments and recommendations. When the FCE is done, the evaluator's work is done.

APPENDIX

FCE Model: Joule FCE by Valpar (continued)

What is the cost to purchase your system? Are there any ongoing fees?	Value Package, $13,495; Premium Package, $26,995. On-site staff training and all trainer are expenses-included in package prices. All systems include a full set of boxes, weights, fine motor test, software, training for up to 9, trainer expenses, 1 year service support, and software upgrades. Premium package also includes materials handling station work simulation equipment and computer. No mandatory per-assessment fees or programs. Optional service support for $395/y.
Is the system "mobile" to allow testing in multiple locations?	Joule has a portable equipment package option. With the notebook computer and portable equipment package, Joule FCEs and postoffer, prehire screens can be administered virtually anywhere.
Is there Web access to the report?	Valpar does not post FCEs on our Web site. However, because Joule reports print out in Word documents, they could be easily placed on a facility's Web site for retrieval by a referral source.
Is there certification of the FCE evaluator, and, if so, at what cost?	Evaluators submit their first 2 FCEs for feedback, quality assurance review, and certification. Thereafter, evaluators may obtain annual recertification by submitting 1 FCE for review. Joule software contains a HIPAA-compatible method of data export that eliminates all identifying information. Certification and recertification are strongly recommended but optional. The cost is included in the $395 service support package and covers all evaluators from 1 facility.

Abbreviations: FCE indicates functional capacity evaluation; PT, physical therapist; OT, occupational therapist; and HIPAA, Health Information Portability and Accountability Act.

FCE Model: JTECH Medical Assessment System and
FCE Training Courses

Contact Information:	**JTECH Medical** **470 Lawndale Dr, Suite G,** **Salt Lake City, UT 84115** **Telephone: (800) 985-8324**
What are the qualifications of the FCE evaluator (eg, PT, OT)?	The JTECH FCE system does not require specific medical licensure. Scope of practice guidelines are determined by the states. We attempt to follow and recommend FCE training based on those guidelines.

FCE Model: JTECH Medical Assessment System and
FCE Training Courses (continued)

Training: How long; what is the process; is continuing education in your FCE method required (please describe)?	We teach that training of the FCE process is ongoing. The initial seminar consists of a self study learning component and a weekend hands-on training seminar, although we have also taught 4-day seminars that include job analysis and postoffer evaluation training (these are not currently offered but may be reintroduced at a later date). Participants are encouraged but not required to return and take advantage of our refresher rate and attend the seminar again. Many attendees state that they learn more the second time around because there is so much information to assimilate. Attendees are required to submit a written test within 30 days of attending the seminar and to submit an FCE report within 6 months. A passing score on each is required to receive certification. No continuing education or recertification requirements.
What is the FCE test length?	Our FCE test philosophy is based on testing for required work abilities or to determine functional capabilities for unemployed workers. Therefore, the length of the FCE is determined by the needs of the evaluator, the referral, the job, and the subject. While there is no set length or order in which tests are administered, evaluations typically take 4 to 8 hours for 1-day tests but may take longer if the evaluee is tested over multiple days. The format is at the evaluator's discretion.
Is a history included as part of the FCE?	We encourage the evaluator to take a detailed history and to avail himself or herself of the medical records and job analysis/description before the FCE so that these can be reviewed ahead of time as well. The Tracker software provides for the input of these findings.
Is a musculoskeletal examination included as part of the FCE?	We strongly encourage the evaluator to perform a detailed, defensible, and injury-specific musculoskeletal examination before commencing with functional testing. The JTECH FCE system uses computerized instruments with automatic data input to complete the musculoskeletal examination. Manual data entry of findings can also be used with a software-only program. The software records and calculates reliability and validity of testing.

APPENDIX

FCE Model: JTECH Medical Assessment System and
FCE Training Courses (continued)

What psychometric tests, if any, do evaluees complete? How are they used?	We teach several psychometric tests that have been published in peer-reviewed medical literature, and students are taught to limit these to the area(s) injured. Tests include the Ransford Pain Drawing, McGill Pain Questionnaire, visual analog pain scales, numeric pain scales, the Revised Oswestry Low Back Disability Questionnaire, the Neck Disability Index, the Shoulder Rating Questionnaire, the Shoulder Pain and Disability Index, the Spinal Function Sort, the Hand Function Sort, and many others. The Tracker FCE system enables the evaluator to report findings of these and many other psychometric tests an examiner may choose to use in the comprehensive software program.
Is aerobic testing performed? Which protocol? If not, how is aerobic endurance addressed?	Aerobic testing can be performed as part of our FCE but is not required. It is encouraged when the job demands have an aerobic demand, especially material handling situations or environmental challenges. All of the protocols we teach are submaximal tests. The primary methods taught in JTECH seminars are maximum aerobic power tests using a step bench or a treadmill. Aerobic tests results are also integrated in the software program.
How is material handling tested? How is lifting frequency determined?	We advocate the use of several standardized lifting evaluations but leave the decision to the evaluator. We use the Snook and Ciriello normative data for occasional frequency lifting and adhere to box dimensions and frequencies that were used to create these normative data. We use the PILE test (Mayer et al) for frequent lifting, and evaluators who use other material handling tests, such as the EPIC Lifting Evaluation, are able to do so and report their findings with the Tracker system.
What size box is used for lifting? Does the box have cutouts or handles?	The type of box used is at the discretion of the evaluator. In our seminar, we demonstrate the use of standard 14- and 9-in boxes with cutouts and a dowel handle for 1-handed lifts. Larger or smaller boxes or boxes without handles are used to simulate specific job demands.

FCE Model: JTECH Medical Assessment System and
FCE Training Courses (continued)

How are non–material handling abilities determined, including movement and sustained positional tolerance? How is frequency determined?	We separate activities and positional tolerances. Both can be tested directly and through distraction, using repetition for movements like reaching and time for positional tolerances. Frequency for positional tolerances is determined by the length of time the posture or combination of postures is demonstrated. For activities, it is determined by time performing the activity or repetitions demonstrated. Frequency is estimated by the evaluator as being occasional, frequent, or constant, depending on the sustained and/or repetitive tolerance of the activity during direct observation or distracted observation activities. The software program features tools to assist with the assessment and recording of tasks.
What hand-related testing is performed in non–hand-specific FCEs (eg, grip, pinch, dexterity)?	Hand tests are at the discretion of the evaluator. Standardized tests are taught that include 5-position grip tests, rapid-exchange grip tests, sustained grip tests with fatigue calculations, and pinch tests (tip, lateral, and palmar). Other custom tests may be created and administered by the evaluator, such as thumb to tip of middle, ring, or little finger for a musician. Dexterity tests are also left up to the evaluator. Tests taught in the FCE seminar include the Purdue Pegboard standard tests, the Minnesota Rate of Manipulation standard tests, and the Bennett Hand and Tool Dexterity Test (standardized). Any test, standard or otherwise, may be included and documented in the Tracker system.
How flexible is your model? Can an evaluator vary the length and breadth of the test protocol?	The Tracker system is very flexible. Any medical test, standard or otherwise, can be included in the system. The evaluator is, therefore, able to construct the test any way he or she chooses. The software in the Tracker system can be used with many other FCE models to document whatever evaluation components are used.
Do you offer "special" protocols (eg, upper extremity FCE, fatigue-related)? What are they, and how do they differ from your "routine" FCE?	We allow the user to determine which tests are appropriate for the FCE. Our objective with the Tracker system is to provide tools to help the examiner determine the ability of the subject in relation to job requirements and physical demand levels. We do not believe in a "one size fits all" FCE. The evaluator has the ability, using the protocol function in the system, to create whatever protocol he or she wants for repetitive use. This is an excellent way of designing and administering postoffer evaluation test protocols.

APPENDIX

FCE Model: JTECH Medical Assessment System and
FCE Training Courses (continued)

Does your model use specialized equipment, meaning items most therapists would not routinely have in the clinic?	Our FCE software program allows therapists to use a variety of standardized tools and equipment for examining the subject. Data can be entered into the software automatically with the use of our computerized musculoskeletal assessment tools or manually from the use of analog tools as the FCE progresses. We also provide a wide range of computerized musculoskeletal and functional testing equipment to streamline the documentation process, as well as a comprehensive job simulation and lifting station. The system as whole has no specific equipment requirements. Our clinical consultants work closely with clinicians to determine needs.
What research supports the test-retest and interrater reliability of your FCE system?	As an FCE system rather than a model, there is no research regarding interrater or intrarater reliability of the system as a whole. Incorporated into the system are tests and tools that have research to support each test. The bibliography for these data is also incorporated into the software and the report of findings. Because of the flexibility of the evaluation system (every client is tested differently depending on the injury and the job), it would be impossible and pointless to conduct a reliability study on the system as a whole.
What research supports the construct and/or predictive validity of your FCE system?	There is no research regarding the construct and or predictive validity of the system as a whole. Our system used peer-reviewed, published protocols to support the validity of each of the tests that are incorporated in the system and the bibliography for these is available. Again, because of the flexibility of the evaluation system, it would be impossible and pointless to conduct a validity study on the system as a whole.
What separates your FCE system from the rest? In other words, why should a clinician choose and use your system?	The robustness of the computerized measurement tools is unsurpassed in the industry. The flexibility of the system as far as conducting and reporting the findings of tests, as well as defending the results in the legal arena, is what makes the system very attractive. Our system was designed primarily to simplify documentation and report writing. As such, it can be used with almost any FCE philosophy or model and is not limited to testing for FCE. The system can be used for any musculoskeletal assessment performed in a clinic.

FCE Model: JTECH Medical Assessment System and
FCE Training Courses (continued)

What is the cost to purchase your system? Are there any ongoing fees?	The cost of the JTECH system varies according to the software and/or equipment used by the examiner. It can range from $5000 for a basic manual data entry software package to $30,000 for a computerized system with advanced testing instrumentation and isometric and isoinertial lifting stations. There are no per-report fees or license fees associated with the use of the JTECH system. The ongoing costs associated with the system include optional software and hardware maintenance programs.
Is the system "mobile" to allow testing in multiple locations?	The JTECH system is very mobile. All devices for the musculoskeletal examination fit into one very durable case for transporting.
Is there Web access to the report?	All JTECH reports can be saved as PDF documents, thus allowing easy electronic submission. The report is created and saved by the user in a flexible database format.
Is there certification of the FCE evaluator, and if so, at what cost?	JTECH offers a certification training course that is focused on the process of performing an FCE. Our equipment is featured at our course. Certification on completion of the course for licensed clinicians is $849.00. Continuing education credits are included.

Abbreviations: FCE indicates functional capacity evaluation; PT, physical therapist; and OT, occupational therapist.

FCE Model: The Matheson System

Contact Information:	**The Matheson System** **PO Box 492, Keene, NH 03431-0492** **Phone: (800) 443-7690 or (603) 358-6525** **www.roymatheson.com**
What are the qualifications of the FCE evaluator (eg, PT, OT)?	The training is open to all allied health professionals. Certification requires completion of a relevant previous degree, which includes occupational therapy, physical therapy, medicine, and/or chiropractic. Professionals from other disciplines may also apply but must show proof of additional university-level training in certain health-related areas.

APPENDIX

FCE Model: The Matheson System (continued)

Training: How long; what is the process; is continuing education in your FCE method required (please describe)?	The basic FCE training is a 5-day program. A person who becomes certified is required to reapply for certification every 5 years and to attend "Critical Thinking Skills for Functional Capacity Evaluators" (a 2-day course) and/or reattend the original training program. All participants are encouraged to attend training in as many FCE systems as possible.
What is the FCE test length?	The FCE test length depends on the referral questions asked, the type of evaluation (eg, state disability, federal disability, return-to-work, personal injury, motor vehicle accident), demands of the target job (if one exists), and the environment in which the evaluator works. Typical test length is from 4 to 8 hours. If necessary, testing may be conducted over 2 days.
Is a history included as part of the FCE?	Yes.
Is a musculoskeletal examination included as part of the FCE?	If appropriate, a full musculoskeletal examination can be included. We also use musculoskeletal screening when appropriate.
What psychometric tests, if any, do evaluees complete? How are they used?	We use Spinal Function Sort, Ransford, McGill, Waddell, Dallas, Oswestry, among others. Primary use of these tests is to more objectively compare subjective reports with objective findings.
Is aerobic testing performed? Which protocol? If not, how is aerobic endurance addressed?	Cardiorespiratory endurance is addressed through 1 of 4 protocols: the Modified Bruce, the Modified Balke, the Bench Step Test, or the bicycle protocol.
How is material handling tested? How is lifting frequency determined?	All strength-related tests use dynamic, functional protocols. Evaluators may select their own lift test. Protocols include the EPIC Lift (occasional and frequent protocols), the Progressive Isoinertial Lift Evaluation (a frequent protocol), an isoinertial occasional protocol based on Snook's work, and the WEST Standard Evaluation (an occasional protocol).

FCE Model: The Matheson System (continued)

	Lift frequency is determined by reference to the lift protocol selected.
	Other manual material physical demands are compared with Snook's occasional work unless indicated.
	When greater frequency of lifting or carrying is required at a person's workplace, work-simulation testing can be added, making use of progressive work circuits and continuous heart-rate monitoring.
What size box is used for lifting? Does the box have cutouts or handles?	The box used depends on the protocol selected. Boxes are 8 or 15 lb. One has cutouts for hand grip; the other has handles.
How are non–material handling abilities determined, including movement and sustained positional tolerance? How is frequency determined?	Distraction-based testing is used throughout the testing day to track positional tolerances. "Longest duration" and "total duration" are calculated. Observed tolerances include sitting, static standing, dynamic standing, neck flexion, and trunk flexion. *Position of preference* during breaks is also tracked.
	Short-duration tolerances are evaluated through a variety of standardized tests including (but not exclusive to) the Valpar 9, Complete Minnesota Dexterity Test, the Matheson Bench, the WEST 7 Bus Bench, and the Matheson Panel System.
	Determination of frequency is based on a decision tree process. A Viewpoint paper is provided to students in this regard. Longer tolerances (ie, frequent and constant) require longer periods of observation and less symptomatic response.
What hand-related testing is performed in non–hand-specific FCEs (eg, grip, pinch, dexterity)?	Hand testing includes grip strength, pinch, medium grasp, gross grasp, sensation, fine finger dexterity, medium finger dexterity, and light handling. We make use of normative and MTM (criterion-referenced) testing.

FCE Model: The Matheson System (continued)

How flexible is your model? Can an evaluator vary the length and breadth of the test protocol?	The Matheson model is to train evaluators to think rather than simply how to use standardized tests. Having said that, the evaluator is trained to use a battery of standardized tests to assess physical effort, reliability of reports of pain and disability, and physical abilities in the format that best addresses the unique needs of each case. The evaluator is free to expand or contract the length of the evaluation to maximize the predictive validity of the result.
Do you offer "special" protocols (eg, upper extremity FCE, fatigue-related)? What are they, and how do they differ from your "routine" FCE?	None of our FCEs are routine. Each is tailored to the needs of the case in question.
Does your model use specialized equipment, meaning items most therapists would not routinely have in the clinic?	Virtually all of the tests used in our model are found in the typical well-equipped clinic. All tests can be purchased through a wide variety of suppliers.
What research supports the test-retest and interrater reliability of your FCE system?	The system itself does not have interrater reliability statistics. The individual tests that comprise the Matheson protocol are based on published, peer-reviewed studies. Two primary components of the Matheson protocol (EPIC Lift Capacity Evaluation and the Spinal Function Sort) are extensively studied, showing excellent interrater reliability. We encourage our evaluators to use tests that are "industry standard" tests.
What research supports the construct and/or predictive validity of your FCE system?	At this stage, there is limited information on predictive validity. Research on a primary component of our system (EPIC Lift Capacity Evaluation) has some research in this regard. Furthermore, true validity in our field relates in large part to whether such findings were eventually taken as fact at a level of "extreme scrutiny." As such, references to multiple Supreme Court cases wherein the Matheson evaluator's opinion was taken are available on request.

FCE Model: The Matheson System (continued)

What separates your FCE system from the rest? In other words, why should a clinician choose and use your system?	Our system is not for everyone. A therapist selecting our system should be interested in performing as a "thinking evaluator." The evaluator should be willing to challenge the tests used, research the history and publications pertaining to each of their protocols, and delve into detail on the specific issues of each case.
What is the cost to purchase your system? Are there any ongoing fees?	The basic training is $1450. Once the initial training is completed, reauditing the course is relatively inexpensive, at $100/d (2-day recertification every 5 years). With the exception of recertification every 5 years, there are no ongoing fees. The cost of equipment depends on how well-equipped the clinic already is. A brand new clinic would typically purchase between $10,000 and $15,000 of equipment and software.
Is the system "mobile" to allow testing in multiple locations?	Yes.
Is there Web access to the report?	Yes, once compiled by the evaluator, the report can be distributed electronically, scanned for inclusion in an electronic system, or saved as a hard-copy document.
Is there certification of the FCE evaluator, and, if so, at what cost?	Students who have completed the basic training may continue to become certified. The Matheson certification designations are CWCE (Certified Work Capacity Evaluator) and CFCE (Certified Functional Capacity Evaluator). Certification requires completion of field work, a formal application package, and review of field-work by an independent committee. The administration fee is approximately $200.

Abbreviations: FCE indicates functional capacity evaluation; PT, physical therapist; and OT, occupational therapist.

APPENDIX

FCE Model: MediGraph FCE RFC-DOT

Contact Information:	Thomas A. Kane, PT MediGraph Software telephone: (800) 804-6334 email: tkane@medigraphsoftware.com
What are the qualifications of the FCE evaluator (eg, PT, OT)?	PTs and OTs are most qualified.
Training: How long; what is the process; is continuing education in your FCE method required (please describe)?	Training occurs as part of a home-study course. The applicant must take a test to obtain certification. Continuing education for the FCE is not offered, primarily owing to the peer-reviewed status of this procedure. Altering the method would not adhere to the parameters as established in the literature, invalidating the results.
What is the FCE test length?	4–5 hours.
Is a history included as part of the FCE?	History may be included as part of the comment section, but does not have a bearing on the outcome of the examination. The results of the examination are produced as a consequence of data collection.
Is a musculoskeletal examination included as part of the FCE?	A visual inspection is not required. The movements included as part of the examination are intended to establish function, not a diagnosis.
What psychometric tests, if any, do evaluees complete? How are they used?	There are no psychometric tests included that have a bearing on the results of the FCE. However, MediGraph contains more than 65 outcome instruments that may be provided to the client and included in the "Comments" section of the report.
Is aerobic testing performed? Which protocol? If not, how is aerobic endurance addressed?	Aerobic capacity is included as part of the ambulation evaluation. A treadmill is required.
How is material handling tested? How is lifting frequency determined?	Material handling (eg, holding, grasping) is defined using a specific protocol that also examines manual dexterity. Lifting frequency is defined by the DOT.

FCE Model: MediGraph FCE RFC-DOT (continued)

What size box is used for lifting? Does the box have cutouts or handles?	A standardized lifting box with handles is used.
How are non–material handling abilities determined, including movement and sustained positional tolerance? How is frequency determined?	Non–material handling is included as part of the sensory/dexterity testing. Frequency is not determined.
What hand-related testing is performed in non–hand-specific FCEs (eg, grip, pinch, dexterity)?	All 3 of the parameters are tested (grip, pinch, and dexterity).
How flexible is your model? Can an evaluator vary the length and breadth of the test protocol?	By design, the model is not flexible. Using an objective, standardized, pre-established, peer-reviewed assessment depends on data collection. The MediGraph FCE uses an objective criterion that has withstood the scrutiny of peer review and eliminates subjectivity. The subjective nature of nonpublished FCEs leads opposing parties (plaintiff and defendant) to question the "impressions" of the examiner. By eliminating the impressions and biases inherent in the performance of these evaluations, the results are reproducible and reliable.
Do you offer "special" protocols (eg, upper extremity FCE, fatigue-related)? What are they, and how do they differ from your "routine" FCE?	The FCE is standardized using pre-established standards.
Does your model use specialized equipment, meaning items most therapists would not routinely have in the clinic?	No. The MediGraph FCE does not require special equipment. MediGraph Software does not sell equipment. Therapists may use the equipment that is already in their facility or purchase the equipment from any common vendor.

APPENDIX

FCE Model: MediGraph FCE RFC-DOT (continued)

What research supports the test-retest and interrater reliability of your FCE system?	The results of the MediGraph FCE were published in *Spine* and in the *Clinical Journal of Pain* for validity and reliability. While many FCEs include published components as part of their testing, the actual results of the testing have not withstood the examination of peer review.
What research supports the construct and/or predictive validity of your FCE system?	The results of the MediGraph FCE were published in *Spine* and in the *Clinical Journal of Pain* for validity and reliability.
What separates your FCE system from the rest? In other words, why should a clinician choose and use your system?	The MediGraph FCE is a peer-reviewed procedure. While clinical judgment and assessments remain the cornerstone of the intervention process, a higher, more objective standard must be applied when determining functional status. As with the American Medical Association *Guides to the Determination of Permanent Impairment,* standardization enables the clinician to eliminate the inherent biases that can alter the outcome of these tests. As medicine and physical therapy move toward the outcome-based model, the importance of objective assessment cannot be overstated. Having established the reliability and validity of the FCE used by MediGraph distinguishes this procedure from the other nonpublished FCEs that involve estimating. Also, many FCEs use coefficient of variation (CV) to determine effort of the participant. The *APTA Journal* published an article in 1998 equating this practice of CV determination to bordering on unethical, because there was no published literature to establish the validity or reliability of this method. Eventually, the provider of an FCE will appear as an expert witness. Eliminating the subjective nature of the FCE process insulates the practitioner from the defense or plaintiff representatives who disagree with the outcome of the procedure. While many FCEs include testing that has been published, the results or outcome of the testing has not been published. The results of the MediGraph FCE have been reviewed, and their reliability and validity are established.

FCE Model: MediGraph FCE RFC-DOT (continued)

What is the cost to purchase your system? Are there any ongoing fees?	The MediGraph FCE costs $25 per examination. There are no up-front costs or enrollment fees.
Is the system "mobile" to allow testing in multiple locations?	The FCE is mobile because it is self-contained and is designed to be performed with generic equipment (eg, treadmill, balance beam, lifting box).
Is there Web access to the report?	The reports are stored in the provider's hardware, with Internet-based backup.
Is there certification of the FCE evaluator, and if so, at what cost?	There is no cost for the certification. Each evaluator must pass a written test to obtain a certificate.

Abbreviations: FCE indicates functional capacity evaluation; PT, physical therapist; OT, occupational therapist; and DOT, *Dictionary of Occupational Titles.*

FCE Model: OccuCare Systems and Solutions

Contact Information:	**Jim Mecham, MS, OTR/L, AEP** **8400 Lakeview Parkway, Suite 750** **Pleasant Prairie, WI 53158** **(800) 340-5143** **jmecham@occucare.net** **www.occucare.net**
What are the qualifications of the FCE evaluator (eg, PT, OT)?	OccuCare primarily trains licensed or registered PTs and OTs in performing our FCE method. We have trained athletic trainers in regard to the functional aspects of our FCE method, based on requests from other companies to have them trained; however, they are not trained to perform musculoskeletal testing.

APPENDIX

FCE Model: OccuCare Systems and Solutions (continued)

Training: How long; what is the process; is continuing education in your FCE method required (please describe)?	The software we offer is more than just FCE software. There are 6 different testing methods in the software. With that said, there are 2 course options: a 3-day in-depth course in regard to performing the OccuCare FCE testing method and a 4-day course in regard to implementing a full industrial rehabilitation program with 2 days of the 4-day course focusing specifically on performing FCEs. Both of these courses are approved for CEUs by the American Occupational Therapy Association and multiple state PT associations. To maintain the level of reliability needed for FCE testing, all testers have to be trained by one of our many trainers throughout North America.
What is the FCE test length?	The FCE is a standard 3- to 4-hour test, and posttest FCE documentation can be completed within 15 minutes using the FCE software.
Is a history included as part of the FCE?	Yes, a history is included in the FCE. This is gathered from medical records, from interview of the client, or both.
Is a musculoskeletal examination included as part of the FCE?	Even though a musculoskeletal examination has been shown to not correlate with function, certain states require this in their FCE testing for the purposes of determining disability. Musculoskeletal examination is an option within the FCE software, and this option includes upper and lower extremities, distal upper extremity, and spinal goniometric or dual inclinometric measurements per the American Medical Association guide to impairment ratings.
What psychometric tests, if any, do evaluees complete? How are they used?	The evaluees have the option of performing any of the following 4 psychometric tests for the purpose of determining the client's Reliability of Pain reports and these are: McGill pain questionnaire, Ransford Pain Drawing, Oswestry Low Back and Neck disability questionnaire.
Is aerobic testing performed? Which protocol? If not, how is aerobic endurance addressed?	Aerobic testing is performed based on testing protocols in which the client is asked to perform multiple lifting tasks to not only determine aerobic capacity using Borg ratings of perceived exertion and heart rate but also to determine frequent lifting abilities.

FCE Model: OccuCare Systems and Solutions (continued)

How is material handling tested? How is lifting frequency determined?	Occasional material handling is tested using a kinesio-physical/observational approach with a possibility of 10 different occasional material handling tests being done if considered job-specific. Frequent material handling testing is done with a 75% kinesiophysical approach and a 25% psychophysical approach while using observational methods with some of the useful approaches used in the EPIC and PILE lifting protocols. We have taken some of the valid and reliable research aspects of both of these protocols and incorporated them into our frequent material handling decisions. Frequent lifting is not a calculated ability but a demonstrated ability based on the aforementioned criteria.
What size box is used for lifting? Does the box have cutouts or handles?	The recommended box for lifting testing is the Haussmann Package Carton Weight box with 2 levels of cutout handles and the closing lid.
How are non–material handling abilities determined, including movement and sustained positional tolerance? How is frequency determined?	Non–material handling abilities are determined through repetitive testing methods of each non–material handling test needed. We have developed what we call our bio-mechanical decision-making charts, which point a tester to the correct decision in regard to a patient's ability to perform various non–material handling tests. Based on testing protocols and the decision charts, the evaluator makes a decision about whether the client is able to perform the non–material handling activity on an avoid, occasional, frequent, or continuous basis.
What hand-related testing is performed in non–hand-specific FCEs (eg, grip, pinch, dexterity)?	If the FCE is a job-specific FCE, multiple grip, pinch, gross motor, and fine motor tests are performed. If the test is not an upper extremity test, these tests are performed specifically for evaluating sitting abilities in regard to distraction-based testing. The specific testing methods incorporated into the FCE include 3-trial grip, 5-span grip, rapid-grip exchange, key pinch, palmar pinch, tip pinch, Purdue Pegboard, Moberg pick up test, Box and Block, and Minnesota Manual Dexterity Test.

APPENDIX

FCE Model: OccuCare Systems and Solutions (continued)

How flexible is your model? Can an evaluator vary the length and breadth of the test protocol?	We feel we have the most flexible testing method on the market. We have developed the FCE to increase the individual test's validity by allowing the clinician to vary the length, breadth, and type of testing as to improve the content validity as much as possible. We are strong believers that the validity and reliability of an FCE play off of each other and that testers need to increase their individual test content validity by correlating the test to specific job-related testing.
Do you offer "special" protocols (eg, upper extremity FCE, fatigue-related)? What are they, and how do they differ from your "routine" FCE?	The FCE testing method and the software offered for this method offer one FCE testing protocol. There are no special protocols in regard to specific variations of an FCE. The software, however, recognizes if ultimately you are performing a special protocol, ie, disability FCE, upper extremity FCE, job-specific FCE, and the end report automatically adjusts to report this type of FCE.
Does your model use specialized equipment, meaning items most therapists would not routinely have in the clinic?	The testing equipment that is recommended in the FCE testing methods we teach and within the software we offer is basic equipment that is available on the open market. We do not have proprietary equipment that testers are required to purchase. The typical equipment purchase for new clinics is $1500.00 in basic open market equipment.
What research supports the test-retest and interrater reliability of your FCE system?	A previous version of our FCE showed average to good test-retest and interrater reliability. We did not publish these findings at the time as we were developing the Web-based software. We are presently in the depths of 4 reliability studies on the present Web-based FCE system method. Two of these studies are being performed independently, and two are being performed by OccuCare.
What research supports the construct and/or predictive validity of your FCE system?	We are presently in the depths of a massive construct and predictive validity study with the hopes of publishing peer-reviewed articles in early 2009.

FCE Model: OccuCare Systems and Solutions (continued)

What separates your FCE system from the rest? In other words, why should a clinician choose and use your system?	What separates us is that our system is not just an FCE testing system. It is a software system and training program that helps clinicians and clinics implement a full industrial rehabilitation program in which FCEs are only one aspect of the overall system. We have found that financially successful programs need to have a full menu of industrial rehabilitation products to offer each patient. The software has 6 different industrial rehabilitation testing methods, and even though it has more testing methods than any other system on the open market, it is less expensive to implement. In regard to the FCE test offered within the scope of the whole software, this is different in that it uses basic therapy equipment that is available on the open market, the posttest FCE documentation can be completed in 15 minutes, the reports are generated immediately, and there are no per-test fees. Last, OccuCare makes upgrades to the FCE software 4 times per year based on newly released evidence-based testing methods. So you can be sure the testing you perform incorporates the latest research.
What is the cost to purchase your system? Are there any ongoing fees?	The average cost per company to implement the 6 different testing methods with training is $7500.00. The many clinics throughout North America that have implemented this system have begun making a significant profit within 6 months. There is a flat-rate, per-use fee of $2000.00.
Is the system "mobile" to allow testing in multiple locations?	Because the system is Internet-based, an FCE could be performed with this software system anywhere in the world as long as the clinician is able to connect to the Internet. We also have mobile options in regard to equipment.
Is there Web access to the report?	This is the only way the report is accessible. It can then be saved as a "paper" version on your computer and ultimately printed but is always accessible via the Internet.
Is there certification of the FCE evaluator, and, if so, at what cost?	We offer certification, but it requires clinicians to submit samples of what their reports look like after they have completed 15 FCEs. They are then put through to a committee of certified evaluators who make sure they meet FCE testing procedures and protocols.

Abbreviations: FCE indicates functional capacity evaluation; PT, physical therapist; OT, occupational therapist; and CEU, continuing education unit.

FCE Model: Physiotherapy Associates

Contact Information:	**855 Springdale Dr** **Suite 200, Exton, PA 19341** **telephone (610) 644-7824; www.physiocorp.com**
What are the qualifications of the FCE evaluator (eg, PT, OT)?	Physical and/or occupational therapist.
Training: How long; what is the process; is continuing education in your FCE method required (please describe)?	Therapist is required to attend a 2-day seminar (14.0 hours [CEUs]), which focuses on providing a comprehensive understanding of the FCE process and the integral test components that comprise our FCE. The training focuses on actual test administration, report writing, marketing, etc. Clinicians are required to submit reports to peer review before release.
What is the FCE test length?	On average 1 day; 4 hours; on occasion 2-day testing is requested.
Is a history included as part of the FCE?	Before any functional testing, the evaluator shall perform an initial 1:1 interview. The components of the intake history shall include subjective history; medical history; social, ADL, and functional status profile; educational history; work history; and job analysis.
Is a musculoskeletal examination included as part of the FCE?	Yes. Clients who are referred for an FCE shall undergo a musculoskeletal assessment appropriate to the diagnosis. The depth and breadth are often determined by the diagnosis, other areas of impairment noted during the interview, and the customary screening practices of the profession. The evaluators shall perform an initial assessment based on their training, standards of practice, and local and national licensure laws. The purposes are to: ■ Screen client to determine the appropriateness of the assessment ■ Identify safe performance ■ Confirm medical stability ■ Confirm contraindications ■ Quantify physical impairment The assessment will include the following: ■ Range of motion and flexibility measurements ■ Manual muscle testing

FCE Model: Physiotherapy Associates (continued)

	■ Soft-tissue screen
	■ Sensory and sensation testing
	■ Regional neurological testing
	■ Postural screen
	■ Waddell nonorganic screen (low back only)
	■ Skin quality
	■ Volumetric and/or circumference edema measures

What psychometric tests, if any, do evaluees complete? How are they used?	Ransford Pain Drawing; McGill Pain Questionnaire; Numeric Pain Rating; Oswestry Low Back Questionnaire; Dallas Pain Questionnaire; Waddell Subjective Questionnaire; and the Waddell Objective testing.

The psychometrics are used by the examiner to assist in determining the reliability of the client's subjective reports and perception of disability and to assist in identifying behavioral factors that affect a person's functional abilities. The psychometrics are given as a battery of tests to assess perceived pain and disability, to assist the evaluator in evaluating the presence or absence of nonorganic findings. |
| **Is aerobic testing performed? Which protocol? If not, how is aerobic endurance addressed?** | Yes, a single-stage treadmill test. |
| **How is material handling tested? How is lifting frequency determined?** | All clients referred for an FCE and who need their strength capacities (lifting, carrying, and pushing/pulling) determined will undergo a series of materials handling testing on a gradual basis in accordance with the individual's needs and/or abilities per medical diagnosis. All clients will be attached to a pulse rate/heart monitor during testing. In addition, the use of the *Dictionary of Occupational Titles* (DOT), which classifies jobs by strength, is commonly used (US Department of Labor, 1991, p. 1012; US Department of Labor 1986, pp. 101–102). In this system, "occasionally," "frequently," and "constantly" describe activities or conditions that exist up to one third of the time, from one third to two thirds of the time, and for two thirds or more of the time, respectively.

For the purposes of strength testing conducted, jobs will be grossly classified in 3 categories (National Institute |

APPENDIX

FCE Model: Physiotherapy Associates (continued)

	for Occupational Safety and Health [NIOSH] Work Practices Guide for Manual Lifting): ■ Occasional lifting: occasional or continuous lifting less than once per 3 minutes ($<$ 20 lifts/hour and $<$ 160 lifts/8-h shift) ■ Frequent lifting: lifting $\geq$1 times per 3 minutes for a period up to 1 hour (20–60 lifts/h and 160–480 lifts/8-h shift) ■ Constant lifting: lifting $\geq$1 times per 3 minutes continuously for 8 hours ($>$ 60 lifts/h and 480 + lifts/8-h shift).
What size box is used for lifting? Does the box have cutouts or handles?	Box sizes may include the following: 8 $\times$ 12 in; 10 $\times$ 10 $\times$ 14 in; or 12 $\times$ 12 $\times$ 14 in. Boxes have cutouts.
How are non–material handling abilities determined, including movement and sustained positional tolerance? How is frequency determined?	To establish an individual's physical/functional capacities for performing non–materials handling activities/tasks (work postures) static and repetitive (balancing, climbing, stooping, bending, crouching, kneeling, reaching, handling, fingering, feeling, sitting, standing, walking, and crawling), the practitioner must determine the appropriate physical demands and/or specific job functions to evaluate. Most FCEs include testing the physical demands as identified by the US Department of Labor. To establish and/or determine an individual's present and safe mobility/movement and work postures, capacities are identified as defined by the Department of Labor DOT Standards relative to a specific job or for the purposes of job placement within the individual's demonstrated abilities. How long do we test for each? How long one assesses body mobility (non–material handling tasks) will be driven by the client's reported functional limitations and job demands. Physiotherapy's position on the use of frequency ratings is as follows: Initial reliance will be given to use of the DOT frequency terms described above. When possible, evaluators will rate a client's physical abilities not only with respect to the above rating scheme, but will also add information (if and when appropriate) providing maximal levels of concurrent ability, ie, "Mr Jones is capable of occasional sitting for periods not to exceed 1 hour in succession. He can return to sitting after a period of 10 minutes."

FCE Model: Physiotherapy Associates (continued)

For evaluation purposes, evaluators will implement the following frequency guidelines when rating tested clients:

- Extrapolation
  - In extrapolating to a full workday, transfer the period of actual performance time to 1 of 4 choices for frequency.
    - 20 min = 1/3 h
- Occasional

  Frequent
  - Client performed at a constant pace for the entire period but is at or near limit.
- Constant
  - If client performed activity for 20 minutes and self-reports no limitation with activity, it is a reasonable assumption to think that the client can perform activity on a continuous basis.
- Avoid
  - Client is unable to perform the activity, cannot safely attempt, or discontinues the activity immediately for known medical reasons or limitations.

What hand-related testing is performed in non–hand-specific FCEs (eg, grip, pinch, dexterity)?	Grip, pinch, fine and gross motor dexterity testing using the Minnesota Rate of Manipulation and Purdue Peg Board and/or other appropriate test when necessary.
How flexible is your model? Can an evaluator vary the length and breadth of the test protocol?	Yes, examiner is encouraged to customize test protocols to the specifics of the job or occupation being tested.
Do you offer "special" protocols (eg, upper extremity FCE, fatigue-related)? What are they, and how do they differ from your "routine" FCE?	No.
Does your model use specialized equipment, meaning items most therapists would not routinely have in the clinic?	No specialized equipment outside of unilateral/bilateral lift/carry boxes, pinch/grip dynamometer, push/pull cart, and shelving unit.

FCE Model: Physiotherapy Associates (continued)

What research supports the test-retest and interrater reliability of your FCE system?	Our system is regarded as being highly reliable in that our staff is trained to follow specific standardized written testing protocols/standards to ensure that procedures and results are dependable across examiners. We have not done any individual research.
What research supports the construct and/or predictive validity of your FCE system?	Our FCE system is valid and can be used as a predictive tool of measurement. Our test measures what it intends to measure and/or define in terms of the individual's present physical/functional capacities. Also, the standardized tools that are used in our systematic approach have already been validated and are well supported in the literature and are considered acceptable tools of practice.
What separates your FCE system from the rest? In other words, why should a clinician choose and use your system?	Our systematic approach to FCE/testing is functionally driven; it measures what it is intended to measure. We use a standardized protocol of progressive functional testing to objectively measure an individual's current physical abilities to perform critical job tasks. The emphasis in on the individual's ability vs disability.

Physiotherapy Associates FCE approach embodies the professional value system endorsed by the American Psychological Association, American Physical Therapy Association, and NIOSH, which states that evaluation must address these 5 hierarchical components:
Safety
Reliability
Validity
Practicality
Utility |
What is the cost to purchase your system? Are there any ongoing fees?	Generally, the range of cost for equipment is ~ $1500–$2500.
Is the system "mobile" to allow testing in multiple locations?	Yes.
Is there Web access to the report?	No.

FCE Model: Physiotherapy Associates (continued)

Is there certification of the FCE evaluator, and, if so, at what cost?	All clinicians who successfully complete the course receive certification; they are then placed on a registry. Annual recertification (online) is required to maintain certification and position on the registry.

Abbreviations: FCE indicates functional capacity evaluation; PT, physical therapist; OT, occupational therapist; CEU, continuing education unit; and ADL, activities of daily living.

FCE Model: Quest–TBS (The Blankenship System)

Contact Information:	**Quest Medical Group, Inc** **PO Box 214** **West Jordan, UT 84084** **Telephone: (800) 248-8846; Web: www.questmedusa.com** **e-mail: info@questmedusa.com**
What are the qualifications of the FCE evaluator (eg, PT, OT)?	Licensed to practice medicine, physical therapy, or occupational therapy in the states/provinces granting and/or issuing the licenses.
Training: How long; what is the process; is continuing education in your FCE method required (please describe)?	**Quest-TBS FCE Evaluator Self-Study Certification Course:** A self-paced study course with video and electronic media covering the topics of Quest-TBS methods and protocols as they are applied to FCE, POET, work-hardening, athletic training, rehabilitation progress monitoring, and forensic FCE. Successful completion of the course, with a final examination, is required for certification and continuing education units. **Quest-TBS FCE Evaluator Certification Seminar:** A live interactive seminar and instructional course in a classroom setting, covering the same FCE topics as the self-study course over a 2-day period. Successful completion of the course, with a final examination, is required for certification and continuing education units. **Quest-TBS FCE Clinical Internship:** A 1.5-day FCE training, one-on-one with a Quest Premier Partner, covering the planning and implementation of FCEs using the Quest-TBS method, protocols, software, and measurement equipment. Quest-TBS FCE Evaluator certification is required for this instruction.

APPENDIX

FCE Model: Quest–TBS (The Blankenship System) (continued)

What is the FCE test length?	The standard total body Quest-TBS FCE is 3–5 hours, depending on if collected data are input manually or via computerized gauge interfaces. Several Quest-TBS FCE protocols have been developed, along with the standard total body FCE, that can be performed for different situations and/or different questions that need to be answered regarding the patient or injured worker. The Quest-TBS FCE consists of the following: 1. Intake process 2. Impairment evaluation process 3. Work assessment process 4. Reliability profile 5. FCE report
Is a history included as part of the FCE?	Yes, as part of the Quest-TBS intake process that is conducted before the FCE.
Is a musculoskeletal examination included as part of the FCE?	Yes. The musculoskeletal examination can document significant anatomic and functional deficits that can automatically preclude some work activities.
What psychometric tests, if any, do evaluees complete? How are they used?	There are 11 psychometric tests listed that can be used in TBS FCE, that can be used/completed before the FCE. For a Quest-TBS Standard FCE, the following psychometric tests (or pain/disability questionnaires) are used: 1. Numeric Pain Scale 2. Visual Analogue Pain Scale 3. Ransford Pain Drawing 4. Non Organic Symptoms Questionnaire 5. Dallas Pain Questionnaire (Activity Questionnaire) 6. McGill Pain Questionnaire The psychometric tests completed by evaluees give information of the patients' perspective of their pain, symptoms, and their disability. The tests are used to compare with other tests performed in the FCE to see if the information provided is appropriate or inappropriate and in or out of proportion to the patient's medical impairment.

FCE Model: Quest–TBS (The Blankenship System) (continued)

Is aerobic testing performed? Which protocol? If not, how is aerobic endurance addressed?	An aerobic fitness test is not performed during the FCE. Heart rate is tracked all the way through the FCE, and Quest-TBS has heart rate criteria for each of the tests. If a test has to be stopped owing to high heart rate, poor cardio-vascular fitness is a problem and a recommendation can be made to improve that so work ability can be improved.
How is material handling tested? How is lifting frequency determined?	Tests are performed to document the patient's ability to perform material handling activities and follow the 12 standard postures for the *Dictionary of Occupational Titles* (DOT) and lifting frequencies for the DOT. Material handling tests are performed using a lifting shelf system and lifting boxes.
What size box is used for lifting? Does the box have cutouts or handles?	Standard box is $12 \times 12 \times 8$ in. It has cutouts for hands to allow for a variety of lifting styles and job simulations. A box without handles is also available to test appropriate patients when there is a question about a precise job match. An overhead box is also available to use for overhead lifting tests and one-arm carrying tests such as a tool box carry simulation.
How are non–material handling abilities determined, including movement and sustained positional tolerance? How is frequency determined?	Non–material handling (NMH) ability is part of the TBS FCE testing process. The NMH activities referenced are the activities documented in the DOT. While there are no published data relative to NMH or databases from which to draw, 2 methods are used in the TBS FCE process for obtaining data for the NMH activities: 1. Make professional judgments based on all collected and available data. Use RMT, extrapolations, and associated tests to identify proper NMH frequency for most NMH activities. 2. Test for balancing, crawling, stair climbing, and ladder climbing if necessary. 3. Test long enough period that you feel the results are accurate within a reasonable degree of confidence. 4. Test Constant Test if insufficient data are available for all of the activities for the frequencies needed.

FCE Model: Quest–TBS (The Blankenship System) (continued)

What hand-related testing is performed in non–hand-specific FCEs (eg, grip, pinch, dexterity)?	Simple Grasp: Simple grasp is observed throughout the FCE. These observations give the evaluator the information necessary to indicate whether the patient has "simple grasp" capability. Purdue Pegboard: Is a test that also provides additional information about simple grasp. Grip Tests: Maximum grip, 5-position grip, rapid-exchange grip, fatigue test Pinch Tests: Key, tip, and palmar
How flexible is your model? Can an evaluator vary the length and breadth of the test protocol?	Yes, it is flexible. Several Quest-TBS FCE protocols have been developed along with the standard total body FCE that can be performed for different situations that can be modified if necessary to answer the questions needed to be answered regarding the patient or injured worker the FCE is being performed on.
Do you offer "special" protocols (eg, upper extremity FCE, fatigue-related)? What are they, and how do they differ from your "routine" FCE?	Yes.
Does your model use specialized equipment, meaning items most therapists would not routinely have in the clinic?	The Quest-TBS FCE is flexible in the fact that therapists can use equipment they may already have in their facility or acquire from Quest Medical Group or other equipment provider to use in performing manual or computerized FCE. Quest-TBS also offers its own equipment that therapists also have the opportunity to purchase.

What research supports the test-retest and interrater reliability of your FCE system?	Narro P. Clarke E, et al. *The Sensitivity and Specificity of the Blankenship FCE System's Indicators of Sincere Effort* [thesis]. North Georgia College & State University Library; 2001.
	 ■ Blankenship reliability (Evaluator's Opinion)
	   – Sensitivity: 76.6%
	   – Specificity: 89.5%

What research supports the construct and/or predictive validity of your FCE system?	Narro P, Clarke E, et al. *The Sensitivity and Specificity of the Blankenship FCE System's Indicators of Sincere Effort* [thesis]. North Georgia College & State University Library; 2001.
	 ■ Blankenship validity criteria
	   – Sensitivity: 80.0%
	   – Specificity: 84.2%

FCE Model: Quest–TBS (The Blankenship System) (continued)

What separates your FCE system from the rest? In other words, why should a clinician choose and use your system?	■ Quest-TBS has the best and most thorough research-supported system that includes standardized, accepted, and peer-review test protocols to support the individual tests that are used in the Quest-TBS FCE process. ■ Quest-TBS Reliability Profile determines whether the FCE results are reliable and can be used for medical and vocational planning. It determines whether the patient being tested is demonstrating a pattern of cooperation with the FCE process that affects the results. ■ Validity Profile is part of the Reliability Profile that helps determine whether the patient is exerting a sincere level of effort on the functional tests. Based on the number of criteria passed will determine valid or invalid FCE results. ■ Defensible in court. ■ Quest-TBS FCE software provides ease of documentation and creates efficiency by performing all the calculations and producing reports. Quest-TBS FCE software also allows flexibility by allowing users to enter test results by keyboard or incorporate Quest-TBS computerized gauges or interfaces. ■ Flexible. Quest-TBS is designed to grow with a user's practice.
What is the cost to purchase your system? Are there any ongoing fees?	Once a health care professional is Quest-TBS FCE certified, he or she can start performing FCEs manually with no additional costs or ongoing fees. The cost of a system depends on the option requested. Prices can range from $5000 for software to $57,000 for a full turnkey system. The average purchase price is $26,000 for a practitioner purchasing the software with the system interface. This combination allows precise and accurate data collection from various gauges and then automatically feeds the information into the FCE report, which also is automatically generated (although the evaluator can customize the report).
Is the system "mobile" to allow testing in multiple locations?	Quest-TBS systems can be configured and modified to meet the needs of the practitioner, client, or patient. It can easily be configured to be portable to test off-site or in multiple locations.

FCE Model: Quest–TBS (The Blankenship System) (continued)

Is there Web access to the report?	A sample report is available by request from Quest Medical at samplereport@questmedusa.com.
Is there certification of the FCE evaluator, and, if so, at what cost?	Yes (see above.) The price is configured depending on stand-alone training, bundled with software, or bundled with equipment. Quest Medical Group is happy to work with practitioners and organizations to define the best Quest-TBS FCE setup and configuration and quote accordingly.

Abbreviations: FCE indicates functional capacity evaluation; PT, physical therapist; OT, occupational therapist; and RMT, repeated movement testing.

FCE Model: Saunders FCE Method–In House (Applies only to FCE Method used at Saunders Therapy Centers Clinics, Twin Cities, MN)

Contact Information:	Saunders Therapy Centers Twin Cities, MN
What are the qualifications of the FCE evaluator (eg, PT, OT)?	PT or OT plus intensive apprentice-like training and ongoing peer-review between staff members at different clinic locations.
Training: How long; what is the process; is continuing education in your FCE method required (please describe)?	Training is apprentice-like and consists of reading the *Saunders FCE Method* book, reading samples of FCE reports, watching evaluators perform an evaluation, performing an evaluation *with* a seasoned evaluator, then ongoing peer review of FCE reports.
What is the FCE test length?	18 hours or custom, as requested. Consists of a 2-hour baseline evaluation on 1 day, followed by two 8-hour days for endurance testing—total over 3 consecutive days.
Is a history included as part of the FCE?	Yes.
Is a musculoskeletal examination included as part of the FCE?	Yes.
What psychometric tests, if any, do evaluees complete? How are they used?	PACT Spinal Function Sort, rating gives perceived abilities score and is used to compare with actual abilities as observed by evaluator.

FCE Model: Saunders FCE Method–In House (Applies
only to FCE Method used at Saunders Therapy Centers
Clinics, Twin Cities, MN) (continued)

Is aerobic testing performed? Which protocol? If not, how is aerobic endurance addressed?	True endurance related to specific job demands is tested on 2 consecutive 8-hour days (this is not necessarily aerobic, unless aerobic is a job demand).
How is material handling tested? How is lifting frequency determined?	Maximum/baseline abilities are tested in a variety of positions (bimanual floor to knuckle height, knuckle to shoulders, shoulder to overhead, single hand with bucket, floor to shoulder height) by starting at 10 lb and adding weight in 5- to 10-lb increments until observable changes in client's ability to control the weight (indicating difficulty with the weight) occur *or* client refuses to continue. We do not stop solely on symptom complaints unless observable changes correlate with the complaints. We do not insist that clients continue, however, if we do not observe changes. We explain our criteria for stopping that particular test and allow the client to choose whether to follow our recommendation. In our report, we indicate the reason for discontinuing, whether symptoms were present, and whether our observations of difficulty correlated with reported symptoms. We also report on whether observations of difficulty and symptom reports were consistent throughout the entire test. Lifting frequency is determined during the two 8-hour days of actually observing frequent and occasional lifting.
What size box is used for lifting? Does the box have cutouts or handles?	14-in square boxes with cutouts are used for the maximum/baseline lifting tests, but during subsequent endurance testing, we use a box(es) that approximates actual on-the-job lifting requirements. If no specific job requirements are given (eg, if the client does not have a specific job to return to and more "generic" lifting capabilities are desired), we use standard boxes and/or generic material handling cardboard boxes we have "palletized" and ask clients to handle them, as in a typical warehouse setting. True endurance related to specific job demands is tested on two consecutive 8-hour days.

FCE Model: Saunders FCE Method–In House (Applies
only to FCE Method used at Saunders Therapy Centers
Clinics, Twin Cities, MN) (continued)

How are non–material handling abilities determined, including movement and sustained positional tolerance? How is frequency determined?	True endurance related to specific job demands is tested on 2 consecutive 8-hour days. Depending on the job requirements, we incorporate more or less sitting, standing, bending, etc, to answer any specific question posed by the referral source. If no particular question is asked, we include intermittent positional tolerances throughout the two 8-hour days sufficient to determine occasional and frequent abilities.
What hand-related testing is performed in non–hand-specific FCEs (eg, grip, pinch, dexterity)?	For non–upper extremity testing, only grip strength is tested. For upper extremity testing, we do, at a minimum, the following: Purdue Pegboard test for fine manipulation, 9-hole peg test, Minnesota Manual Dexterity test, grip strength, pinch strength, and Lafayette Hand Tool Dexterity test.
How flexible is your model? Can an evaluator vary the length and breadth of the test protocol?	Our method is designed to be very flexible to specifically answer referral sources' questions.
Do you offer "special" protocols (eg, upper extremity FCE, fatigue-related)? What are they, and how do they differ from your "routine" FCE?	Our method is designed to be very flexible to specifically answer referral sources' questions.
Does your model use specialized equipment, meaning items most therapists would not routinely have in the clinic?	No, in fact, our method uses common equipment and actual job objects as much as is feasible and/or necessary to approximate actual job requirements to accurately, through direct observation, try to answer the referral sources' questions.
What research supports the test-retest and interrater reliability of your FCE system?	We have performed test-retest and interrater reliability tests in house, sufficient to show reliability of our system. We have not published these results.

APPENDIX

FCE Model: Saunders FCE Method–In House (Applies
only to FCE Method used at Saunders Therapy Centers
Clinics, Twin Cities, MN) (continued)

What research supports the construct and/or predictive validity of your FCE system?	We have not performed validity tests but believe that the philosophy of our system (of testing actual endurance/ repeatability over two 8-hour days) leads naturally to a more valid test. Feedback from our referral sources over several years has supported that belief.
What separates your FCE system from the rest? In other words, why should a clinician choose and use your system?	See www.saunders-therapy.com/industrial.html#fce.
What is the cost to purchase your system? Are there any ongoing fees?	We do not sell our system. A book can be purchased on the basic principles, but we do not certify or otherwise guarantee proficiency in anyone other than our own employees using the method.
Is the system "mobile" to allow testing in multiple locations?	Not applicable.
Is there Web access to the report?	No.
Is there certification of the FCE evaluator, and, if so, at what cost?	Not applicable.

Abbreviations: FCE indicates functional capacity evaluation; PT, physical therapist; and OT, occupational therapist.

For more information, go to: www.saunders-therapy.com/industrial.html#fce.

FCE Model: WorkAbility Systems

Contact Information:	**Rick Wickstrom PT, CPE, CDMS (Rick@WorkAbility.US) WorkAbility Systems, Inc 7665 Monarch Court Suite 109 West Chester OH 45069 Phone (513) 821-7420**
What are the qualifications of the FCE evaluator (eg, PT, OT)?	Only PTs and OTs are permitted to administer comprehensive FCE evaluations. These guidelines are consistent with recommendations by the Ohio BWC task force on FCEs. Other instructional courses are offered. Interested persons should contact Mr Wickstrom.
Training: How long; what is the process; is continuing education in your FCE method required (please describe)?	PTs and OTs who administer comprehensive and job-specific FCEs must complete a minimum of 3 days of specialized training (18 CEUs) that includes the following courses: ■ WorkAbility Fitness Applications (6 CEUs) ■ WorkAbility Job Analysis Applications (6 CEUs) ■ WorkAbility FCE Applications (6 CEUs) PTs and OTs who receive direct FCE referrals from WorkAbility Network or participate in our WorkAbility eJob Match licensing arrangement receive quality assurance and ongoing mentoring support to help further refine examination-administration and report-writing skills. Supervising PTs or OTs for injured workers referred by WorkAbility Network are minimally expected to be trained and equipped to provide a basic WorkAbility Fitness Screen. WorkAbility Network has established a Web-based video analysis process to verify competency of evaluators who administer WorkAbility Lift/Carry Strength tests. It is also possible to make arrangements for a WorkAbility Systems trainer to come to a clinic and for a person to complete an internship with a WorkAbility Trainer at a WorkAbility Regional Center.

FCE Model: WorkAbility Systems (continued)

What is the FCE test length?	Comprehensive FCE for job search: $\sim 4.0 \pm 0.5$ hours Job-specific FCE: $\sim 2.5 \pm 0.5$ hours.
Is a history included as part of the FCE?	Yes, a comprehensive history is performed.
Is a musculoskeletal examination included as part of the FCE?	Yes, a comprehensive examination is done.
What psychometric tests, if any, do evaluees complete? How are they used?	None are required; however, the FCE examiner may administer certain psychometric tests when requested and appropriate to screen for complicating job placement factors or recommend follow-up by other professionals. Examples of psychometric tests that have been administered during a WorkAbility FCE examination include the Fear Avoidance Beliefs Questionnaire, PBI Symptom Survey, Beck Depression Inventory, Beck Anxiety Index, PHQ-9 Nine Symptom Checklist, the Health and Work Performance Questionnaire (HPQ), Wide Range Achievement Test (WRAT), Wonderlic Personnel Test, CAP*CAT Temperament Factor Scale, and Career Scope.
Is aerobic testing performed? Which protocol? If not, how is aerobic endurance addressed?	Yes, for many years, we have administered the Siconolfi Submaximal 10-in Step Test and encouraged FCE examiners to make accommodations for evaluees by lowering the step's height if necessary for evaluees with functional leg weakness or more significant deconditioning. We have recently made further adjustments to the step test protocol to lower the standard administration height to 8 in and adjust the metronome pacing to keep the MET level consistent with first and second stages of the original Siconolfi method. The folding step recommended for this test is designed for administration at 8- and 2.5-in heights and is sturdy enough for obese persons who weigh up to 500 lb.

FCE Model: WorkAbility Systems (continued)

How is material handling tested? How is lifting frequency determined?	A kinesiophysical model of testing is used to determine materials handling strength in different vertical zones. Commonly tested lift and carry strength tests include Overhead Lift Strength (30 in ⇔ lift the tote just above head height), Chest Lift Strength (30 in ⇔ 48 in hand-hold destination), Pallet Lift Strength (30 in ⇔ 6 in hand-hold destination), Knee Lift Strength (30 in ⇔ 18 in and hand-hold destination), and Carry Strength (50-ft distance with hands at or above waist level). The aforementioned lifting strength tests may be adjusted based on job-specific lift zone requirements or accommodated to determine accommodation needs of the test subject. Our WorkAbility Method offers complete flexibility to lifting in any combination vertical destination, given that painter's tape is used to provide a visual mark on the wall at the level to which the tote pan must be elevated or lowered. The ACGIH TLVs for lifting or other ergonomic tools may be used by FCE examiners to justify recommended safety limits for job redesign when an evaluee's ability does not match the job-specific lifting demands.

Frequent Lift tests are commonly administered for the Chest Lift (30 in= ⇔ 48 in) and Pallet Lift (30 in ⇔ 6 in). The subject must complete 5 cycles within 30 seconds. The average of Frequent Chest Lift and Frequent Pallet Lift is used for job search applications. The most relevant measures are used or selected for job match comparisons.

There is much confusion in the literature about what terms such as *occasional, frequent,* and *constant* mean in terms of number of repetitions. To operationally define these terms better for WorkAbility Functional Capacity Evaluation and Job Analysis applications, we have chosen to operationally define these terms using language that corresponds more closely with the ACGIH TLV categories for materials handling. Contact Mr Wickstrom for more information.

FCE Model: WorkAbility Systems (continued)

What size box is used for lifting? Does the box have cutouts or handles?	The highly mobile Ergo-Totes Set meets the dimensional requirements of the testing process. Most of the lift strength tests are done using the 1-handled Ergo-Tote that is exactly 10 lb and is approximately the size of a box of standard paper (15 × 12 × 10 in). The cutout handles on this tote are blocked by the 1-handled attachment intentionally during our standard tests, so that the subject has to handle the load without handles or cutouts. This 1-handled Ergo-Tote will easily hold the 8 unmarked 5-lb weight bags, which are included with the Ergo-Totes Set. There is an identically sized Ergo-Tote that has 2 cutout handles that nests with the 1-handled Ergo-Tote if testing with additional weight is necessary or a job-specific test must be simulated with handle cutouts. A folding 8-in step is used in combination with painter's tape applied to the wall to adjust the vertical dimensions of each lift.
How are non-material handling abilities determined, including movement and sustained positional tolerance? How is frequency determined?	Finger dexterity, manual dexterity, and agility are rated by skill level or aptitude, based on the ratio between the subject's performance time on timed work samples and the industrial time standard determined by the MODAPTS system of work methods time analysis. For example, the Total-Body Dexterity Test is a versatile work sample that can be administered in a seated or stooped work posture during the Forward Manipulation tests (right- and left-handed tests); while kneeling, crouching, or sitting on a low step during the PAT Lower Manipulation Test (right- and left-handed tests); and while reaching overhead when the PAT Total-Dexterity Tester is positioned at 72 in on a door hanger during the PAT Upper Manipulation Test (right- and left-handed). Work tolerances such as standing and walking, sitting, reaching above shoulder level, twisting and turning the head, bending over and stooping, climbing steps, climbing ladders, and kneeling and squatting are rated by endurance based on observation of the subject's performance on work samples that require these work abilities. This rating requires professional judgment based on consideration of multiple factors.

APPENDIX

FCE Model: WorkAbility Systems (continued)

What hand-related testing is performed in non–hand-specific FCEs (eg, grip, pinch, dexterity)?	The WorkAbility Systems FCE includes many tests of upper extremity function. Commonly administered strength tests include grip strength (right and left), 3-point pinch strength (right and left), arm lift strength (right and left), shoulder strength (right and lift), and horizontal pull strength (both hands). Placing and return tests are administered using the Grooved Pegboard Test for the right and left hands. The Grooved Pegboard Placing Test evaluates finger dexterity, whereas the Return Test evaluates motor coordination. The PAT Total-Body Dexterity Tester evaluates manual dexterity for turning with the right vs left hands. The Turning Test with the Minnesota Manual Dexterity Test is also used to evaluate manual dexterity with one or both hands.
How flexible is your model? Can an evaluator vary the length and breadth of the test protocol?	Nearly all of the functional tests may be administered with accommodated work postures if the subject has a work performance barrier that limits ability to complete the standard protocol. The evaluator has the flexibility to select only testing components that are applicable to the subject's health impairments, job demands, or referral questions.
Do you offer "special" protocols (eg, upper extremity FCE, fatigue-related)? What are they, and how do they differ from your "routine" FCE?	With certain types of health conditions that involve fatigue, we have the flexibility to repeat functional testing components over multiple days. Usually this is done while the subject is participating in a work conditioning or hardening program. We are usually able to identify complications related to fatigue or provocation of symptoms during a single-day examination by monitoring cardiorespiratory signs and symptoms during the examination. Fatigue complications may be identified by comparing strength and submaximal step test results at the beginning of the examination with dynamic lift-carry test performance and changes in baseline symptoms and vitals at the end of testing.
Does your model use specialized equipment, meaning items most therapists would not routinely have in the clinic?	Yes, it has been our experience that some additional equipment is required that is not routinely available in most clinics. The following additional equipment is needed to conduct a postoffer Workability Fitness Screen and postinjury work capacity evaluation: 1. Set of 2 inclinometers (to measure spine active range of motion)

FCE Model: WorkAbility Systems (continued)

	2. Metronome (Submaximal Step Test)
	3. Grooved Pegboard Test (finger dexterity/motor coordination test)
	4. Minnesota Manual Dexterity Test (manual dexterity test)
	5. Adjustable pull strap and carabineer hook for measuring of job pull forces, arm lift strength, shoulder strength, and horizontal pull strength
	For comprehensive FCEs or upper extremity FCEs, we use the PAT Total Body Dexterity Ring to evaluate tolerance of awkward postures such as kneeling, stooping, and reaching overhead. We also recommend a pulse oximeter to monitor cardiopulmonary response to endurance tasks.
What research supports the test-retest and interrater reliability of your FCE system?	Many of the original FCE protocols developed by physical therapist Rick Wickstrom in the late 1980s and early 1990s were translated into Dutch and adopted into the Ergo-Kit FCE System that has seen in widespread use in the Netherlands. The FCE protocols and equipment originally developed by Wickstrom have undergone further refinement during the past 15 years in an Ohio-based statewide WorkAbility Network of independent physical and occupational therapy providers. A partial list of supporting references for the WorkAbility FCE Method includes:

- ACGIH. *Threshold Limit Values (TLVs) for Lifting.* TLVs and BEIs Book. 2007.
- Bryden PJ, Roy EA. A new method of administering the Grooved Pegboard Test: performance as a function of handedness and sex. *Brain Cognition.* 2005;58:258–268.
- Gouttebarge V, Wind H, Kuijer PP, Sluiter JK, Frings-Dresen MH. Intra- and interrater reliability of the Ergo-Kit functional capacity evaluation method in adults without musculoskeletal complaints. *Arch Phys Med Rehabil.* 2005;86:2355–2360.
- Gouttebarge V, Wind H, Kuijer PP, Sluiter JK, Frings-Dresen MH. Reliability and agreement of 5 Ergo-Kit functional capacity evaluation lifting tests in subjects with low back pain. *Arch Phys Med Rehabil.* 2006;87:1365–1370.
- Hamilton A, Balnave R, Adams R. Grip strength testing reliability. *J Hand Ther.* July–September 1994:163–170.

APPENDIX

FCE Model: WorkAbility Systems (continued)

	■ Mathiowetz V, Kashman N, Volland G, Weber K, Dowe M, Rogers S. Grip and pinch strength: normative data for adults. *Arch Phys Med Rehabil.* 1986;6:69–72.
	■ Ruff RM, Parker SB. Gender and age specific changes in motor speed and eye-hand coordination in adults: normative values for the Finger Tapping and Grooved Pegboard tests. *Percept Mot Skills.* 1993;76(3 pt 2): 1219–1230.
	■ Siconolfi SF, Garber CE, LaSater TM, Carleton RA. A simple, valid step test for estimating maximal oxygen uptake in epidemiologic studies. *Am J Epidemiol.* 1985;121:382–390.
	■ Wickstrom RJ. Intra-tester reliability and normative data for hand-wrist manipulation with the JAMAR Physical Agility Tester (PAT). Unpublished study. 1994.
	■ Wickstrom RJ. Normative data for strength, coordination and dexterity of entry-level workers. Unpublished study. 2002.
	■ Wickstrom RJ. Test-retest reliability of workability fitness screen tests. Poster presented at: APTA Combined Sections Meeting; February 15–18, 2007; Boston, MA.
	■ An inter-rater reliability study of lift/carry strength tasks is being conducted in collaboration with Dr Kari Dunning from the University of Cincinnati.
What research supports the construct and/or predictive validity of your FCE system?	■ Ijmker S, Gerrits EH, Reneman MF. Upper lifting performance of healthy young adults in functional capacities evaluations: a comparison of two protocols. *Occup Rehabil.* 2003:13:297–305.
	■ Rustenberg G, Kuijer PPFM, Frings-Dresen MHW. The concurrent validity of the ERGOS Work Simulator and Ergo-Kit with respect to maximum lifting capacity. *J Occup Rehabil.* 2004;14:107–118.
What separates your FCE system from the rest? In other words, why should a clinician choose and use your system?	1. The WorkAbility FCE System is completely mobile for providing service at multiple clinics or job-specific work capacity evaluations at work-site locations.
	2. The reports are easily understood, customer-friendly, and Web-accessible.
	3. The System provides more comprehensive assessment of upper extremity cumulative trauma disorders (such as carpal tunnel syndrome), including the innovative, PAT Total Body Dexterity Tester patented by Rick Wickstrom, PT, CPE, TWD.

FCE Model: WorkAbility Systems (continued)

	4. PTs and OTs who receive direct FCE referrals from WorkAbility Network or participate in our WorkAbility Systems FCE Maintenance service receive quality assurance and ongoing mentoring support to help further refine examination-administration and report-writing skills.
	5. The WorkAbility FCE System is readily adaptable to a wide range of occupational health and industrial rehabilitation screening applications.

What is the cost to purchase your system? Are there any ongoing fees?	The start-up cost for a complete set of mobile FCE equipment to perform a comprehensive FCE is ~ $2995 for WorkAbility providers and $3395 for out-of-network providers (plus applicable sales tax and shipping). Therapy providers may already have some equipment in place that satisfies our protocol.
	The start-up cost for a complete set of mobile equipment to perform a WorkAbility Fitness Screen is ~ $1835 for WorkAbility providers and $2138 for out-of-network providers (plus applicable sales tax and shipping). Therapy providers may already have some equipment in place that satisfies our protocol.
	Training tuition (3 days) is ~ $585 per person for WorkAbility providers and $815 for out-of-network providers.
	The WorkAbility eJobMatch License (FCE template and Web-based reporting for job analysis and work-ability progress updates, roundtable participation, and telephone support) is $500 for a single location for WorkAbility Network providers and $995 for out-of-network providers.

Is the system "mobile" to allow testing in multiple locations?	Yes, the WorkAbility FCE System is completely mobile to support service at multiple clinic or work-site locations. Only a single trip using a luggage carrier is required to transport all recommended equipment items to and from the rear compartment of a car and testing locations. All recommended components have been carefully selected to withstand rugged use that is inherent to mobile testing applications.

APPENDIX

FCE Model: WorkAbility Systems (continued)

Is there Web access to the report?	Yes, WorkAbility Network launched the Web-based WorkAbility eJobMatch to support global access for worker-job match and job safety analysis.
Is there certification of the FCE evaluator, and, if so, at what cost?	Yes, WorkAbility Network has established a certification program for therapists who demonstrate work-site therapy expertise. Therapists must satisfy the following competency requirements to receive a certificate of designation as a Certified WorkAbility Therapist (CWT):

1. Completion of *WorkAbility SAW/RTW Consulting Applications* training modules (6 CEUs)
2. Completion of *WorkAbility Fitness Screen Applications* training modules (6 CEUs)
3. Completion of *WorkAbility Functional Capacity Applications* training modules (6 CEUs)
4. Completion of a comprehensive applied ergonomics course (eg, Ohio BWC's *Ergonomics Applied* course is free to Ohio BWC providers)
5. Satisfactory performance on a minimum of 2 case referrals that demonstrate competency in WorkAbility Fitness Screening, job analysis, and progress reporting.

Training tuition for the 3-day WorkAbility Certification Series (1,2, and 3) is ~ $585 per person for WorkAbility providers and $815 for out-of-network providers.

We insist that our FCE providers have an ergonomics background because it is necessary to formulate a meaningful assessment with job-specific FCEs.

There is no initial or ongoing credentialing fee for supervising PTs or OTs who are employed by WorkAbility therapy providers. Certification fees are $300 each for initial credentialing and $75 each for annual renewal for out-of-network therapists.

Abbreviations: ACGIH TLVs indicates American Conference of Governmental Industrial Hygienists Inc threshold limit values; CEUs, continuing education units; FCE, functional capacity evaluation; MODAPTS, modular arrangement of predetermined time standards; PAT, Physical Agility Tester; PT, physical therapist; and OT, occupational therapist.

APPENDIX

FCE Model: WorkSTEPS/XRTS

Contact Information:	**Larry Feeler, PT, CEAS; CEO, WorkSTEPS** **Lfeeler@grandecom.net; (432) 366-9541**
What are the qualifications of the FCE evaluator (eg, PT, OT)?	PT, OT, some physicians.
Training: How long; what is the process; is continuing education in your FCE method required (please describe)?	2 days with required recertification every 2 years; recertification can be done online; pretest and posttest for certification.
What is the FCE test length?	From 30 minutes to 8 hours depending on individual diagnosis, consistency of effort, and performance time needed to best determine measured ability and limitations.
Is a history included as part of the FCE?	Yes.
Is a musculoskeletal examination included as part of the FCE?	Yes, customized to the injured part or systems based on diagnosis.
What psychometric tests, if any, do evaluees complete? How are they used?	A variety of common pain questionnaires are used for the comprehensive and upper extremity FCEs. The EMIS Pain Validity Test is used as a psychometric test to detect sincerity of effort. We believe that psychometric testing should also include appropriate physical assessments like Waddell Symptom Exaggeration testing, sincerity-of-effort testing using the peer-reviewed published XTRS bilateral hand strength assessment, etc.
Is aerobic testing performed? Which protocol? If not, how is aerobic endurance addressed?	Yes; YMCA step test, Bruce treadmill protocol, others if these are not tolerated, if possible, based on diagnosis; heart rate monitored and documented throughout all test activities, especially regarding endurance and cardio fitness level for the specific job in question; information automatically calculated and reported in test report.

FCE Model: WorkSTEPS/XRTS (continued)

How is material handling tested? How is lifting frequency determined?	NIOSH boxes and incremental lift protocol for 4 postures, as well as push, pull, and carry if job-related, followed by actual job tasks using virtual equipment; human performance laboratory with operating drilling rig floor, 18-wheeled vehicle, and >1000 simulations to cross-validate strength and motion requirements to successfully perform job-specific tasks; cross-validation to standard measures like grip, lift, and pull, compared with WS largest industrial database results in standardization of data required for specific job tasks, ie, safe performance to be a beverage truck driver.
What size box is used for lifting? Does the box have cutouts or handles?	Normally the 14-in NIOSH box for 3 lifts and the standard 8-in box for overhead; handles at 4 and 12 in from floor.
How are non–material handling abilities determined, including movement and sustained positional tolerance? How is frequency determined?	All Department of Labor DOT parameters such as balance and climbing are performed a specific time, while pain, heart rate, motion, and complaints are monitored. A simple check system allows for all information affecting performance to automatically be reported and, based on performance, classified as unable, occasional, frequent, or constant. Typically, we evaluate only job- or disability-related tasks.
What hand-related testing is performed in non–hand-specific FCEs (eg, grip, pinch, dexterity)?	We have a hand-specific FCE, but in the non–hand-specific evaluation, the clinician performs 5 position grip tests, 3 trials in position 2, key, tip and Palmer. Sensory testing may be performed, as well as any job-specific tasks entailing hand activities. If there is a sincerity-of-effort question, our peer-reviewed published bilateral hand strength assessment is used. A clinician who sees a problem and wants to expand may pick any number of hand musculoskeletal evaluation procedures from a menu, all with automated reporting (eg, Minnesota Rate of Manipulation, Volumetrics, Purdue Pegboard, and Semmes).

FCE Model: WorkSTEPS/XRTS (continued)

How flexible is your model? Can an evaluator vary the length and breadth of the test protocol?	Very flexible. Evaluators may easily vary the length and breadth of the test protocol. If the knee is evaluated, there are specific knee musculoskeletal tests that must be performed. The same is true for all other body parts that may be individually assessed. If the patient proves to be sincere, the test progresses very quickly to functional and job-related measures. If the patient appears questionable as far as sincerity, the test moves to validation-of-effort components that may also be performed rather quickly. The protocols follow current literature and research for consistency of product nationwide, but clinicians can also customize the test if there are particular specialty tests in the menu they want to include related to the diagnosis or job.
Do you offer "special" protocols (eg, upper extremity FCE, fatigue-related)? What are they, and how do they differ from your "routine" FCE?	We have an entire upper quadrant FCE that has standard measures for the head and neck, shoulders, elbows, wrists, and hands. There are some required measures based on diagnosis, but a variety of well-recognized standardized tests and additional evaluation procedures are also available to allow therapists to customize and expand the test based on their individual preferences, all with automated calculations, correlations, and reporting. Fatigue-related testing is the true job-related function performed in the same posture and at the same pace, repetition, and distance as performed at work (carried out to physiologic safe limit or stabilization phase). The noncompliant or questionable patient would likely not be willing to participate much in these activities and would move to psychometric pain-validity testing and sincerity-of-effort testing.
Does your model use specialized equipment, meaning items most therapists would not routinely have in the clinic?	No, although it will accommodate information from devices such as isokinetics and isometrics, and therapists may add specialty tests from a variety of commonly used devices; the protocols may be performed in their entirety with a few items common to almost any medical clinic. The model allows for consistency of product without large upfront equipment costs.

FCE Model: WorkSTEPS/XRTS (continued)

What research supports the test-retest and interrater reliability of your FCE system?	Most of the parameters of the tests are the established recognized standards published in the literature. Such literature supports the test-retest reliability of grip with a Jamar, the use of bubble inclinometry, goniometry, Purdue Pegboard, etc. Reproducibility of NIOSH box lifting and other strength measures is common to the industry. We have test-retest and interrater reliability research findings that are all statistically significant but have not been published for proprietary reasons. WS has the largest human database in the entire United States. We have a peer-reviewed published study regarding sincerity of effort. Our database, with consistency measures built into it, includes >40 measures on more than 1 billion people. The consistency of healthy subjects compared with thousands of patients with a variety of diagnoses studied in the FCE is scientifically revealing. Since all measures are collected automatically, all parameters are subject to ongoing investigation. We believe that reliability should be subordinated to the more important issue of whether the patient was fully compliant during the test. We use distraction-based benign tests that fairly and scientifically identify sincerity of effort during testing.
What research supports the construct and/or predictive validity of your FCE system?	We have an entire bibliography of literature with cross-references to each protocol correlated to the predictive value of the FCE system. We have many outcome studies not published for proprietary purposes. Two recent studies are currently submitted. The basic principle of science is reproducibility. If certain measured inconsistencies are noted, 2 corresponding sets of empirical data are collected to prove or disprove statistically the sincerity of effort. Peer-reviewed published EMIS "Pain Validity" testing and peer-reviewed published sincerity-of-effort testing using 2 identical sets of distraction-based empirical measures. Three pending sincerity-of-effort studies that are completed and being prepared for publication.

FCE Model: WorkSTEPS/XRTS (continued)

What separates your FCE system from the rest? In other words, why should a clinician choose and use your system?	Our extensive database and proprietary research; the flexibility of the musculoskeletal evaluation to collect certain measures specific only to the diagnosis; complete automation where therapists simply measure and document and do not have to interact with or proof the results. Once data entry is complete (Windows format), a number of menu-driven reports are automatically available at any time. This automation makes same-day reporting possible. All measures are automatically calculated and correlated with other measures and results tabulated. All industrial FCEs include job-specific testing from the WS ergonomic library available to the WS network. The model does not allow clinician bias, manipulation of measured data, or labeling or unjustified "impressions" of the patient. The software allows customized subjective explanations and requires objective sincerity-of-effort testing if certain inconsistencies are noted. Once data are entered, there is instantly a menu of 4 reports, including a billing statement that automatically correlates time spent on each parameter, a comprehensive report that describes the tests and the expected results, a less complicated report that summarizes the results of each test parameter, and finally a job summary report that was designed by physicians based on their needs and ease of reading that is typically 1–2 pages. This report is very popular because it "tables" all pertinent information in regard to pain, sincerity of effort, things not tolerated, job-related and essential function capability, and recommendations, if needed.
What is the cost to purchase your system? Are there any ongoing fees?	$500 per year for postoffer testing and the FCE product; per test royalty fee of $35 for up to 3 hours and $45 for tests >3 hours.
Is the system "mobile" to allow testing in multiple locations?	As long as therapists can take grip, pinch, boxes, inclinometers, their minds, and their hands, they can perform the WorkSTEPS test in its entirety.

FCE Model: WorkSTEPS/XRTS (continued)

Is there Web access to the report?	Yes.
Is there certification of the FCE evaluator, and, if so, at what cost?	There is certification of FCE evaluators. The cost of the course is $150.

Abbreviations: FCE indicates functional capacity evaluation; NIOSH, National Institute for Occupational Safety and Health; PT, physical therapist; and OT, occupational therapist.

FCE Model: WorkWell Systems*

Contact Information:	**WorkWell Systems: Provider Network** **11 E Superior Street, Ste 370** **Duluth, MN 55802** **Phone: 866 WWS WORKS (866) 997-9675** **Fax: (218) 728-6454** **network@workwell.com**
What are the qualifications of the FCE evaluator (eg, PT, OT)?	Licensed/registered PT/OT
Training: How long; what is the process; is continuing education in your FCE method required (please describe)?	Two 8-hour days of FCE training with WorkWell faculty member. Therapist takes pretest and posttest; must demonstrate understanding of the philosophy and method presented; successfully participate in performance of an FCE; participate in writing an FCE summary report. Annual certification is required to be a member of WorkWell's Quality Provider Network (WQP), which includes proof of professional license renewal, malpractice insurance, continued employment at a facility that owns the WorkWell FCE, and 2 recent FCEs for review by quality assurance therapist.
What is the FCE test length?	1-day FCE, 3–4 hours 2-day, FCE 4–5 hours

FCE Model: WorkWell Systems* (continued)

Is a history included as part of the FCE?	Yes. A history must be included in WorkWell's FCE. This gives the therapist the opportunity to understand the mechanism of injury, treatment, current status, etc.
Is a musculoskeletal examination included as part of the FCE?	Yes. A preliminary musculoskeletal examination must be performed as part of WorkWell's FCE. The preliminary examination will identify contraindications to functional testing and identify potential physical limitations that may influence the functional testing. Correlation of the physical limitations with the functional limitations will be used as reliability indicators.
What psychometric tests, if any, do evaluees complete? How are they used?	Self-report instruments available for integrating into the WorkWell FCE include OREBRO Musculoskeletal Pain Screening Questionnaire, Fear Avoidance Beliefs Questionnaire, Oswestry Disability Index, Neck Disability Index, and Roland Morris Disability Questionnaire. Clinicians choose the most appropriate questionnaire(s) to use. The goal of introducing self-report questionnaires is to identify which clients are at risk for developing long-term disability. In addition, the questionnaires should complement the history, physical examination findings, and functional activities to provide a more complete picture of the client. The Spinal Function Sort (SFS) is another instrument used in the WorkWell FCE. The SFS gives the client's perception of his or her abilities, which can then be compared with actual performance during testing.
Is aerobic testing performed? Which protocol? If not, how is aerobic endurance addressed?	Yes, 6-Minute Walk Test (6MWT). The 6MWT is used as it evaluates global and integrated responses of all systems during exercise. It is performed before the material handling activities in the FCE. Cardiovascular response is monitored throughout all FCE test items, including heart rate, respiratory rate, and blood pressure. The client wears a heart rate monitor for continuous monitoring.
How is material handling tested? How is lifting frequency determined?	Standard material handling activities include waist to floor, waist to crown, front carry, and static push/pull. Optional material handling activities are dependent on the client's ability to perform front carry and dependent on job requirements. These may include short carry, right carry, left carry, dynamic push/pull, or others.

FCE Model: WorkWell Systems* (continued)

	Most standardized material handling activities in WorkWell's FCE require 5 repetitions be performed safely before progressing to the next level. Activities are dynamic functional lifts/carries with the exception of static push/pull. Static push/pull force is determined from the average of 3 safe maximum pushes/pulls.
	Determining the frequency of material handling activities throughout the workday combines quantitative and qualitative observations using the kinesiophysical observation method.
What size box is used for lifting? Does the box have cutouts or handles?	12 × 12 × 12 weight crate with handles at top of crate.
How are non–material handling abilities determined, including movement and sustained positional tolerance? How is frequency determined?	Standardized non–material handling activities include elevated work weighted and unweighted, forward bend standing, sitting, standing, walking, crouch, kneel, and stair climbing. Optional non–material handling activities are dependent on diagnosis, referral question, and job requirements and include ladder climbing, crawling, forward bend sitting, rotation, high level balance, and other job-related activities. For the standardized activities, WorkWell developed a standardized method of testing for each activity; frequency combines quantitative and qualitative observations. For job-related activities, method and frequency are determined by the job requirements.
What hand-related testing is performed in non–hand-specific FCEs (eg, grip, pinch, dexterity)?	Standardized testing requires grip and hand coordination. Pinch is optional, unless related to diagnosis or job requirement.
How flexible is your model? Can an evaluator vary the length and breadth of the test protocol?	WorkWell offers a standardized 1-day core FCE and a standardized 2-day FCE. Flexibility is provided to incorporate diagnosis-specific activities, referral-specific activities, and job-related activities. These are easily added to the standard battery of test activities. Other modified or abbreviated formats can be performed as well.

FCE Model: WorkWell Systems* (continued)

Do you offer "special" protocols (eg, upper extremity FCE, fatigue-related)? What are they, and how do they differ from your "routine" FCE?	WorkWell standardized FCE protocols include 1-day core FCE, 2-day FCE, hand, upper quarter, lower quarter, low back, and disability. What differs with each is the length of testing time and the activities tested.
Does your model use specialized equipment, meaning items most therapists would not routinely have in the clinic?	Some pieces of equipment required in the WorkWell FCE are not typically found in a PT/OT clinic unless the clinic offers industrial/occupational health services. These include adjustable shelving unit, $12 \times 12 \times 12$ weight crate, force dynamometer for push/pull, overhead work wall system, hand coordination boards, unilateral weight carry box, and industrial ladder.
	Some pieces of equipment required in the WorkWell FCE are typically found in a PT/OT clinic. These include hand grasp dynamometer, weights, heart rate monitor, blood pressure cuff and stethoscope, stop watch, and stairs.
What research supports the test-retest and interrater reliability of your FCE system?	Brouwer S, Reneman MF, Dijkstra PU, Groothoff JW, Schellekens JMH, Goeken LNH. Test-retest reliability of the Isernhagen Work Systems FCE in patients with chronic low back pain. *J Occup Rehabil.* 2003;13.
	Gross DP, Battie MC. Reliability of safe maximum lifting determinations of a FCE, *Phys Ther.* 2003;82:287–295.
	Isernhagen SJ, Hart DL, Matheson LM. Reliability of independent observer judgments of level of lift effort in a kinesiophysical FCE. *Work.* 1999;12:145–150.
	Brouwer S, Reneman MF, Meinema A, Dijkstra PU, Geertzen JHB, Groothoff JW. Test-retest reliability of the IWS FCE in healthy adults. *J Occup Rehabil.* 2004;14:295–305.
	Reneman MF, Dijkstra PU, Westmaas M, Goeken LNH. Test-retest reliability of lifting and carrying in a 2-day FCE; *J Occup Rehabil.* 2002;12:269–275.
	Reneman MF, Jaegers SMHJ, Westmaas M, Goeken LNH. The reliability of determining effort level of lifting and carrying in a FCE. *Work.* Winter 2002.

FCE Model: WorkWell Systems* (continued)

	Smith, RL. Therapists' ability to identify safe maximum lifting in low back pain patients during FCE. *J Orthop Sports Phys Ther.* 1994;19.
	Hart DL. Test-retest reliability of the static push/pull test for FCE. *Phys Ther.* 1998;68:824.
What research supports the construct and/or predictive validity of your FCE system?	Brouwer S, Dijkstra PU, Stewart RE, Goeken LNH, Groothoff JW, Geertzen JHB. Comparing self-report, clinical examination and functional testing in the assessment of work-related limitations in patients with chronic low back pain. *Disabil Rehabil.* 2005;27:999–1005.
	Gross DP, Battie MC. Construct validity of a kinesiophysical FCE administered within a worker's compensation environment. *J Occup Rehabil.* 2003;13:287–295.
	Gross DP, Battie MC. The prognostic value of FCE in patients with low back pain, part I: timely return to work. *Spine.* 2004;29:914–919.
	Gross DP, Battie MC. The prognostic value of FCE in patients with low back pain, part II: sustained recovery. *Spine.* 2004;29:920–924.
	Kiujer W, Gerrits EHJ, Reneman MF. Measuring physical performance via self-report in healthy young adults. *J Occup Rehabil.* 2004;14:77–87.
	Matheson LN, Isernhagen SJ, Hart DL. Relationships among lifting ability, grip force, and return to work. *Phys Ther.* 2002;82.
	Reneman MF, Bults MMEE, Engbers LH, Mulders KKG, Goeken LNH. Measuring maximum holding times and perception of static elevated work and forward bending in healthy young adults. *J Occup Rehabil.* 2001;11.
	Reneman JF, Fokkens AS, Dijkstra PU, Geertzen JHB, Groothoff JW. Testing lifting capacity: validity of determining effort level by means of observation. *Spine.* 2005;30.
	Reneman MF, Joling CI, Soer EL, Geoken LNH. FCE: ecological validity of three static endurance tests. *Work.* 2001;16:227–234.

FCE Model: WorkWell Systems* (continued)

Reneman MF, Jorritsma W, Schellekens JMH, Goeken LNH. Concurrent validity of questionnaire and performance based on disability measurements in patients with chronic non–specific low back pain. *J Occup Rehabil.* 2002;12:119–129.

Gross DP, Battie MC. Factors influencing results of functional capacity evaluations in workers' compensation claimants with low back pain. *Phys Ther.* 2005;85: 315–322.

What separates your FCE system from the rest? In other words, why should a clinician choose and use your system?	What differentiates WorkWell FCE is our evidence-based protocols, expert training, and the support we offer after purchase. The following are provided to all WorkWell Quality Providers:

1. Clinical, marketing, and technical support at no charge provided 7:00 AM to 5:00 PM, Central time, 5 days a week. Clinicians talk with therapists experienced in FCEs.
2. Critiquing of FCEs at no charge
3. Internet-based software for documentation; no charge for the software or training. There is a $10 charge per FCE documentation.
4. Business opportunities are brought to WQP including FCE referrals from national insurer companies WorkWell has a working relationship with as well as prework screens from national employer contracts. In 2005–2007, WorkWell brought $4.7M in direct revenue to WQP.
5. Access to Provider Resource Center for prepared marketing presentations, vendor discounts, and answers to common clinical questions
6. Discounts on program training and courses: 3 courses developed specifically for WorkWell Providers: "Advanced FCE for the Experienced Clinician," "Putting Ergonomics Into Practice," and "Growing Your Business"
7. Research on behalf of providers. International research team committed to ongoing improvement process to assure providers are using the most up-to-date, researched-backed protocols. FCE v.2 was the result of WorkWell establishing a task force comprised of international faculty, researchers, and experts.

APPENDIX

FCE Model: WorkWell Systems* (continued)

	8. Marketing Tool Kit to assist local marketing efforts 9. Market Survey tool available to determine your market need 10. Analytics tool available to assist in identifying customer ROI (return on investment)
What is the cost to purchase your system? Are there any ongoing fees?	Cost is dependent on whether the facility already has a WorkWell FCE-trained therapist on staff, whether the facility is part of a company with other locations, how many therapists are trained, number of locations, etc. Typical cost including the 2 days of training with a WorkWell faculty member is $2500–$9000. Equipment needs are additional and variable per location. Ongoing fees include annual WQP membership of $350–$595 to continue to receive all benefits and business opportunities available.
Is the system "mobile" to allow testing in multiple locations?	WorkWell's FCE is portable. A mobile equipment option is available, which is lightweight and easily transported in a carrying case. WorkWell's FCE can be used in multiple clinical locations by purchasing a license for the copyrighted FCE materials for the locations. If FCE testing is performed at the employer site, home, or other nonclinical location, no additional copyright license is needed.
Is there Web access to the report?	Yes, there is Web access to WorkWell's FCE summary report.
Is there certification of the FCE evaluator, and if so, at what cost?	Each FCE OT/PT evaluator must complete FCE training with a WorkWell faculty member, pass pretest and posttest, demonstrate understanding of WorkWell's method, perform a WorkWell FCE, and write an FCE Summary Report as part of initial FCE certification. Initial certification is included as part of the training fee. No recertification is required.

Abbreviations: FCE indicates functional capacity evaluation; PT, physical therapist; and OT, occupational therapist.

* WorkWell Systems FCE was formerly known as Isernhagen Work Systems FCE. WorkWell owns all materials and copyright privileges related to the name and research regarding Isernhagen Work Systems FCE.

INDEX

Page numbers for figures and tables appear in italics.